THE SURVIVAL MEDICINE HANDBOOK

DOOM AND BLOOM™ MEDICAL

A DOOM AND BLOOM™ GUIDE

THE SURVIVAL MEDICINE HANDBOOK

Third Edition

THE ESSENTIAL GUIDE FOR WHEN MEDICAL HELP IS NOT ON THE WAY

JOSEPH ALTON MD

AMY ALTON ARNP

DISCLAIMER

All information in this book is meant for educational and entertainment purposes only and does not constitute medical advice or the practice of medicine. No provider-patient relationship, explicit or implied, exists between the publisher, authors, and readers. This book does not substitute for such a relationship with a qualified provider.

As many of the strategies discussed in this volume would be less effective than proven present-day medications and technology, the authors and publisher strongly urge their readers to seek modern and standard medical care with certified practitioners whenever and wherever it is available.

The reader should never delay seeking medical advice, disregard medical advice, or discontinue medical treatment because of information in this book or any resources cited in this book.

Although the authors have researched all sources to ensure accuracy and completeness, they assume no responsibility for errors, omissions, or other inconsistencies therein. Neither do the authors or publisher assume liability for any harm caused by the use or misuse of any methods, products, instructions or information in this book or any resources cited in this book.

Illustrations by Usman Aziz, Jeff Meyer, Joe Alton

Photographic images by Amy Alton, Shutterstock

Printed in the United States of America

ISBN-13: 978-0988872554

ISBN: 0988872552

DEDICATIONS

This book is dedicated to my wife Amy, whose positive attitude and sunny disposition truly puts the "Bloom" in "Doom and Bloom". She is the person who first made it clear to me that this book was both possible to write and needed by those who want to be medically prepared in times of trouble.

JOSEPH ALTON, M.D.

I dedicate this book to my husband Joe, whose selfless attitude and compassion for his patients over the years has never wavered. He is unceasing in his efforts to help those who want to learn how to keep their loved ones healthy, in good times or bad.

AMY ALTON, A.R.N.P.

Additionally, we both dedicate this book to those who are ready to take responsibility for the health of their loved ones in times of trouble. We salute your courage in accepting this assignment; have no doubt, you will save lives.

JOSEPH ALTON, M.D. AND AMY ALTON, A.R.N.P.

"DO WHAT YOU CAN, WITH WHAT YOU HAVE, WHERE YOU ARE."

THEODORE ROOSEVELT

ABOUT JOSEPH ALTON, M.D. AND AMY ALTON, A.R.N.P.

Joseph Alton practiced as a board-certified Obstetrician and Pelvic Surgeon for close to 25 years before retiring to devote his efforts to preparing families medically for any scenario. A Life Fellow of the American College of Obstetrics and Gynecology and retired Fellow of the American College of Surgeons, he is a contributor to many well-known preparedness magazines and is a keynote speaker at preparedness conferences throughout the country on the subject of medical readiness. A member of MENSA, Dr. Alton collects medical books from the 19th century to gain insight on off-grid medical strategies.

Amy Alton is an Advanced Registered Nurse Practitioner and a Certified Nurse-Midwife. She has had years of experience working in large teaching institutions as well as smaller, family-oriented hospitals. She is a designer of quality first-aid and trauma medical kits at store. doomandbloom.net and lectures frequently on disaster medical supplies. Amy has extensive medicinal herb gardens and works to include natural remedies into her strategies.

Dr. and Ms. Alton are devoted aquaculturists and cultivate aquaponic, raised bed, and container gardeners. As "Dr. Bones and Nurse Amy", they host the top ten survival website **www.doomandbloom.net** and produce video and radio programs under the Doom and Bloom™ label.

Dr. and Ms. Alton have a simple mission: To put a medically prepared person in every family for any disaster. They know that, to accomplish their mission, the average person must learn to use all the tools in the medical woodshed. The Altons are convinced that a medically-prepared family will have the best chance to succeed, even if everything else fails.

PREFACE

+++

THE THIRD EDITION

When we first embarked on the adventure of writing the first edition of this book, "The Doom and Bloom™ Survival Medicine Handbook", we were overwhelmed by the challenge that confronted us. There was already a wealth of information about the occasional injury on a wilderness hike. Few books, however, considered the possibility of a setting so remote or devastated that no hope of modern medical care existed. Even books meant for use in third world environments often ended their chapters by exhorting their readers to get to modern medical care as soon as possible.

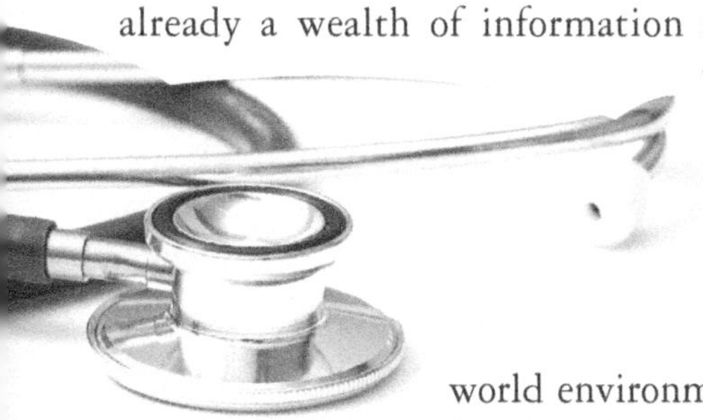

We realized that we were in uncharted territory. One issue was a disaster that overwhelmed the capability of emergency services to respond to all that needed help. Another issue was when a catastrophe prevented ready and able resources from reaching the scene, as when flood water wash out roads. Standard first aid books struggled to provide answers for when medical help existed but was unavailable to those that required it.

A third issue was the truly major catastrophe that isolated a family from modern medicine for the long term. Trained personnel would not likely exist in this scenario at all.

So the question was: What can a mother or father do in this circumstance? How could they deal with injuries or sickness? What could we, a doctor and nurse practitioner, do to improve their family's chances of surviving and staying healthy?

We decided that a how-to manual in plain English was the best option. We had to put together a strategy for each medical issue that we felt the family "medic" would encounter in times in trouble. It had to be simple. It had to make use of limited resources in a sustainable manner.

The book also had to be realistic. This part was the hardest. It's difficult for people to believe that a head injury or a gunshot wound to the chest may not be survivable. Certainly, no one wants to return to a time when pregnancy was a major cause of death. It's painful to think about, but we must face the hard truth that there are circumstances where we may be able to comfort but not to save.

In researching the third edition, we looked at every individual medical problem likely to confront the medically responsible person in the family. How could we teach a non-medical person to approach that problem in an effective but simple way? We considered what medical supplies they would need, how to use them, and how to replace them with natural alternatives when needed. More importantly, we figured out ways to do something even more important: How to prevent medical problems.

It wasn't easy to write a medical book that didn't tell you to seek the nearest hospital or clinic when an emergency occurs. Many times, we had to dig back into our collection of 19th century medical books to find methods that would be useful in grid-down situations. We realized that many of these methods weren't superior to what modern medicine has to offer; as a matter of fact, some were downright obsolete. Despite this, we found a number of our ancestors' strategies that might be useful in a future calamity.

When the first book was published, we expected that, perhaps, a couple of hundred people might obtain a copy. Well, it turned out that tens of thousands bought it, and the second edition sold three times the number. We underestimated the number of people that were concerned about the risk of both natural disasters and man-made ones, such as terrorist attacks.

This third edition covers more issues than the second, and covers almost every subject in more detail. Every section has been updated or amended in some way. The one thing that isn't changing is the title. We didn't know whether the word "handbook" applied to so large a book. After all, it could still be carried in one hand. After looking at the book series "*Handbook of the Birds of the World*", where *each* of the 16 volumes was the page count of the third edition, we decided to keep the title as is.

We hope that this book will serve as a useful reference for the average family. The person that accepts responsibility for their family's medical well-being in uncertain times is a very special person. We hope that we have provided a tool for their goal: To keep it together, even when everything else falls apart.

TAKING RESPONSIBILITY

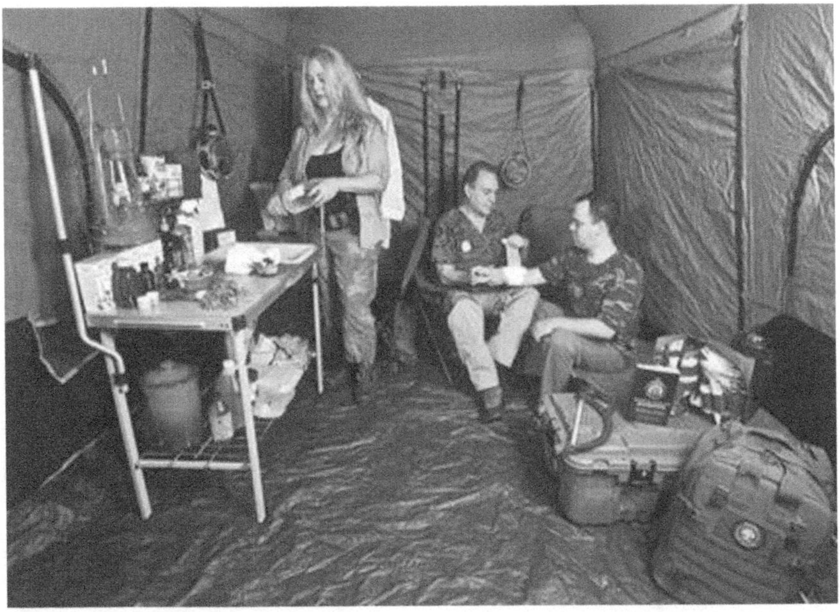

Most outdoor medicine guides are intended to help you manage emergencies in austere scenarios. An "austere" setting is one where modern help is unavailable due to its remoteness. It can also pertain to the aftermath of a disaster or other situations where you are "off the grid". Certainly, modern medical care isn't readily available on an ocean voyage or wilderness hike. You can probably even say the same of trips to urban areas of some underdeveloped countries.

There are medical strategies for these mostly short term scenarios that are widely published, and they are both reasonable and effective. An entire medical education system exists to deal with limited wilderness or disaster situations, and it is served by a growing industry of supplies and equipment. You expect that the rescue helicopter is already on the way and, in normal times, you're probably right.

Let's consider your goals when an emergency occurs. The primary objectives of "wilderness" or "disaster" medicine are to:

1. Evaluate any injured or ill individuals.
2. Stabilize their condition.
3. Transport them to the nearest modern medical facility.

This series of steps makes perfect sense, doesn't it? After all, you're not a doctor; somewhere, there are facilities that have a lot more technology than you have in your backpack. Your priority is to get patients out of immediate danger and then ship them off to others with the skills to treat them.

This will not only benefit the patient, but allow you to continue on your wilderness adventure. Transporting the injured person may be difficult to do (sometimes very difficult), but you still have the luxury of being able to "pass the buck" to those who have more knowledge, technology and supplies. Sounds reasonable? Of course it does.

One day, however, there may come a time when a pandemic, civil unrest, or terrorist attack may precipitate a situation where the miracle of modern medicine may be unavailable. Indeed, not just unavailable, but a circumstance so extreme that the potential for access to modern facilities no longer exists.

We refer to this type of long-term scenario as a "collapse". In a collapse, you will have more risk for illness and injury than on a hike in the woods, yet little or no hope of obtaining more advanced care than you, yourself, can provide. It's not a matter of a few days without modern technology, such as after a hurricane or tornado. Help is not coming. Period. Therefore, where the "buck" stops for the foreseeable future is...you.

Few are prepared to deal with the harsh realities of a long-term survival situation. To go further, very few are willing to even entertain the possibility that such an occurrence is possible, not to mention the tremendous burden that might be placed upon them.

Even for those stalwarts that are willing, there are few, if any, books that provide any strategies for this drastic turn of events. Yet, there are many natural and man-made disasters. The likelihood of your exposure to one, at some point in your life, may not be as small as you think. It stands to reason, therefore, that it might be a wise thing to obtain some medical knowledge and supplies.

Almost all handbooks (some quite good) on wilderness or third world medicine will usually end a section with: "Go to the hospital immediately". Although this is excellent advice for modern times, it won't be very helpful in an uncertain future when the hospitals might all be out of commission. We only have to look at Hurricane Katrina in 2005 to know that even modern medical facilities may be useless if they are understaffed, undersupplied, and overcrowded.

The majority of the citizens in New Orleans became, involuntarily, their own medical care providers in the aftermath of the storm; With medical assistance teams overwhelmed, no one was coming to the aid of one injured or ill individual when thousands needed help simultaneously. Each household became the "end of the line" when it came to its own well-being.

When this situation is thrust upon a head of household, certain adjustments can increase the chances of staying healthy. Medical supplies must be accumulated to deal with varied emergencies. Medical knowledge must be obtained, shared, and assimilated.

The acquired medical supplies and skills have to fit the mindset that you must adopt in a true disaster: That things have changed for the long term, and that you might be the highest medical asset your family has.

This is an enormous responsibility. Many, when confronted, will decide that they cannot bear the burden of being in charge of the medical care of others. Others, however, will find the fortitude to wear the badge of survival "medic". These individuals may have some medical experience, but most will simply be fathers and mothers who understand that someone must be appointed to handle things when medical help is not on the way.

If this reality first becomes apparent when a loved one becomes deathly ill, the likelihood that you will have the training and supplies needed to be an effective medical provider will be close to zero. This is a sure way to make certain that, when everything else fails, you will, too.

This book is meant to educate and prepare those who want to ensure the health of their loved ones. If you can absorb the information here, you will be better equipped to handle 90% of the emergencies that you will see if the power goes down. As well, you will have a realistic view of what medical issues are survivable without modern care.

These realities may place you between a rock and a hard place. Over time, you will certainly have to make difficult decisions. With this book, we hope to give you the tools to arrive at choices that will help you successfully treat injuries and disease.

All the information contained in this book is meant for use in a situation where modern medicine no longer exists. If your leg is broken in five places, it stands to reason that you'll do better in an orthopedic hospital ward than with a splint made out of two sticks and strips of a T-shirt.

In addition, the strategies discussed here are not the most effective means of taking care of certain medical problems. In fact, some of them are straight out of the last century. They adhere to the philosophy that something is better than nothing. In a catastrophe, that "something" might just get you through the storm. As Theodore Roosevelt once said, "You must do what you can, with what you have, where you are".

Hopefully, society will never be poised on the brink of collapse. This book is a weapon against, not an argument for, an end of the world scenario. Even if we never encounter a long-term survival situation, however, this book will still have its uses. Natural catastrophes such as Hurricane Katrina will always rear their ugly heads.

These events are inevitable at one point or another, and will tax even the most advanced medical delivery systems. Medical personnel will be unlikely to be readily available to help you if they are overwhelmed by mass casualties.

Even a few days without access to health care may be fatal in an emergency. The information provided here will be valuable while you are waiting for help to arrive. With some medical knowledge and supplies, you may gain precious time for an injured loved one and aid in their recovery.

An important caveat: In most locales, the practice of medicine or dentistry without a license is against the law. None of the recommendations in this book will protect you from liability if you implement them where there is a functioning government and legal system. Consider obtaining formal medical education if you want to become a healthcare provider in a pre-collapse society. All it takes is time, energy, and dedication.

Although you will not be a physician after reading this volume, you will certainly be more of a medical asset to your family, group, or community than you were before. Among other things, you will have:

- Learned to think about what to do when you become the end of the line in terms of your family's well-being.
- Considered preventative medicine and sanitation.
- Looked at your environment to see what plants might have medicinal value.
- Put together a medical kit which, along with standard equipment and drugs, includes traditional medications and natural remedies.
- Thought about how to improvise in an austere setting.

Most importantly, you will have become medically prepared to face the uncertain future. And, after all, wasn't that your goal when you first picked up this book?

WHAT THIS BOOK ISNT...

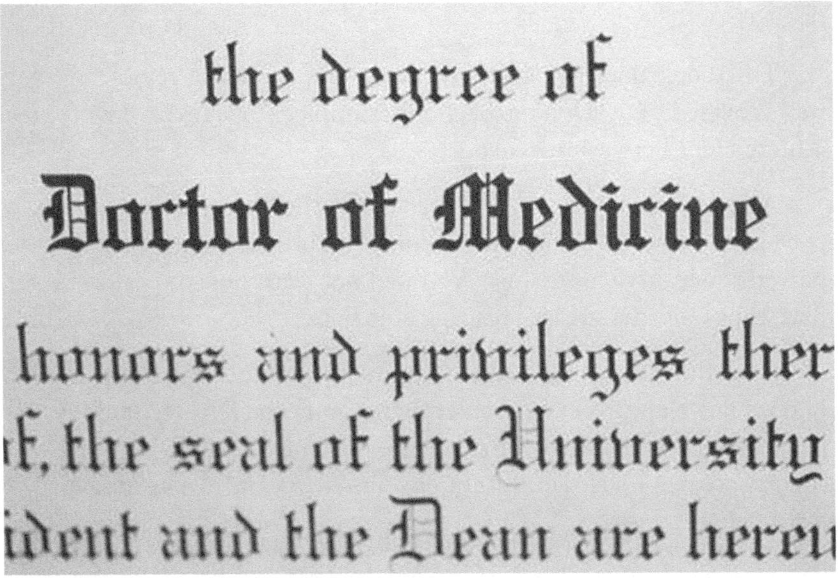

To be honest, this book will not meet the needs of certain people. If you are already a doctor or formally-trained medical professional, you may feel that some of the information in this book is below your pay grade.

You would be right; this book is not primarily intended for you. It is meant for the non-medical professional who is concerned about keeping their family healthy when trained personnel such as you are no longer around.

This book might have some use, however, for the flexibly-minded medical pro. In a long-term survival situation, medical personnel will not have the luxury of transport capability and will have to adjust their mindset to fit a more austere setting. This book is written entirely in that mindset.

It's also important for medical professionals to realize that, although they may be experts in particular aspects of medicine, no one knows it all. Family doctors don't know how to do major surgery and surgeons don't know how to treat diabetes. Paramedics don't do daily nursing care on open wounds and nurses aren't experts at patient transport in the field. This book may be able to fill some holes in their knowledge database.

This book does not claim to be a comprehensive review of every topic covered in it. Don't expect, for example, 50 pages on how to treat athlete's foot between its covers.

As well, this book is not meant for the person who expects to perform advanced medical procedures in the wilderness or any other power-down survival setting. You will not learn how to perform a cardiac bypass off the grid by reading this book.

If nothing else, this book is meant to provide realistic solutions. It does not claim to cure problems that only modern technology will help. Having said this, we firmly believe that it will help you deal with the majority of issues you might encounter in your role as medic.

This book adheres to the philosophy of integrating natural and conventional medical methods. If you are dead set against one or the other, you will not be happy with this book. This book often bucks the conventional medical wisdom; at the same time, it is skeptical of claims that a particular substance is a cure-all for every disease.

This book looks objectively at what is likely to be of benefit in emergency situations with limited supplies. It is meant to be a reference that will give you the best chance of maintaining the long-term health of a family or community in times of trouble.

TABLE OF CONTENTS

+++

INTRODUCTION

✚ ✚ ✚

THE NEW NORMAL

Since the last edition of this book was published, the natural and man-made disasters humanity has endured have been too numerous to count. Floods, tornadoes, hurricanes, heat waves, blizzards, and other weather events have caused major damage and loss of life. Terrorist attacks and active shooter events have become more commonplace. International tensions have elevated and may lead to a major confrontation in the future.

It's hard to witness recent events without a vague sense of foreboding. Regardless of your political beliefs, somewhere in the back of your mind you know that things are not the same as when you were a child. There are more extreme weather events. There are more open declarations of hostility and violent acts almost everywhere, sometimes by organized groups and other times by the unhinged and deranged.

Despite our current predicament, those who prepare for the consequences of these happenings are looked upon with amusement and, sometimes, suspicion. The general population associates them with reality show contestants that dress in camouflage and live in bunkers. In other words, not quite normal.

But recent events suggest that there is a new normal. What is it? To determine this, let's define "normal". Let's say a man with a microphone and a press badge comes up to you. He says:

"Excuse me, sir (or madam), may I ask you a question? Are you normal?"

Seems like such a simple question, doesn't it? Who believes that they're not normal? You'd probably give the man with the mike a strange look and walk on. The truth, however, is that the answer is not as simple as it seems.

What, exactly, are "normal" people? The word "normal" has several definitions, but we'll focus on two:

1) "Standard, average or conforming to the group", and…
2) "Sane".

"Normal" people have certain characteristics that would match the above. You'd agree that "normal folks" need a level of organization in their life. They don't want a lot of clutter, so they make sure to keep no more than 3 days' supply of food in the pantry. They wait until the gas tank is nearly empty to refill it, and have no medical supplies other than a few Band-Aids and some aspirin in the medicine cabinet.

Whenever there's a crisis, whether it's national (the 9/11 attacks) or personal (losing a job), they see before them just a bump on the road. When they stumble, they pick themselves up, brush the dirt off, and continue on their way as if nothing had happened.

Normal folk don't feel that there are lessons to be learned by current events. A major storm is just a news story or a chance to play some board games with the kids. A terrorist attacks elicits a response only if it's close to home. Despite the risks, no action is taken. This is because normal people depend on others to resolve all their problems.

They pay taxes, so they believe the government will step in and give them a helping hand whenever they need it. The support could be in the form of food stamps in hard times, swift emergency responses in natural calamities, or intervention in areas of civil unrest. Most people believe wholeheartedly that help will always be on the way.

The greater the role of government in daily life, the more the population depends upon it. Given the definitions of normal we mentioned earlier, this attitude certainly is standard and conforms to the group, but is it sane?

Let's take the case of essential personnel for a municipality. This would include police officers, firefighters, emergency medical techs, etc. These are the emergency responders that "normal" folks expect will help them out of a crisis. But what would really happen?

In surveys performed in several cities' police precincts and fire stations, many public servants we depend upon have indicated that they won't report for duty in the case of a truly serious catastrophe. The same goes for many doctors, nurses, and paramedics.

Unthinkable? To some, perhaps; however, the professionals that we count upon to rescue us in times of trouble also have wives, husbands, parents, and children. Who do you think they will rush to protect in a horrendous emergency: you or their own families? This is just a simple fact of life, not a criticism of the brave men and women who keep us safe in normal times.

In the aftermath of Hurricane Katrina, the New Orleans Police Department surveyed those law enforcement officers who did not report for duty. Although some, indeed, were victims of the catastrophe, most cited their families as the reason for their absence. To expect them to leave their loved ones and do their duty might be a "normal" expectation of some in our society, but it certainly isn't "sane".

So how do "normal" people become "sane" people? By realizing that society can be fragile and there are events that may occur to send the world into disarray. Once things happen that knock us off-kilter, a downward spiral will make life difficult. Certainly, it will be a challenge for all, but less so for those who prepare beforehand for disasters and unrest. That small minority is known as the preparedness community, or "Preppers".

Preppers are what we call people who stockpile food and supplies for use in a societal upheaval. They also take time to learn skills, largely lost to modern city dwellers, which would be useful if a disaster took away the grid. They are few and far between, comprising perhaps three per cent of the population. Yet, they will be the vanguard of a movement if a collapse occurs.

What types of events could cause a collapse to happen? There are various scenarios that could lead to times of trouble: Flu pandemics, terrorist attacks, solar flares, and economic collapse are just some of the possible calamities that could befall a community, a region, or even a country. The likelihood of any one of these life-changing occurrences may be very small, but what is the chance that your or your children will *never* be affected by one of these events over the course of a lifetime? Not so small, perhaps.

The preparedness community understands that there could be storm clouds on the horizon. Unlike the oblivious majority, they face perilous circumstances with action, not disbelief. It can be argued, therefore, that they are the "normal" ones. Even though they may not "conform to the group", they are a lot more "sane" than their fellow citizens.

Instead of facing an uncertain future with fear and desperation, the preparedness community uses the opportunity to learn new skills that could get them through any catastrophe. Many of these were common knowledge to their ancestors, such as growing food and using natural products for medicinal uses. They were just lost somewhere in the river of time.

By learning things that are useful if the power goes down, they increase the likelihood that they and their loved ones will succeed if, heaven forbid, everything else fails. If a calamity transpires, they will be prepared for the worst, even while hoping for the best.

Some documentaries have portrayed the preparedness community as paranoid. You can see them on various media clad in camouflage, armed to the teeth, and hunkered down in some foxhole. For the grand majority, however, this could not be farther from the truth.

Those that are self-reliant are not eagerly waiting for some terrible series of events to bring society down. They want nothing more than to die at age 100, with their grandchildren whispering in their ear: "Gee, Grandpa, what are we going to do with all these supplies?"

They view their preparations as insurance. You buy health insurance, but that doesn't mean you want to get sick; you buy life insurance, but you certainly don't want to die. Being prepared is insurance as well. Instead of paying money for something that isn't tangible, you're buying food, medical supplies, and other things that will ensure that you and your loved ones will do well regardless of what slings and arrows life may throw at you.

The road to self-reliance is a long and winding one. It will take some of your time and some of your energy to become self-sufficient. It will take some of your money, as well, to accumulate things that will be useful in obtaining a head start to success in dark times. This can be done frugally; a 50 pound bag of rice, for example, is still about $20 at the time of this writing.

Many of the products that will be useful in a collapse scenario can also be improvised. A bandanna and a stick will be almost as good a tourniquet as a high-tech, commercially manufactured one. Look at what you have in your home and consider the ways that household items could be modified for use in a disaster.

A realistic assessment of your medical supplies will give you a good idea of how prepared you are for an unforeseen event. Where are you deficient? What purchases or improvisations will offer you the best opportunity to be ready? What skills would be useful to learn? You'll find the answers in this book.

Benjamin Franklin once said: "When the well is dry, we learn the worth of water". The same can be said for many aspects of modern technology. If you are thrown into a situation where there is no electric power, how many items in your house will be useless? Quite a few, we suspect.

Thus, it stands to reason that, among other things, you should consider the ways that you will produce power. For most people, there are a few standard batteries in a drawer somewhere. This may get you a few hours' worth of flashlight or radio use, but what then? It's important to have a strategy that will give you a steady supply of at least minimal power. Switch to rechargeable batteries and get a solar battery charger so that you'll have a renewable power source at all times. Consider the various other options, such as propane gas, wind power, and solid solar panels with marine batteries and inverters.

You don't have to be an industrial engineer or an extremely wealthy person to put these together; just some motivation and perhaps a little elbow grease, and you'll be on your way.

This volume is meant to help you begin your journey to medical preparedness. You won't be a physician after reading this. We promise you, however, that you will know more about assuring your family's medical well-being and become a better asset to those you care about.

If you begin to prepare for difficult times, and maintain a positive attitude, you will be an example for others in your family or community. If they see that preparing for disasters just makes good old common sense, they might start to prepare as well. Imagine an entire community, or even a nation ready to deal with life's untoward events. In that circumstance, "conforming to the group" would actually be "sane", and we would live in a truly "normal" world.

SECTION 1

✚ ✚ ✚

PRINCIPLES OF MEDICAL PREPAREDNESS

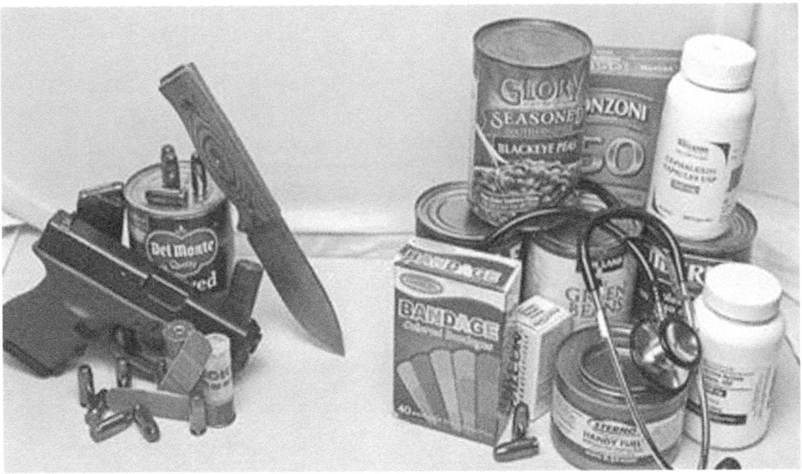

Public Perception of Preparedness (L) vs. Actual Preparedness (R)

HISTORY OF PREPAREDNESS

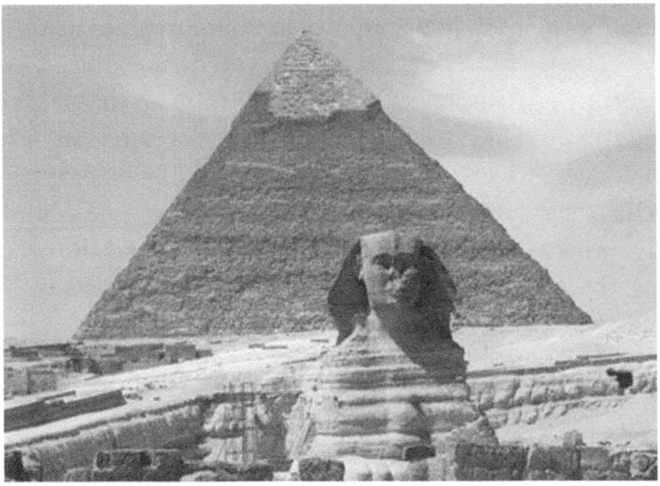

Some say that preparedness has its origin in the animal kingdom. Squirrels, foxes, chipmunks, and various other animals store food to get through lean times. Even though it is instinctual behavior, they are assuring their survival in a fashion that we can all learn from. When human beings realize that tough times are on the way, a relatively small percentage will start preparing, and these people are the ones that will be successful in times of trouble.

Preparedness is just the human way to store those nuts for the coming winter. We prepare to ensure that there will be food, medical supplies, and all the other things we need to survive. In a true survival setting, most of these necessities will be hard or impossible to obtain. By putting some time, effort, and money into accumulating tangible items, we will be able to ensure our well-being if the worst happens. We certainly don't want disasters to occur, but we want to be ready for them.

Although it is wise to be prepared, gathering supplies is not just a sign of intelligence. Preparedness signifies a well-developed sense of self-preservation and even social responsibility. Those who can weather the storm can help their neighbors and their communities to survive.

Preparedness is an achievable goal, and one that doesn't require accomplished outdoor skills or great wealth to achieve. Anyone, regardless of their station in life, can be successful if they dedicate themselves to this objective.

We all, in the back of our minds, are concerned about the massive calamity: The perfect storm, solar flares, terrorist attacks, economic collapse, or any of a number of events could turn our fragile civilization into a nightmare. These events are horrific, to be sure, but "the end of the world" doesn't have to be nationwide or worldwide; it can just as easily be personal. The loss of a family member or one's employment can easily throw a family into disarray. By storing food and other essential items, the "personal apocalypse" can be a bump in the road instead of the end of the road.

The preparedness community has a long history; in fact, as far back as biblical times. When the Hebrew Joseph was in the Egyptian Pharaoh's jail, he was known for his ability to interpret dreams. After hearing about this ability, Pharaoh sent for the young man, and asked him about a recurring dream that the Egyptian leader was having. In the dream, there were seven fat, healthy cattle. There then came seven thin, diseased cattle which devoured the healthy ones.

Joseph took this to mean that Egypt would experience seven years of plenty followed by seven years of famine. He recommended that the Pharaoh spend the next seven bountiful years accumulating grain; in that way, the people would be fed during the subsequent lean years. This was done, and Egypt was prosperous during a famine that left all of its neighbors destitute and starving. This was the very first recorded instance of "prepping". By following Joseph's recommendation to accumulate supplies, we can be a prosperous Egypt instead of its unfortunate neighbors.

In the millennia since the time of Joseph, there have been many instances where disaster has been averted by the practice of preparedness. Farmers, for example, stored grain by erecting silos and "cribs". In this way, they got through long winters or the occasional crop failure.

Every army that crossed into enemy territory learned to stockpile supplies in advance; if they didn't, they would find themselves starving and vulnerable in a hostile land, much like what happened during Napoleon's retreat from Russia.

In every instance, those who prepared for times of crisis had a head start on everyone around them. Over time, municipalities learned to store food, water, and medical supplies for natural disasters specific to their areas, such as tornadoes in the Midwest or hurricanes on the East and Gulf coasts.

This is a wise move, but leads to complacency on the part of those who now believe that the state is responsible for their long-term care in a major disaster. As a result, backcountry skills that ensured success for our ancestors have fallen by the wayside.

Just as cities have plans of action for emergencies, so should the average family. The plans of mice and men (and municipalities) often go astray, so having a personal preparedness plan will give you that extra bit of security that only self-reliance can bestow. Include your extended family, your neighbors, and those with varied skills and like minds.

Being prepared for catastrophes is not political. It makes such common sense that you can say it's "anti-political". Preparedness crosses racial, ethnic, religious, and even national boundaries. It's not right-wing or left-wing. It's about a diverse group of people with the same goal: The continuation of the species, and a life that is worth living.

MEDICAL PREPAREDNESS

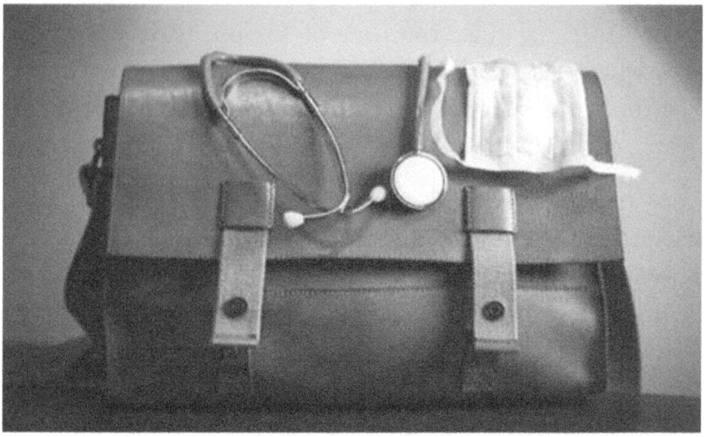

The focus of this book is medical preparedness: The ability to deal with sickness and injuries in tough times. Of course, anyone wishing to survive must first have food, water, and shelter. There is no question that a full stomach and protection from the elements will be the top priority. So what's next on the list?

After gathering food and building a shelter, many prepared individuals consider personal and home defense to be the most important priority in the event of a societal collapse. Certainly, defending oneself is important, but have you thought about defending your health?

In a situation where power might be down and normal methods of filtering water and cleaning food don't exist, your health is as much under attack as the survivors in the latest zombie apocalypse movie. Infectious diseases may run rampant and it will be a challenge to maintain sanitary conditions. Simple activities of daily survival, such as chopping wood, will commonly lead to cuts that could get infected. These minor issues, so easily treated by modern medical science, can easily become life-threatening if left untreated in a collapse.

Clearly, you owe it to your family to devote some time and effort to obtain medical knowledge and supplies. You may be an accomplished outdoorsman; you may have plenty of food and your share of defensive weaponry. That's commendable, but what would you say to a member of your family who becomes ill or injured? Take two bullets and call in the morning?

There will likely be a lot more diarrheal disease than gunfights at the OK corral. History teaches us that, in the Civil War, there were more deaths from dysentery than there were from bullet wounds. Some survivalists' motto may be "Beans and Bullets", but we say "Beans and Bandages, then Bullets".

It's a hard reality that you will eventually be responsible for healing the sick and treating wounds. Someone has to make the commitment to learn how to treat medical issues and store medical supplies; in other words, to volunteer as family medic in times of trouble.

If you accept the role of medic, you will be taking a genuine first step towards assuring your family's survival in dark times. The materials you store will always be there if the unforeseen happens, and the knowledge you gain will be there for the rest of your life. In this book, you'll learn, and be surprised by, how long the shelf lives are for many medical supplies. Their longevity will be one of the factors that will give you confidence when moving forward. Also, don't ignore the value of medical supplies as barter items in times of trouble.

There's another perk besides the tangible benefits of medical supplies: knowledge. We encourage you to learn, not just about standard drugs and treatments, but also about natural remedies and alternative therapies that may work against a particular problem. We can't vouch for the effectiveness of every claim that a certain herb will cure what ails you. We can say, however, that our family has an extensive medicinal garden and that it might be a good idea for your family to have one also. Many herbs that have medicinal properties grow like weeds, so a green thumb is not required to cultivate them. Many of them don't even require full sun to thrive.

It's important to understand that some illnesses will be difficult to treat if modern medical facilities aren't available. It will be hard to do much about those clogged coronary arteries; there won't be many cardiac bypasses performed. However, by ensuring that your storage includes nutritious foods, you will give your family the best chance to minimize some major medical issues. Start them off healthy and you'll have the best chance to keep them healthy.

For the survival medic, an ounce of prevention is worth, not a pound, but a ton of cure. If you can prevent a medical problem from happening, you'll save a lot of supplies and extend the life of your storage. You'll also save a lot of headache and, perhaps, some heartache as well.

We're not asking you to do anything that your great-grandparents didn't do as part of their strategy to succeed in life. In a collapse, we'll be thrown back to an era without manufactured pharmaceuticals and intensive care units. We'll be left with the methods our ancestors used to stay healthy. For this reason, we included as many natural remedies as possible in this book. Many of them will be mainstays in how you deal with medical issues after a true disaster.

Some members of our family wonder why we spend all our time trying to prepare people medically for catastrophes. Like most "normal" people, they are totally certain that there is no scenario that could take away, even for a while, the wonders of high technology. After all, they see the hospital on their way to work and they have health insurance, what could happen? As such, our family is truly puzzled when they read our books and articles. They tell us that we can't turn everyone into doctors, so why we should try?

So we asked ourselves: Are we trying to turn you all into doctors? No, there's too much to learn in one lifetime. We often come across things we're not sure about, even as medical professionals. That's what medical books are for, so make sure that you put together a good survival library you can refer to when necessary. You'll be glad you did.

But it's time to admit the truth. We are, indeed, trying to turn you into something: a medical asset to your family and community. We firmly believe that, even if you have not undergone a formal medical education, you can learn how to treat the majority of problems you will encounter in an off-grid setting. You can, if you absolutely have to, be the end of the line with regards to the medical well-being of your people.

USING ALL THE TOOLS IN THE WOODSHED

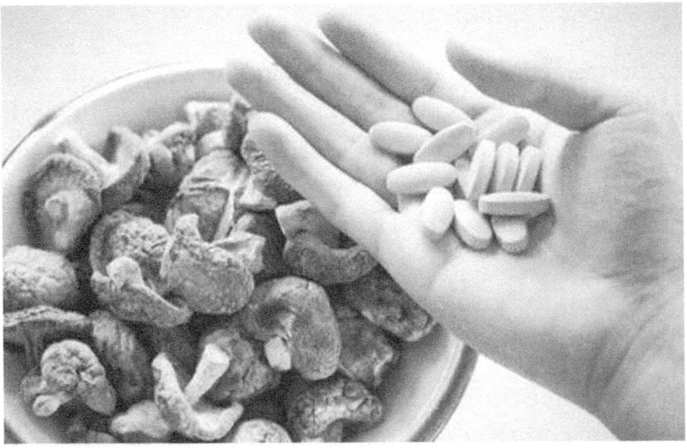

Most average citizens have a relationship with a conventional healthcare provider, but a growing number regularly see alternative healers as well. Both of these professionals have much to offer in the maintenance of our medical well-being; yet, these two disciplines are often at odds with each other. This ill feeling has always made little sense to us, and it makes even less sense if we find ourselves off-grid due to a disaster.

In survival, having an inflexible attitude towards one branch of medicine or another may be hazardous to your health. If you are a proponent of alternative medicine, there isn't much that herbal therapy will do to set a broken leg. On the other hand, if you're an advocate of conventional medicine, what will you do when those pharmaceuticals you stored run out? Both of the above are likely events in a truly austere setting.

Therefore, this book is not geared, like most books, only towards standard medical treatment, but includes natural healing options. It isn't, however, solely a book on natural remedies either. Those of you who are completely against one or the other will probably be unhappy with the opinions registered here. If this is the case, have you thought about *why* you are so dead set against one or the other?

We once had a conventional doctor challenge us to find an illness, any illness, which a natural remedy will cure or prevent. We have also heard an herbalist challenge researchers on the benefits of the vaccine that eliminated Smallpox from the world. In each case, no amount of evidence budged either practitioner from their notion that the other was a "quack" or a "profiteer".

This intransigence saddens us. Why not use all the tools in the medical woodshed? Not doing so is like entering a fistfight with one hand tied behind your back. If you are going to have a long-term strategy for medical self-reliance in an austere setting, you must integrate the practice of medicine to include all methods. The pharmaceuticals may run out but the odds are there may be plants in your own backyard that have medicinal benefits. We call this approach "integrative medicine". With integrative medicine, you will incorporate all of the various options available to you.

If we ever enter truly bad times, we will have to do a lot of improvising. Having commercially made supplies is great, but conventional items and even some natural ones will run out over time. This is where it makes sense to put together a sustainable medicinal garden. Yes, gardening is a skill that the medic should learn if they want to succeed in their role. More on this later.

Besides having more options, you have more flexibility. Your approach to a patient can change, based upon what the problem is and how serious it is. If you break your arm, for example, you will first turn to traditional medicine to set the bone and splint it. Afterwards, however, you might add other approaches to strengthen your immune system and speed the healing process.

This method of treating the whole patient is termed "the holistic approach". In holistic medicine, you emphasize the need to look at multiple aspects of health, including the physical, nutritional, emotional, lifestyle, and social. This practice helps your patients recover from the mental stress associated with their injury as well as the physical.

Spirituality and Survival

Since time immemorial, we have incorporated spirituality into survival. Shamans and Medicine Men used a society's belief system in their therapies as much as medicinal plants. Even today, we say prayers for the sick and some use items like St. Christopher medals to ward off injury and sickness.

Atheists will put it all down to superstition, but we should remember the part that spirituality plays in the recovery from an injury or illness. For many, it plays a very important role in fostering the healing process.

This isn't just a personal observation; studies show that cancer patients with a positive attitude supported by spirituality experience longer survival times and a better quality of life.

Spirituality may be your friend in another way, as well. It might strengthen your resolve in the face of adversity. U.S. prisoners of war in Vietnam tell stories about how their personal beliefs gave them a sense of hope and carried them through a dire situation.

Never underestimate the power of positive thinking and spiritual peace in disasters. Remember that you, as the medical caregiver, will be in charge of your family's emotional well-being as well as their physical health. You can bet that you'll encounter episodes of anxiety and depression in these situations much more often than bullet wounds.

We say this not to endorse a specific religion, philosophy, or ritual, but to encourage you to reach inside yourself. There is an inner strength there that many folks don't know they have. If you have what it takes to be an effective medic, it will be most apparent in a crisis. If you're medically *and* spiritually prepared, you're better prepared to handle an emergency. Consider it just another weapon in the arsenal.

Here's our message to colleagues in every medical discipline: Both alternative and traditional medical professionals should have respect for and encourage cooperation with each other. Few are deliberate "quacks" or "profiteers" and both have much to contribute. Each should be willing to learn about the other and incorporate all that is useful from every possible avenue. Together, they can work to ensure a healthy society in good times or bad.

WHAT IS SURVIVAL MEDICINE?

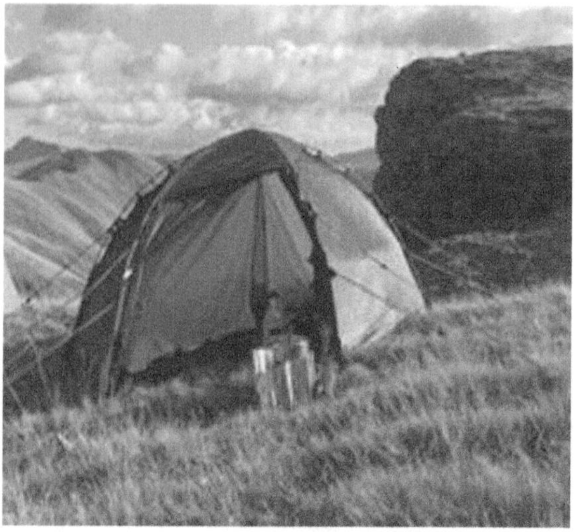

Wilderness Medicine

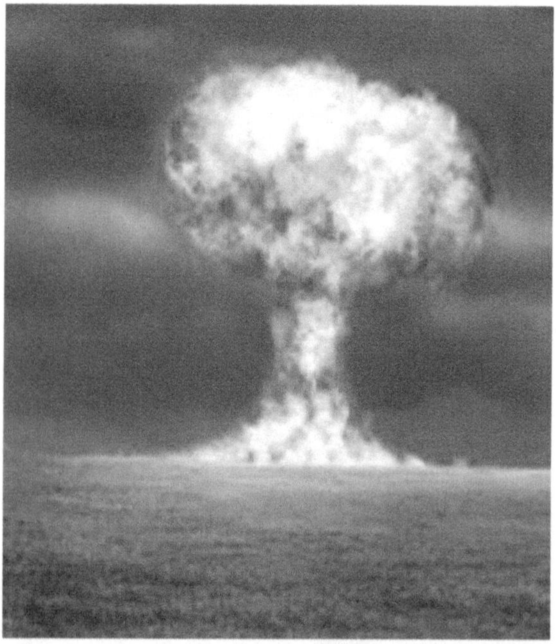

Survival Medicine

Almost every book on "survival medicine" is actually a book on standard emergency medicine. So what is emergency medicine and how does it differ from true long term survival medicine? Emergency medicine involves medical strategies geared towards wilderness hikes, maritime expeditions, and sojourns in underdeveloped countries. In these cases, modern care, training and facilities exist but are not readily available. With some resourcefulness, however, they can eventually be accessed. There is no shortage of excellent resources on this subject, some of which we mention in the reference section of this book.

The basic assumption in emergency medicine is that trained doctors and modern hospitals are a possibility, just not at hand. You, as temporary caregiver, will be responsible for stabilizing the patient. That means not allowing the injury or illness to get worse. It doesn't mean, however, that your responsibility will extend to the entire course of the medical problem.

Your primary goal is the evacuation of the patient to modern medical facilities, even though those facilities might be hundreds of miles away from your current location. Once you have transferred your patient to the next highest medical resource, your duty has been discharged and you can go on your way. Emergency Medical Technicians or military corpsman might recognize this strategy as "Stabilize and Transport".

Although following the principles of emergency medicine has saved countless lives, this approach is different from what we call "long term survival medicine". In a long term collapse, there is no access to modern medical care, and there is no potential for such access in the foreseeable future. As President Harry Truman used to say, "The buck stops here". The arrow that says "here" is pointing at *you*.

As a result of this turn of events, you go from being a temporary first-aid provider to being the caregiver at the end of the line. You are now the highest medical resource left, whether you have a medical diploma or not.

This fact will lead you to make adjustments to your medical preparedness plan. As the caregiver in an off grid setting, you need more than just first aid training. You need knowledge about long term wound care, epidemic infections, chronic medical conditions, and much more. You will also need more supplies, and these will need to be more comprehensive than you'd find in the average first aid kit.

How to get the kind of training that you would need? Medical training and education for non-physicians can include wilderness medicine classes, Emergency Medical Technician and even Military Medical Corps training. Unfortunately, these courses presuppose that you are rendering care in the hope of later transporting your patient to a working clinic, emergency room or field hospital. In other words, "Stabilize and Transport". If you can make the commitment, this training is very useful to have. We admit that it's much more likely that you'll experience a short term absence of medical assistance than a long term one.

Despite this, you must plan for the possibility that you'll be completely on your own one day. That includes medically, so the way you think must be modified when intensive care units and emergency rooms might be inaccessible. You won't have the luxury of passing the sick or injured individual to a formally trained provider, so you must learn how to diagnose and treat medical problems. Most importantly, you must expect to be there from start to finish.

You will also have to understand how to treat certain chronic medical conditions. Even a paramedic is unlikely to know how to deal with an abscessed tooth or a thyroid problem. Many of these issues are treated with drugs and procedures that may no longer be available.

Therefore, you must learn methods that will work in a power-down scenario; you may even have to reach back to older strategies that modern medicine might consider obsolete. If a scenario takes you off the grid, you must make do with what you have on hand to treat an injury or illness. Using a combination of time-honored remedies, improvisation, and prudent utilization of supplies, you should be able to treat the grand majority of problems you might face in a true disaster.

Although all of this might seem daunting, there is enough information in this book to make you more competent in handling medical issues in times of trouble. That confidence will come as a result of having planned for both short term disasters and long term ones. When you know what to do in any scenario, you will feel that quiet resolve that comes with the knowledge that you *can* do the job. You'll be up to the challenge that stands before you.

THE IMPORTANCE OF COMMUNITY

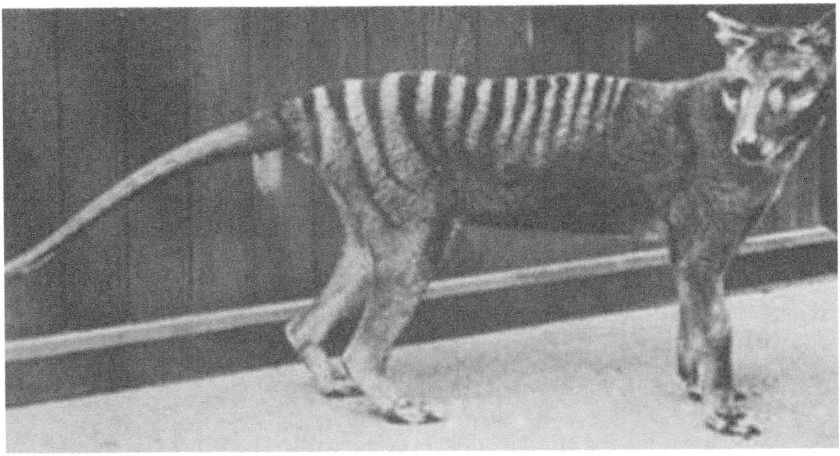

Let's suppose that a calamity has occurred, and you have survived. The power grid is down, and is unlikely to be up again for years. You, however, have prudently stored food, medical supplies, farming and hunting equipment, and are safe in your shelter. You are a fine, young, strapping individual with no medical issues and are reasonably intelligent. Unfortunately, you also haven't the slightest idea what the first thing is that you should do to ensure your future survival.

The very first way to help assure your medical well-being is very basic. Don't be a lone wolf! The forlorn creature in the above photograph is a Thylacine, sometimes called a Tasmanian wolf. Why did we choose this animal instead of a majestic red or gray wolf? Because the Tasmanian wolf is extinct, and, if you try to go it alone in a long-term disaster, you will be too.

The support of a survival group, even if it's just your extended family, is essential if you are to have any hope of keeping it together when things fall apart.

There will be activities that you would find hard to imagine in an austere setting. You will have to stand watch over your property. You will have to lug gallons of water from the nearest water source. You will have to chop wood for fuel. Pick up a full 5 gallon bucket with water or some logs and walk 100 yards with it (after staying up all night standing outside your house) and you'll get the feel of what you might have to go through on a daily basis. Believe me, it would be a miserable existence if you had to do it alone.

Being the sole bearer of this burden will negatively impact your health and decrease your chances of long-term survival. Exhausted and sleep-deprived, you will find yourself an easy target not only for marauding gangs, but marauding bacteria as well.

Since your immune system weakens when exposed to long-term stress, you will be at risk for illnesses that a well-rested individual could easily weather. Division of labor and responsibility will make a difficult situation more manageable.

You can imagine how much more possible this will be if you have a group of like-minded individuals helping each other. You can't possibly have all the skills needed to do well by yourself, even if you're Daniel Boone.

For example, we are medical professionals that are also Master Gardeners for our state, ham radio techs, and raise tilapia as a food fish. Sounds like we have some skills, but neither of us have done any carpentry or raised livestock. Neither have we ever been in charge of the security of others. There are those, however, who *have* done these things, but could use some of the skills we possess.

Put enough people together with differing skills, and you have put together, even in the middle of a city, a village. A village filled with people that will help each other in a crisis. A rugged individualist might be able to eke out a meager existence in the wilderness alone, but a society can only be rebuilt by a community.

There's no time like the present to communicate, network, and put together a group of like-minded people. How many? The right number of able individuals to assemble for a mutual assistance group will depend on your retreat and your resources. The ideal group will have people with diverse skills but similar philosophies. Unless you are already in such a community, you may feel that it is impossible to find and put together a group of people that could help you in times of trouble.

Luckily, that isn't the case. Whether online at places like American Preppers Network (APN) or Americans Networking To Survive (ANTS) or in person at your local civic club or church, there are others who feel like you do. Start there and we guarantee you will find others that share your concerns.

It's not enough to just be in a group, however. The people in that group must have regular meetings, decide on priorities, and be ready to set things in motion. Put together a Plan A, a Plan B, and a Plan C. Have several plans in place for different turns of events. Keep lines of communication open so that all your group members are kept informed.

PRACTICE WHAT YOU PREACH

We mentioned the importance of community in a grid-down environment, but there is another essential part of preparedness. This part is rarely part of the planning process, even for the most self-reliant individual: To optimize your health *prior* to a catastrophe occurring. If you, as medical caregiver, do not set the example of good health and fitness, why should you expect anyone else to? It's time to practice what you preach.

You must accomplish the following personal goals:

- Maintain a normal weight for your height and age
- Eat a healthy diet and store healthy food
- Maintain good hygiene
- Keep physically fit
- Eliminate unhealthy habits (smoking, etc.)
- Manage medical issues in a timely fashion

It's important to "tune up" any chronic medical problems that you might currently have. You'll want to have that blood pressure under control, for example. If you have a bum knee, you might consider getting it repaired surgically so that you can function at maximum efficiency if times get tough.

Those with poor eyesight might consider having corrective procedures such as LASIK performed to obtain the perfect vision that would be so useful in a survival situation. Use modern technology now while it is available; it will improve your chances of doing well in harder times.

Dental problems should also be managed before bad times make modern dentistry unavailable. Remember how your last toothache affected your work efficiency?

In a collapse situation, you will be building shelters, walking long distances to find food, tending fires, and many other activities that will test you physically. Getting fit now will prepare you to accept those challenges. Also, doctors say to eat well and exercise for a reason; make sure you get good nutrition and watch those calories. This doesn't mean that you have to run marathons. Even just a daily walk around the block is going to help keep you active and mobile.

This philosophy is pertinent for your mental health and acuity as well. You can't go for long without food and water, but many people will go without a new thought for years on end. Even just doing crossword puzzles or reading a newspaper will help keep your mind sharp. Remember the old saying that a mind is a terrible thing to waste. Don't waste yours.

If you have bad habits, work to eliminate them. If you damage your heart and lungs by smoking, for example, how will you be able to function in a situation where your fitness and stamina will be continually tested? If you drink alcohol in excess or take drugs, how can you expect anyone to trust your judgment in critical situations?

Paying careful attention to hygiene is also an important factor for your success in times of trouble. Those who fail to maintain sanitary conditions in their retreat will have a difficult time staying healthy. Infections that are usually seen only in underdeveloped countries will become commonplace here off the grid. As such, soap and water become some of the most important supplies you can have for long term success.

Achieving Health Goals

If you don't work to achieve your own health goals, your preparations will be useless. It's hard to make changes in life, especially with regards to your health. There are those who succeed and the vast majority who fail. What separates the two?

Setting a positive goal is important, but getting into a positive mind-set isn't easy. As a result, many people set goals that are just plain negative. An example of a negative goal is to eat less. An example of a positive one is to eat healthier.

To paraphrase Winston Churchill, setting a goal is like wooing a crocodile: You're never sure whether to tickle it under the chin or beat it over the head with a stick. The point is to decide if a negative goal is better than a positive goal. In most cases, it isn't.

Negative goals are tough to reach because you're not learning any new strategies. You're just continually trying to stop or shame yourself when you stray. I'll admit that whacking your hand with a ruler every time you reach for food may have you eating less. Planning out a new diet you can live with, however, will increase the chance for long term success.

Many people see health goals as black or white. Your goal is to lose 50 pounds but you lose only 10. You feel disappointed but the truth is that you're better off than you were. You got healthier but feel like a failure. It's important to see progress for what it is: Progress.

Environmental factors are a big reason for failure to survive after a disaster. If you haven't planned for the environment, you have it a formidable enemy. This goes for your health goals, as well.

For example, let's say you want to quit smoking, but all your friends smoke and it drives you nuts when you're the only one in the room not lighting up. It's hard to resist temptation and it's harder to ask others not to lead you into it. If you don't, however, you're allowing environmental factors to control your failure or success.

Of course, you could replace your friends. It might be the most effective strategy, but it might be more reasonable to replace that cigarette with some nicotine gum. Even better, make a rule that smoking only occurs at certain times of the day or in certain areas (say, outside the house). This doesn't eliminate the issue, but it's taking a step towards controlling some of the factors that cause you to smoke. The end result? You'll achieve the goal of smoking less, your stamina will improve, and your chances of meeting survival challenges increase.

THE PATIENT ADVOCATE

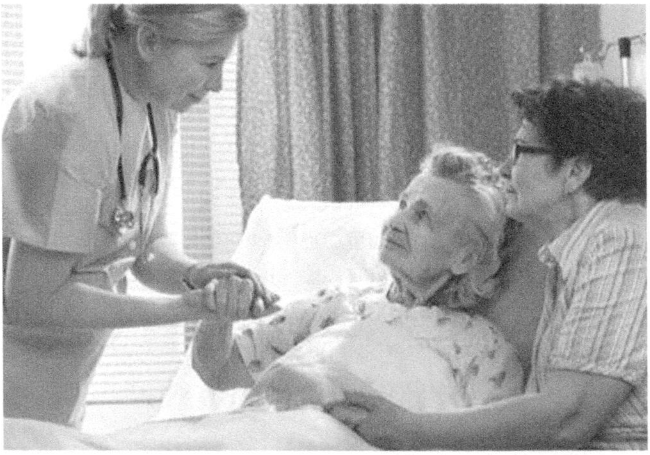

Before we move on, let's talk about an important aspect of patient care. We spend a lot of time in this book talking about medical issues in a disaster, from a violent storm to a complete societal breakdown. However, disasters can also be very personal, such as when you or a loved one suffers a debilitating medical condition in normal times.

In many instances, it is easy for the patient to "fall through the cracks" of a huge medical establishment. This has happened to one of our sons, Daniel. Daniel is a 32 year old who has had severe diabetes since he was nine years old. Due to his disease, he had developed kidney failure and partial blindness, and had been on dialysis and a transplant list for more than a year.

After a number of false alarms, a kidney and pancreas became available as a result of a drunk driver taking the life of a young father as he was riding his bicycle. Daniel underwent transplant surgery at a large city hospital, one of the few in the state that performed this type of procedure.

The good news is that the new organs functioned well from the very start, producing urine and lowering his blood sugars to almost normal levels within 24 hours. Several days after the operation, he was deemed fit enough to leave the Intensive Care Unit and go to a regular floor. This meant that, instead of having a nurse specifically for him, he shared a nurse with several other patients. This is standard operating procedure, and usually has no ominous implications.

However, when we went to see him the day of his transfer, he wasn't looking well. He seemed pale and his abdomen seemed more distended that it did before. There was a drain coming out of his belly, and it was full of bright red blood.

Seeing the blood draining out of his abdomen was concerning. We took Daniel's vital signs earlier than scheduled; and found him to have a racing pulse and a dropping blood pressure. As we were unable to find medical staff, we emptied the bloody drain and watched it rapidly fill up again (and again) in short order. It was clear that he was bleeding internally.

This was late at night, and most visitors had left. Staffing was light, and it took some time to find his nurse, who was attending another patient. Our hackles were raised, and we're not ashamed to admit that we raised a racket. This led an overworked resident to take a look at him. To her credit, she realized that something was wrong, and he returned to the operating room. They wound up removing 3 or 4 liters of free blood from his abdomen before the hemorrhage came under control.

Daniel recovered from this ordeal and, thankfully, his transplanted kidney and pancreas are still functioning. However, thinking about this episode, it was clear to us that it could have ended very badly. If not identified in time, it's very likely that we would have received a call in the morning notifying us that Daniel passed away during the night.

We tell you this story not to gain sympathy or a pat on the back, but to convince you of the importance of being a patient advocate. If you are working to become a better medical asset to your people in hard times, then you must take patient advocacy as serious as learning first aid. You must walk a mile in the shoes of your patient.

You may already see yourself as an advocate for your patient. Indeed, most doctors today feel they know what's best for their patients. As a medic in a disaster, however, you may be overworked and under stress.

This may make it difficult for you to see things from your patient's perspective. Your patient may "fall through the cracks" if you're not careful, simply due to the amount of pressure on you to care for a large survival community.

Consider appointing a family member or other individual to follow a sick patient with you, not necessarily to provide care but to provide support as an advocate. Allow your patient to participate in medical decisions regarding their health and never resent their questions. If they are too weak to do so, communicate your plan of action with their appointed advocate.

Here are the **Three A's of Advocacy**:

1) **Accept** the importance of a patient's rights.
2) **Advise** the patient so that they can be a full partner in the therapeutic process.
3) **Allow** an advocate to be an intermediary if the patient is too weak to actively participate in their care.

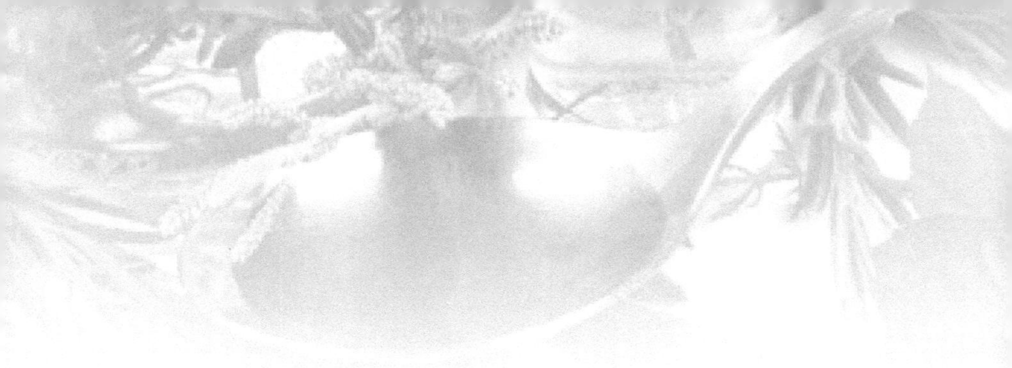

SECTION 2

✚ ✚ ✚

BECOMING A MEDICAL RESOURCE

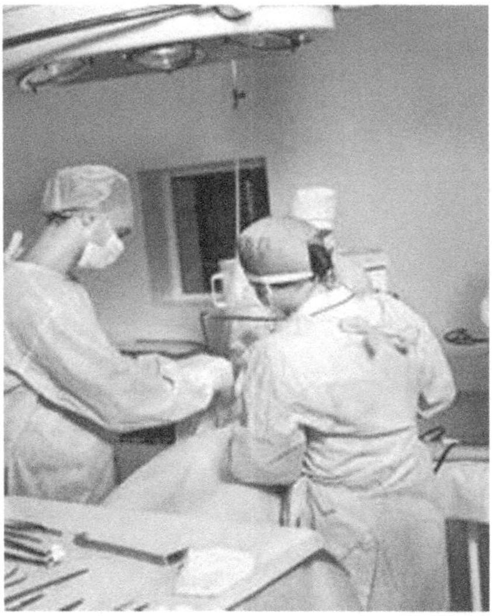

What you won't have

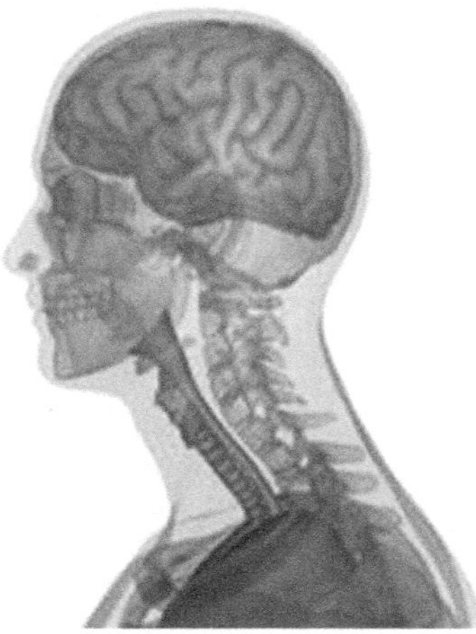

What you WILL have

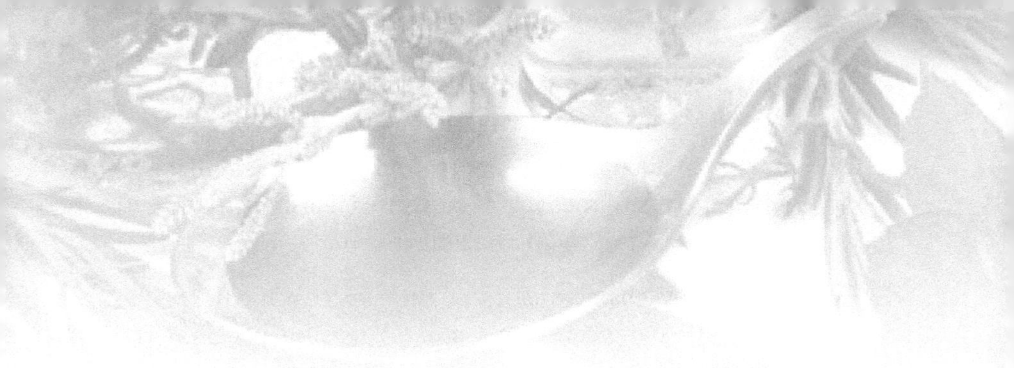

THE SURVIVAL MEDIC

In a long term survival situation, it will be an extremely fortunate family or group that has a physician or other formally trained medical professional among its members. When there is no doctor, however, someone in your group should be assigned the responsibilities of group medic. That person will make the difference between success and failure for a community that has lost access to modern medicine.

The "survival medic" knows that they have been handed a major challenge and that there are some tough decisions ahead. Those who step up and take responsibility for the medical well-being of their loved ones will be special individuals with a special mission.

If you have been chosen to pick up the flag, your first assignment is to get some training. Some of it will be book learning, and some will be hands-on; the more you learn, the more comfortable you will be in your new role.

Start by studying basic first aid and have a good book on family medicine in your library. A good approach would be to learn as much anatomy and physiology as possible. Anatomy is the blueprint of the body; physiology is the operating manual. With a working knowledge of these two subjects, you're in a better position to understand disease and injury. This is essential for you to become a successful medic.

At the same time, research some alternative disciplines such as herbalism. When the commercial medicines run out, you will need a base of knowledge about area plants that may have medicinal benefits. Many times, a successful medic will cultivate favorite herbs specifically for the purpose of having them available for emergencies.

What are some characteristics of the effective medic? The most important is just having common sense. A sensible person with good medical supplies, a few medical books and a willingness to learn can be successful in keeping their family healthy in disasters.

Besides a sensible, practical nature, it helps if you have a calm demeanor. Sick or injured people take comfort from a level-headed caregiver. Another useful attribute of a good medic is the dedication to teach others. One person can't be everywhere at once, and you'll likely find other members of your group eager to learn. Cross-training is extremely important, as the medic might, one day, need a medic.

Confidentiality could be a very important asset to ensure success as a medical resource. You should interview your group members now so that you'll have all the information you need to keep them healthy in times of trouble. Sometimes that information includes things that your patient doesn't want to be made public. You must never disclose anything that would make others see you as untrustworthy. If you don't have the trust of the community you serve, you lose effectiveness as a medic.

There is one last essential characteristic of the successful medic: Self-preservation. This may sound strange to you, but you are an indispensable resource to your entire group. If you frequently place yourself in harm's way, you will eventually find yourself as the patient more often than you or anyone else would like. Always determine if you can care for the victim without placing yourself in undue danger. You must abolish all threats; if someone has a gunshot wound, it stands to reason that there's a guy with a gun out there! Don't become the next casualty.

THE STATUS ASSESSMENT

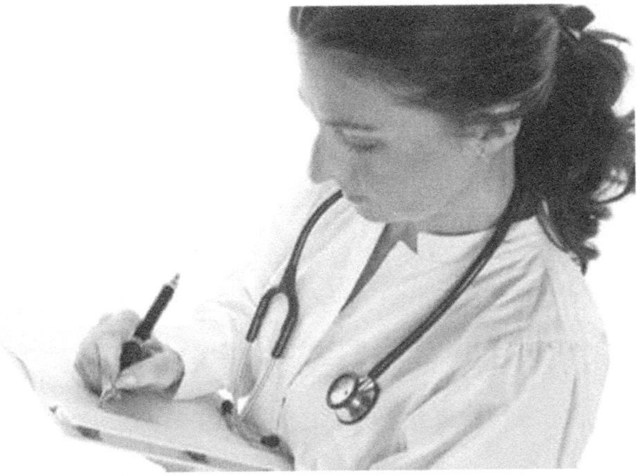

The family medic should assess their level of preparedness well before a disaster occurs. We call this "the status assessment". When performing this assessment, a number of questions must be asked and answered that clarify your job description and your level of readiness.

What Will Your Responsibilities Be?

It goes without saying that, as group medic, you will be responsible for the medical well-being of your survival community. But what does that mean? It means that, as well as being the Chief Medical Officer, that you will be:

Chief sanitation officer: It will be your duty to make sure that sanitary conditions at your camp or retreat don't cause the spread of disease among the members. This will be a major issue in an austere setting, and will cause the most medical issues in any survival group.

Some of your responsibilities will relate to latrine placement and construction, others will relate to the supervision of appropriate filtration and sterilization of water. Assurance of proper preparation of food and cleaning of work surfaces will also be very important, as will be the maintenance of good personal and group hygiene. Elimination of vermin from shelters will decrease the spread of disease.

Careful attention to these details on your part will be an essential part of a program that will keep your family or community healthy.

Chief dental officer: Medical personnel in wartime or in remote locations often report that patients arriving at Sick Call complained of dental problems as often as medical problems. Anyone who has had a bad toothache knows that it affects concentration and, certainly, work efficiency.

You will need to know how to deal with dental issues (toothaches, broken teeth, lost fillings) to be an effective medic in a long term survival setting. Part of your planning, therefore, will be the accumulation of appropriate dental supplies that can handle emergencies you're likely to encounter. More on this later in the book.

Chief counselor: It goes without saying that any societal collapse would wreak havoc with people's mindsets. You will have to know how to deal with depression and anxiety as well as cuts and broken bones. In other words, you're the chaplain.

Therefore, you will have to sharpen your communication skills as much as your medical skills. A good healthcare provider also understands, as mentioned earlier, the importance of confidentiality in all their patient contacts. Having the trust of the members of your group greatly increases your effectiveness.

Medical quartermaster: You've done your job and accumulated medical and dental supplies, but who decides when you break them out and use them? You do.

When will you dispense your limited supply of antibiotics, for example? In a collapse, these items will no longer be produced due to the complexity of their manufacture. Careful monitoring of supply stock and usage allows you to control the ability to handle medical emergencies.

Medical Archivist: You are in charge of writing down the medical histories of the people in your group. Seems like a lot of work? Perhaps, but this record will be useful to remember all the medical conditions that your people have, their allergies, and medications that they might be taking. If your community is large, it would be almost impossible to memorize all of this information.

Also, your histories of the treatments you have performed on each patient are important to put into writing. One day, you might not be there to render care; your archives will be a valuable resource to the person that is in charge when you're not around. Until that day, however, these histories must remain confidential.

Medical education resource: You can't be in two places at once, and you will have to make sure that those in your group have some basic medical knowledge. It's important that they can take care of injuries or illness while you're away. Some injuries require quick action, and the training you impart can save a life.

These responsibilities are many, but may be modified somewhat by the makeup of your group. If you have a pastor or other clergy in your group, they can take some of the burden of counseling away from you. If you have someone skilled in engineering, water treatment, or waste disposal, they might be able to use their knowledge to help maintain sanitary conditions at the retreat, or assure healthy filtered water. Be sure to take whatever help you can get.

What Scenario Are You Preparing For?

It's important to accumulate medical supplies and knowledge that will work in any situation, but what are you actually expecting to happen? Your preparations should be modified to fit the particular situation that you believe will cause modern medical care to be unavailable. There are many possible scenarios that could leave you without access to medical help, and each of them requires some specialized planning. Your readiness to deal with the most likely illnesses or injuries will increase your effectiveness exponentially.

Economic Collapse: If you feel that we are on the verge of an economic collapse, you probably believe that the reliable transport of food from farms to the public will no longer exist (nobody is paying the truckers). In that case, malnutrition will be rampant. Your responsibility as medic would be to make sure that your group's food storage includes everything required to give good nutrition. Stockpiling vitamin supplements, commercial or natural, would be a good strategy in this situation. Even if not taken daily, they may be helpful in preventing diseases caused by deficiencies.

Knowledge of what nutrients are present in local plant life will also be useful. Take the following historical example: In the 1500s, a Spanish exploration party was dying of scurvy (Vitamin C deficiency) in the middle of a forest. Native Americans noted their plight and took pity upon them.

They walked to the nearest pine tree and picked some new green pine needles. They made a tea out of them and nursed the Spaniards back to health. The pine needles happened to be rich in Vitamin C. It's that kind of knowledge that could be as critical to you as it was for them.

Civil Unrest: Certainly, civil unrest is part and parcel of many natural or man-made disasters. In this case, tailor your supplies and training to equip you to deal with possible traumatic injuries. Stock up on bandages and antiseptics. Other specialized equipment such as splints and blood clotting agents would be important in this circumstance.

Pandemic: From the Black Plague to Ebola, many people are concerned about a widespread outbreak of infectious disease that could reach epidemic status. When it affects multiple regions, we call it a "pandemic".

If you're worried about a "super flu" descending on your area, stock up on masks and gloves as well as antibiotic and antiviral drugs. Figure out a quarantine strategy to keep your family isolated from sick individuals. Most importantly, plan out a survival sick room that will help the ill recover while limiting exposure of the healthy to the infection.

Nuclear Meltdown: How about a nuclear reactor meltdown? To take this to extremes, perhaps you live near an army base, a large city, or a nuclear plant and you're concerned about a terrorist group setting off a nuclear bomb. In that scenario, you'll have to know how to protect your group from radiation, and how to build an effective shelter. You'll want medications like Potassium Iodide to counteract some of the long-term effects of radiation on the thyroid gland.

Terrorist Attack: Terror events are part of the "new normal" that we may have to accept in the uncertain future. Most will be an active shooter or a strategically placed bomb. It will be important to carry materials specifically to stop bleeding in mass casualty incidents.

It's clear that your supplies and training should be modified depending on the course of events. Determine specific scenarios that are likely to involve you and plan accordingly.

How Many People Will You Be Responsible For?

Your store of medical supplies should cover the number of persons that you will be responsible for. If you have stockpiled 5 treatment courses of antibiotics, it might be enough for a couple or a sole individual. But it will go fast if you are taking care of 20 people.

Remember that most of those people will be out performing tasks that they aren't used to doing. They will be making campfires, chopping wood and lifting heavy loads. You'll see more injuries like sprains and strains, fractures, lacerations, and burns; you'll need enough supplies to deal with them.

Can you ever have enough medical supplies? They'll get used up faster than you think. Another consideration is that you, almost certainly, will wind up dealing with more survivors than you expected. The biggest mistake that the survival medic will make is the underestimation of the number of people that will appear on their doorstep in times of trouble. You won't turn away *every* person that needs help. As a result, your group will be bigger than you would expect and your medical storage should take this into account.

Let's say that you had more medical supplies than you need. In this unlikely scenario, any "excess" items will always be highly sought after for barter purposes. You might spend your money on buying physical silver and gold, but you won't be able to set a broken bone or wrap a sprained ankle with "precious" metals. Food and medical items will be more valuable than mining stocks in hard times.

The bottom line is simple: Always have more medical items on hand than you think are sufficient for the number of people in your group.

What Special Needs Will You Have To Care For?

The special issues you will deal with depend on who is in your group. The medical needs of children or the elderly are different from an average adult. Women have different health problems than men.

You will have to know if group members have a chronic condition, such as asthma or diabetes. Failure to take things like this into account could be catastrophic. For example, would you be prepared if you found out a group member required adult diapers *after* a calamity occurs?

Be certain to interview all of your group members, so that you won't be surprised that this person has thyroid problems or that person has high blood pressure. All of these variables will modify the supplies and medical knowledge you must obtain. Encourage those with special needs to stockpile medicines and materials that will help keep them well. Encourage them to have a frank discussion with their physician and obtain extra drug prescriptions in case of emergency (and have them filled in advance).

What Physical Environment Will You Live In?

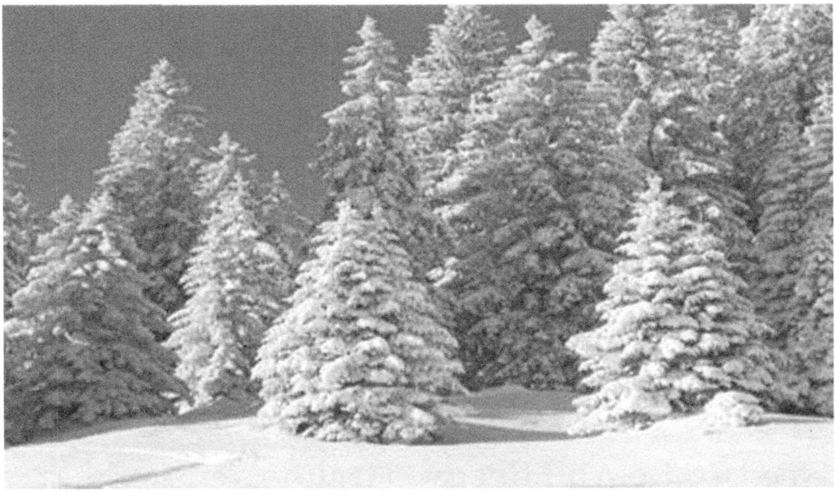

Is your retreat located in a cold climate? If so, you will need to know how to keep people warm and how to treat hypothermia and other complications of exposure. If you're located in a hot climate, you will need to know how to treat heat stroke. Is your environment wet and humid? People who are chronically wet generally don't stay healthy, so you will have to have a strategy to keep your group members dry. Are you in a dry, desert-like environment? If you are, you will have to have a strategy for providing a steady supply of clean water.

Some people live in areas where all of the above conditions exist at one point or another during the year. These considerations might even factor into where you would choose to live if a collapse is imminent.

How Long Do You Expect To Be The Sole Medical Resource?

Some catastrophes, such as major damage from tornadoes or hurricanes, may limit access to medical care for a relatively short period of time. A societal breakdown, however, could mean that there is no availability of advanced medical care for the foreseeable future.

The longer you will be the healthcare resource for your group, the more supplies you will have to stockpile and the more varied those supplies should be. If the catastrophe means a few weeks without medical care, you probably can get away without, for example, equipment to extract a diseased tooth. If it's a true long-term collapse, however, that equipment will be quite important.

Spend some time thinking about all the possible medical issues you might face as the end of the line caregiver for your family. Prepare a plan of action to handle each one. Take precautions to be ready for issues that may occur in the future, such as birth control for a daughter who has not yet reached puberty.

How Do You Obtain The Information You Will Need To Be An Effective Healthcare Provider?

A good library of medical, dental, and nutritional books will give you the tools to be an effective medic. Even if you were already a doctor, let's say a general practitioner, you would need various references to learn how to perform surgical procedures that you ordinarily would send to the local surgeon. If you're a surgeon, you would need references to refresh your knowledge of the treatment of diabetes. Even the most resourceful homesteader can't know everything.

Don't ignore online sources of information. Take advantage of websites with quality medical information; there are thousands of them. By printing out information you believe will be helpful to your specific situation, you'll accumulate a unique store of knowledge that fits your particular needs. We want you to have it in physical form because you never know; one day, the internet may not be as accessible as it is today.

Some information is best absorbed visually. Sites like YouTube have thousands of medically oriented films on just about every topic. Videos range from suturing wounds to setting a fractured bone to extracting a damaged tooth. You will have the benefit of seeing things done in real time, which is always better than just looking at pictures.

The number of medical resources is almost endless; take advantage of them. We have compiled a list of reference books and useful videos at the back of this book. Review them and consider adding them to your library.

How Do You Obtain Medical Training?

There are various ways to get practical training. Almost every municipality gives you access to various courses that would help you function as an effective healthcare provider. Some are time-intensive and costly, but many are not.

EMT (Emergency Medical Technician) Basic: This is the standard for providing emergency care. The courses are set out by the U.S. Department of Transportation, and are offered by many community colleges. The course length is usually several hundred hours.

We know that this represents a significant commitment of time and effort, but it is the complete package short of going to medical or nursing school for years. You will receive an overview of anatomy and physiology, and an introduction to the basics of looking after sick or injured patients.

These programs, however, are based around delivering the patient to a hospital as an end result. As medical facilities may not be accessible in the aftermath of a disaster, they may not be perfect for a long-term survival situation. Having said this, you will still learn a lot of useful information and we highly recommend them.

It should be noted that there are different levels of Emergency Medical Technician. EMT-Basic is the primary course of study, but you can continue your studies and become a Paramedic. Paramedics are taught more advanced procedures, such as placing airways, using defibrillators, and inserting intravenous lines. In remote areas, they might even take on the roles of physicians and nurses to give injections, place casts, or stitch up wounds. These skills are highly pertinent in the aftermath of a disaster.

CERT (Community Emergency Response Team): Most of us will not have the time and resources to commit to such an intensive course of training. For many, a Red Cross First Responder or CERT course is the ticket. These programs cover a lot of the same subjects (albeit in much less detail) and would certainly represent a good start on your way to getting trained. The usual course length is 40-80 hours. Besides the Red Cross, many municipalities also offer the course.

CPR (cardio-pulmonary resuscitation): Of course, the American Heart Association and others provide standard CPR courses. Everyone should take these whether or not they will have medical responsibility in times of trouble. The limitation here is that successful resuscitation from, say, a heart attack, will require patient transfer to an intensive care unit to significantly increase the chance for full recovery.

Wilderness and Other Medical Courses: There are a number of "specialty" courses provided by private enterprises which might be helpful. Wilderness EMT/Tactical EMT courses are programs meant to teach medical care in a potentially hostile environment. Sometimes, they have a prerequisite of at least EMT-Basic.

There are many wilderness "schools" out there, however, that will offer some practical training to non-medical professionals At the very least, they are cognizant that such a disaster scenario could happen, and that your goal of transporting the patient to modern medical facilities might not be an option. It pays to research the schools that provide this training, as the quality of the learning experience probably varies.

Military Training: One course of learning not yet mentioned is military training. Some of the best caregivers in times of trouble will be those who served as medics in the armed forces. If you are eligible to serve, consider it. It's a big decision, but one that may pay dividends down the road.

LIKELY MEDICAL ISSUES YOU'LL FACE

It is important to tailor your education and training to the probable medical issues you will have to treat. In an austere or post-collapse setting, it might be difficult to predict what these might be. Therefore, it's helpful to examine the experience of those who provide medical care in underdeveloped areas. With this information, you will be able to determine what medical supplies will be needed and prepare yourself for the probable emergencies you'll face.

The experiences of medical missionaries over an extended time in a remote area identify likely medical issues that would occur in disaster settings. It wasn't unusual to see the following:

Trauma

- Minor Musculoskeletal injuries (sprains and strains)
- Minor trauma (cuts, scrapes)
- Major traumatic injury (fractures, occasional knife and/or gunshot wounds)
- Burn injuries (all degrees)

Infection

- Respiratory infections (pneumonia, bronchitis, influenza, common colds)
- Diarrheal disease (sometimes a community-wide outbreak)
- Infected wounds
- Minor infections (for example, urinary infections, "pinkeye")
- Sexually transmitted diseases
- Lice, Ticks, Mosquitoes, and the diseases they carry

Allergic reactions

- Minor (bees, bed bugs, or other insect bites and stings)
- Major (anaphylactic shock)

Dental

- Toothaches
- Broken or knocked-out teeth
- Loss fillings
- Loose crowns or other dental work

Women's issues

- Pregnancy
- Miscarriage
- Birth control

The above are just a few of the issues you can expect to encounter in your role as medic.

A short aside here: If you have purchased this volume, you probably have done some research into collapse scenarios which could lead to society unraveling. You have probably been given a great deal of advice as to what to do in this situation or that, but you have never been given this advice:

If you want to be fruitful, don't multiply; at least in the early going of a major collapse.

It should be clear that you are going to need all of your personnel at 110% efficiency. Anyone who has been pregnant knows that there may be a "glow" associated with it, but you sure aren't at peak performance. Even those who are well-prepared for just about any disaster often forget that pregnancies happen, and don't plan ahead for them. When a member of your family or group is unexpectedly with child, you may find it difficult to be mobile when you need to be. As well, your supply of manpower, especially in a small family, has taken a big hit.

Pregnancy is relatively safe these days, but there was a time in the not too distant past where the announcement of a pregnancy was met as much with concern as joy. Complications such as miscarriage, postpartum bleeding and infection took their toll on women, and you must seriously plan to prevent pregnancy, at least until things stabilize.

Condoms are reasonable options, but will become brittle after two or three years. Consider taking the time to learn about natural methods of birth control, such as the Natural Family Planning method. This is a simple method that predicts ovulation by taking body temperatures, and is relatively effective. A discussion of this method and others will take place later in this book.

Don't misunderstand us: We are not saying that you shouldn't rebuild society or follow your personal or religious beliefs. We just want you to understand that your burden, in a collapse, will be heavier if you don't plan for every possibility.

MEDICAL SKILLS YOU'LL WANT TO LEARN

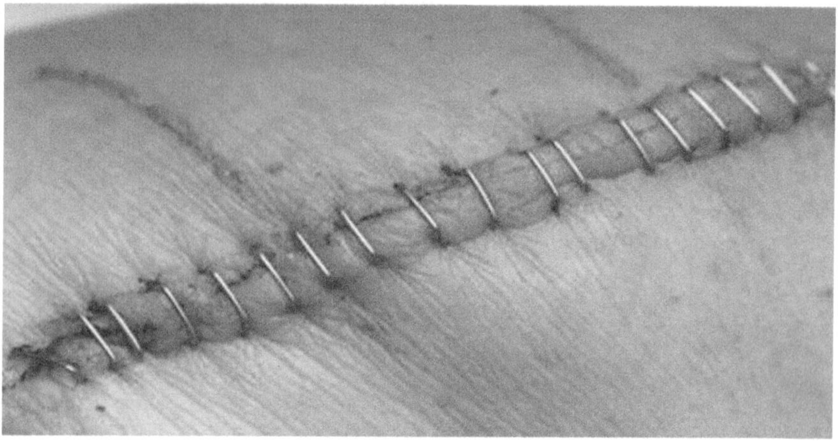

A very reasonable question for an aspiring medic to ask is "What exactly do I need to know?" The answer is: As much as you're willing to learn. Using the previous list of likely medical issues will give you a good idea of the skills you'll need. You can expect to deal with lots of ankle sprains, colds, cuts, rashes, and other common medical issues that affect people in normal times. In addition, you will need to know how to deal with more significant problems, such as a leg fracture. You'll also need to know what medical supplies will be required and how to follow your patient's status until they are fully recovered.

To become an effective medical resource, you'll want to learn how to:

- Take vital signs, such as pulses, respiration rates and blood pressures.
- Place bandages on injuries.
- Clean an open wound.
- Treat varying degrees of burns.
- Perform a normal delivery of a baby and placenta.
- Splint, pad and wrap a sprain, dislocation, or fracture.
- Identify bacterial infectious diseases (such as Strep throat, etc.).
- Identify viral infectious diseases (such as influenza, etc.).

- Identify parasitic/protozoal diseases (such as Giardia, etc.).
- Identify and treat head, pubic, and body lice, as well as bed bug and tick bites.
- Identify venomous snakes and treat the effects of their bites and those of other animals.
- Identify and treat various causes of abdominal, pelvic, and chest pain.
- Recognize and treat allergic reactions and anaphylactic shock.
- Identify and treat sexually transmitted diseases.
- Evaluate and treat dental problems (replace fillings, treat abscesses, and perform extractions).
- Recognize and treat various skin conditions.
- Care for the bedridden patient (treating bedsores, transport considerations).
- Establish basic hygiene, nutrition and sanitary practices (this couldn't be more important).
- Counsel the depressed or anxious patient (you will see a lot of this in times of trouble).
- Insert an IV (EMT classes teach this).
- Close a wound with sutures, staples, glues, or butterfly closures (and, more importantly, when *not to* close a wound).
- Identify the reasons to use different medications, essential oils, and alternative therapies. As well, know the dosages, frequency of administration, and side effects of those substances. This is best accomplished with a copy of the Physician's Desk Reference, a large book that comes out yearly with information on just about every drug in existence, a good herbalism book, and the book you're reading now.

Perhaps the most important medical skill is how to *prevent* injuries and illnesses. You will spend much of your time observing simple things, such as whether your people are appropriately dressed for the weather. You will be required to enforce the use of hand and eye protection during work sessions. You must learn to recognize situations that place your family at risk; if you can do this, you'll avoid many problems.

We know that this is a lot to absorb. Don't feel, though, that learning this information is impossible, or that you can't be an asset if you only learn some of the above. The important thing is to learn enough to treat some of the more common medical issues.

Once you've learned the basics, you'll be able to take care of 90% of the problems that confront you in times of trouble. After that, any additional information you learn will just make you even more effective as a medical resource.

MEDICAL SUPPLIES

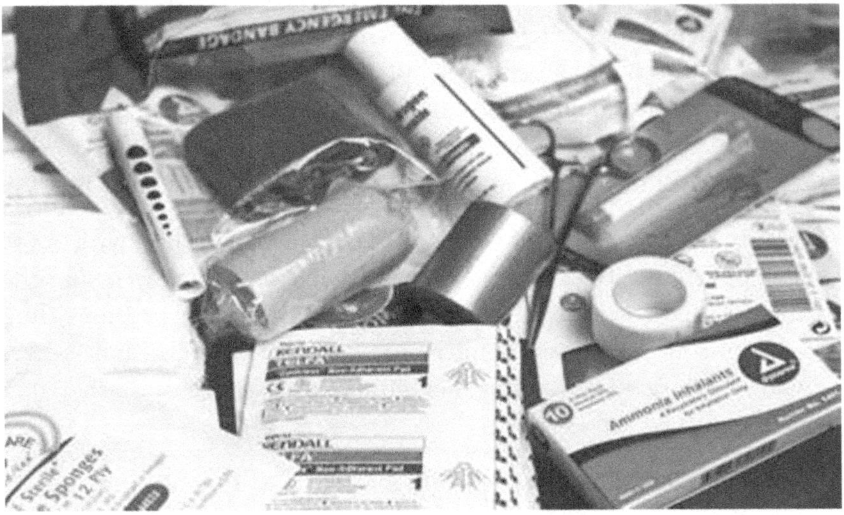

For anyone to do their job properly, they'll need the right equipment. Imagine a carpenter having to use a steak knife as a saw, or a hunter using a pea shooter instead of a rifle. The same goes for the medic. The successful survival caregiver has spent a lot of time and energy (and some money) on accumulating a stockpile of medical supplies. The more the better, since you don't know how long you might have to function without access to modern medical care.

It's important to note that the value of many medical supplies depends largely on the knowledge and skill that the user has obtained through study and practice. A blood pressure cuff isn't very useful to someone who doesn't know how to take a blood pressure. Concentrate first on obtaining items that you can use effectively, and then purchase more advanced equipment as you learn more skills.

Don't forget that many items can be improvised; a bandanna can serve as a sling, an ironing board as a stretcher, or thin fishing line and a sewing needle as suturing equipment. A careful inspection of your own home would probably turn up lots of items that can be adapted to medical use. Look with a creative eye and you'll be surprised at the medical issues you are already equipped to deal with.

The Medic Bag

If you are going to be the medical caregiver for your family or community in times of trouble, you will, hopefully, have accumulated a significant number of medical supplies. You'll find many articles that tell you what to put in a medical kit, but few ever talk about a basic piece of medical equipment that everyone needs: the medical bag that will contain all these supplies.

Without a place to put your medical supplies, they will, most likely, be strewn about in a way that prevents you from accessing the stuff you need when an emergency arises. This wastes precious time when someone's life may hang in the balance. Organization is key; if you're disorganized, you're not going to be effective at the time you're most needed.

One important aspect of choosing a bag that fits your needs is size. Size matters; you should assess your needs to determine which size bag is right for you. The factors that go into this decision include:

- Are you staying in place or on the move?
- How many people are you responsible for?
- How long will you be the medical resource for your family or group?
- Are you in an area that is potentially dangerous?
- What climate should you be prepared for?
- What medical issues will you be most likely to encounter?
- Can you depend on clean water?
- How many medical supplies do you have?

Which medical supplies should every member of your family carry in case you get separated? What are the more advanced supplies that the medic should carry? You might start by having members of your group carry an IFAK (Individual First Aid Kit) whenever they're away from base camp. The family medic carries the advanced items in a larger bag.

The best medic bags are sturdy ones with lots of clear or mesh pockets. These bags have everything you'll need in an emergency in plain sight if packed right, and will avoid the question you never want to ask yourself if someone's injured: "Where'd I put the tourniquet?", or "Where'd I put the burn dressings?" Closed pouches in the bag could be used for non-emergency items, like certain medicines, water filters, etc. Putting your items in groups based on the issues they deal with is also a great idea.

The important thing is to have the medical kit make sense for you. This might mean taking an already packed kit like one of ours and moving things around so that the arrangement seems natural for your purposes.

A medical bag doesn't have to be commercially produced; a tool box or other item that sets up your supplies in an organized way is all that is needed.

Medical Kits

When we speak at various conferences throughout the country, the question we are invariably asked is "What medical supplies should I have stored away?"

Most people will search for an already-complete kit and, indeed, we even design such kits ourselves for our website. Unfortunately, most commercial first aid kits you'll find are fine for a single mishap, but not enough to handle your long term role as family medic.

We're talking about serious medical stockpiles here. There are three levels of medical kits that we will identify and for which we'll list our preferences for content:

- The individual first aid kit, also called an "IFAK"
- The family kit
- The field hospital

The lightest kit is the individual first aid kit or **IFAK**. Every member of a group carries this kit; it allows, in most cases, treatment of some common issues encountered in the wilderness or when traveling. This is especially useful when every member of a group is given some medical training.

In some military services, the IFAK is useful to the combat medic as a source of supply. If a squad member is injured, the medic may first use items from the wounded soldier's kit. This serves as a resource multiplier and allows the corpsman to carry the more advanced equipment in their pack. One example of a useful IFAK item is a tourniquet.

The second kit listed below is the "family kit": This kit is mobile, with the items fitting in a standard large backpack, and will suffice as a medical "bug-out" kit for a couple and their children. It is, in our opinion, the minimum amount of equipment that a head of household would need to handle common emergencies in a long-term survival situation.

A family kit is meant to be sufficient to fully handle injuries and illnesses for a small number of people. This set requires a designated person (probably you) to transport it when changes of location are necessary. A typical item for this kit would be a moldable 36 inch splint.

The third kit is the "field hospital". It will contain everything that you have stockpiled for the long term care of the family or group. This is meant to be all at a place your community would consider to be the hospital or clinic. As such, items here would include a number of cots, dedicated bedding, plastic sheeting, and work surfaces.

Don't feel intimidated by the sheer volume of supplies in the more advanced kits. Few of us have the resources or skills to purchase and effectively use every single item. If you can put together a good family kit, you will have accomplished quite a lot.

Here are the supplies we recommend for each kit. See what makes sense for you to have; use a pen or pencil to fill in the "dot" when you acquire the item:

The IFAK or Personal Kit

- ○ Nitrile Gloves (hypoallergenic), in various sizes for larger group supplies
- ○ Cold packs/Hot packs, instant and/or reusable

- Scalpels and/or Field Knife
- Ace Wraps
- Israeli Bandage or other compression bandages
- Celox or Quikclot hemostatic clotting agents (stops moderate to severe bleeding in wounds)
- Tourniquets (CAT, SOF-T, SWAT, EMT are examples)
- Compressed Gauze (H and H brand is an example)
- Steri-strips or Butterfly Closures and Tincture of Benzoin (to help the strips stick to skin)
- Nail Scissors or Clippers
- Hemostat Clamp 5", Straight or Curved
- 3-0 Nylon or Silk Suture
- Super Glue or Medical Glue
- Tweezers (in various sizes and tips for larger group supplies)
- Penlight and Headlamp
- Bandage Scissors 7.25" Stainless steel (better) or EMT scissors
- Adhesive Bandages, various sizes (non-latex if possible)
- ABD Dressings, in small and large sizes
- Gauze Dressings Sterile and Non-sterile, various sizes
- Non-Stick Sterile Dressings (Telfa type), various sizes
- Roller Gauze Sterile Dressings (Kerlix), various sizes
- Moleskin or Molepad
- Mylar, Solar, or Survival blanket
- Cloth Medical Tape
- Duct Tape
- Triangular Bandage with safety pins, and bandannas
- Ammonia Inhalants
- Antibiotic Ointment or Creams, like Triple, Bacitracin, Neomycin and Bactroban (Rx)
- Alcohol Wipes, Povidone-iodine (Betadine) Wipes, BZK wipes (Benzalkonium Chloride)
- Burn Gel and Hydrocortisone Cream
- Sting Relief Wipes
- Hand Sanitizer
- Lip balm, and Sunscreen
- Ibuprofen Tablets, Benadryl Tablets and Rehydration Packets
- Waterproof Paper and Pencil

All of the above plus the following, quantities will be dependent on the number of people you are medical responsible for. Obtain as much as possible, you may be taking care of more people than you think.

The Family Kit

- First Aid Reference Book (this one is good)
- Headlamps, with extra batteries (for night or poor lighting conditions)
- Instant Glucose and/or Raw Unprocessed Honey
- Chest Seals, Vented, 2 per pack (entry and exit wound coverage)
- Oral Airways (to keep airway open)
- Nasal airways- NPAs (keeps airways open) and Surgical lube
- Soap and/or Dr. Bronner's Castile liquid soap
- CPR Shields
- Safety Pins (large), Rubber Bands and Paper Clips
- Scalpel and disposable blades (lots)
- Neck Collars, various sizes
- Extra Large Absorbent Pads (ABD or other brand)
- Petrolatum/Xeroform dressings in various sizes
- Burn Dressings and Burn Blankets
- Coban or Self-Adhering Wraps
- Liquid Bandage (Like New Skin)
- Medical Tapes, various types (Elastoplast, Silk, and Paper) and sizes (1 inch, 2 inch etc.)
- Skin Tac Liquid Adhesive Barrier (prepares skin for application of tapes, dressings and protects the skin with a hypo-allergenic sticky film) or equivalent Skin Prep Wipes
- Moleskin or Spenco Second Skin Blister kit
- Styptic Pencils
- Eye Cups, Eye Pads, Patches and Eye wash
- SAM splints and Slings
- Blood Pressure Cuff, various sizes (sphygmomanometer)
- Stethoscopes
- Bio Glo Strips (Fluorescein sodium Rx only)- used to stain the eye, and a Cobalt Blue light bulb to shine on the injured eye and allow visualization of cuts or foreign objects

- Cotton Swabs (Q-tips), Cotton Balls, Cotton-tipped applicators, Cotton Rounds
- Face Masks (surgical and N95)
- Chest Decompression Needles
- Tongue Depressors
- Magnifying Glasses
- Extra Batteries
- Glow Sticks
- Multi Tools
- Flashlights
- Paracord 550
- Ring Cutter
- Kelly Clamps, straight and curved in various sizes
- Needle Holders
- Half Circle sewing needles and Silk Thread
- Sutures in many variations, such as:
- Vicryl; 0, 2-0, 4-0 (absorbable)
- Chromic 0, 2-0, 4-0 (absorbable)
- Silk, Nylon and Prolene 0, 2-0, 3-0, 4-0(non-absorbable)
- Sharps Disposal Box
- Suture Removal Tray
- Surgical Staplers and Staple Removers
- Iodoform Sterile Packing Gauze
- Micropore Tape
- Styptic Pencil (stops bleeding from superficial cuts)
- Silver Nitrate Sticks and Cautery Pens
- Saline Solution (several liter bottles), or DIY with recipe in this book
- Irrigation Syringes (60-100 ml is good) and Irrigation Cups (like Zerowet)
- Hair Combs and Brushes (hygiene)
- Nail Files, Foot Files and Heel Creams
- Thermometers (rectal or ear)
- Hot Water Bottles and Ice Bags (both reusable)
- Ziploc Bags, Plastic Wrap
- Aluminum Foil (use to sharpen scissors, by cutting the foil several times)

- Cotton Sheets (100% in white)
- Eye Droppers and Bulb Syringes
- Measuring Spoons and Cups
- Antiseptic Solutions in large and medium quantities (Betadine, Hibiclens, etc.)
- Hydrogen Peroxide 3% and 6-7%
- Rubbing Alcohol
- Enema Bags
- Nutritional Supplements (Boost, Pediasure)
- Vitamins, multi, and Pregnancy Vitamins
- Sunblock
- Lip Balms
- Insect Repellants
- Bactine or equivalent (for cuts and bug bites)
- Fels-Naptha/Zanfel Soap (poison ivy, oak and sumac)
- Poison Ivy Wipes (like Zanfel)
- Hydrocortisone Cream 1%
- Lidocaine Cream or jelly 2.5% (topical anesthetic)
- Dermoplast Spray and Solarcaine Cool Aloe Burn
- Medi-First Burn Spray (analgesic, antiseptic and liquid band-aid all in one)
- Biofreeze Gel or Cold Freeze Spray for intact skin only
- Acetaminophen/Ibuprofen/Aspirin
- Benadryl (Diphenhydramine)
- Epinephrine (Epi-pen, prescription injection for severe allergic reactions)
- Claritin (Loratadine)
- Anti-Nausea Medication (Meclizine hydrochloride 2.5mg tablets)
- Zofran (Rx for nausea and vomiting)
- Ear and Eye Drops
- Cough Syrup and Lozenges/Drops
- Expectorants (to loosen up thick mucus)
- Decongestants (to move mucus out of the respiratory system)
- Vicks Vapor Rub
- Nebulizer, saline, tubing, mask or mouth piece (plus Rx Albuterol single dose liquid)

- Sleep Aids (like Alteril, Tylenol PM, Melatonin, Chamomile or Valerian Tea etc.)
- Fiber Supplements (Metamucil)
- Stool Softeners and Laxatives
- Suppositories and Finger Cots
- Beano or equivalent (to reduce gas formation with certain foods)
- Anti-Diarrheal, Imodium (Loperamide)
- Pepto-Bismol (Bismuth Subsalicylate)
- Heartburn Medications and natural treatments
- Rid Shampoo/Nix Lotion or Creme Rinse and Nix Electric Lice Comb (for lice)
- Oral Rehydration Packs and Gatorade Packets (or make it from scratch)
- Water Purification Tablets
- Emergency Water Bag
- Water Filters, portable and large family size
- Waterproof Matches, lighters and other methods to start fires
- Gold Bond Foot Powder
- Calamine lotion
- Burn Cream (Rx Silvadene), Burn Gel or burn treatments (sprays) with anesthetic
- Colloidal Silver (for external treatments)
- Anti-fungal Cream (Terconazole)
- Anti-fungal Powder (Tinactin)
- Fluconazole 100 or 150mg tablets (Rx antifungal)
- Urinary Pain Reliever (Uristat or AZO tablets)
- Wart Removal cream/ointment/solution/freeze
- Hemorrhoid Cream or Ointment (Preparation H)
- Zinc Oxide cream or ointment
- A & D ointment
- Vaseline
- Muscle Rub (like Icy Hot, Blue Emu, or Arnica salve)
- Tens Unit or equivalent (Muscle Stimulation pain reliever machine)
- Oral Antibiotics (discussed later)
- Radiation Pills, Thyrosafe or equivalent, one box per person (if your area may be exposed to radiation)

- PMS Medication, like Pamprin (which acts as a mild diuretic also), and natural remedies
- Caffeine Pills
- Natural Equivalents of any the above; see natural medicine chapters
- Birth Control Accessories (condoms, birth control pills, cervical caps, etc.)
- Emergency Obstetric Kit (comes as a pack) and Nitrazine strips (pH strips)
- Midwifery Reference Books
- Fetal Electronic Doppler or Fetoscope
- Maxi Pads and Tampons (female use, and tampons for nose bleeds)
- Measuring Tapes
- Paper, pencils, pens and permanent markers

Dental Tray:

- Cotton Pellets and Rolls
- Dental mirror
- Tongue Blades
- Toothpaste and Toothbrushes
- Baking Soda and Peppermint Oil
- Hydrogen Peroxide 3% (oral rinse to treat or prevent gum issues)
- Syringes 12cc Curved tip
- Dental Scraper
- Dental Pick and Toothpicks
- Dental Floss and Dental Wax
- Oral Analgesics
- Canker Sore Tx (like Orajel or Hurricane Gel and Kank-A, and Orabase)
- Clove Bud Oil (anesthetic for toothache)
- Zinc Oxide (make a paste with oil of cloves and you get temporary dental cement), or…
- Commercial dental kits (Den-Temp, Cavit)
- Hank's Solution (used to preserve viability in knocked-out teeth)

- Pill Cups
- Scalpels, disposable
- 4-0 Chromic sutures (absorbable)
- Needle Holder
- Gauze 2 x 2 inches
- Actcel Hemostatic agent (stops dental bleeding, and dissolves naturally)
- Extraction Equipment (several different extractors and elevators)
- Spoon Excavator
- Generic or brand name Ibuprofen
- Gloves, Masks, and Eye protection

Natural Remedy Supplies

- Witch Hazel and Extract
- Bag Balm ointment
- Drawing Salve
- Raw Unprocessed Honey (local is best)
- Cayenne Pepper Powder (see medicinal garden chapter)
- Aloe Vera
- Herbal Teas, Tinctures, Salves, and Essential Oils (see Natural Remedies)
- Neti Pot (use only with sterile solutions) and Diffusers
- Medicinal Herb and Plant seeds (in long-term storage packaging)
- Herbal Medicine Reference Books
- Gardening Reference Books
- Mortar and Pestle
- Graters, Stainless Steel
- Clear and Brown Glass Jars with Lids
- Glass Bottles (various sizes) Green, Brown and Clear with Cork Tops
- Metal Tins, ½ ounce to 4 ounce sizes
- Sealing Wax
- Funnels, Kitchen Mesh Strainers and Cotton Muslin Bags
- Clocks and Kitchen Timers
- Kitchen Scale

- Grain Alcohol and Vodkas (for making tinctures), other spirits as needed
- Copper Distiller (to distill essential oils, etc.)
- Cheesecloth
- Coffee Filters
- Tea Ball Infuser
- Coconut, Olive, Neem, Sesame, Shea Nut, Wheat Germ, Castor, Grapeseed, Soybean Oils
- Vegetable Glycerin, Vitamin E Oil, Steric Acid, Grapefruit Seed Extract, Citric Acid
- White cosmetic clay (Kaolin), makes an excellent poultice base
- Beeswax and pastilles, Cocoa Butter wax and wafers, Shea Butter
- Gelatin or Vegetable Capsules, Capsule Making Machine
- Teapots, Coffee Pots
- Coal Tar Shampoo
- Selenium Shampoo
- Baking Soda and Corn Starch
- Apple Cider Vinegar and White Vinegar
- Epsom Salts
- Sugar, Salt, and Salt Substitutes (part of rehydration formula)
- Cayenne Pepper Powder (for sore throat gargle and to help stop mild-mod bleeding)
- Saline Nasal Spray (or sterile homemade solution)

The Field Hospital

All of the above in larger quantities, plus:

- Extensive medical library
- Pandemic Protective Gear: Face Shields, Tyvek Coveralls, Hoodies, Aprons, Boots, long Gloves, Waterproof Boots
- Goggles, indirect vented
- Treatment Table and Stretches
- Cots or Beds and Chairs
- Bedside Table and Mayo Stands
- Portable Lights and Stands

- Lanterns, Candlesticks and Holders
- Waste Bins and Biohazard bags, trash bags
- Foldable Stretchers
- Heavy Plastic Sheeting, Large Rolls
- Duct Tape, Large Rolls
- Mosquito Netting
- Portable Large Capacity Tent or Shelter
- White 100% Cotton Sheets and Pillow Cases
- Pillows, with waterproof cases
- Blankets, Towels, Patient Gowns
- Basins, Bowls and Washcloths
- Portable Shower or Curtain for privacy and Portable Sinks
- Shampoo and Conditioner
- Hair Clips and Rubber Bands
- Nail Brushes, Emory Boards and Nail Clippers
- Large Capacity Water Filtration Systems
- Water Pitcher and Cups
- Lemon Glycerin Swabs or equivalent
- Disposable Razors, or lots of blades
- Chux or Waterproof Pads
- Bedpans and Portable Male Urinals
- Laundry Soap, Bleach, buckets, mop handle, dedicated laundry scrub brushes
- Clothesline
- Scrub Suits
- Fire Extinguishers
- Extra Reading Glasses in various strengths
- Charting Materials and Forms
- Clip Boards, Pencils and Pens (don't forget the sharpeners)
- Watch with a Second Hand and Stopwatch
- Scales, newborn and adult sizes
- Resuscitation Facemask with one-way valve
- Resuscitation Bag (Ambu-bag)
- Endotracheal Tube/ Laryngoscope (allows you to breathe for patient)
- Portable Defibrillator/ AED (expensive)
- Pulse Oximeter

- O2 Concentrator, tubing, and face mask or nasal cannulas, with portable power source
- Portable EKG monitor (battery operated is preferred)
- Blood Pressure monitors (battery operated, wrist sizes are handy)
- Otoscope and Ophthalmoscope – (instruments to look into ears and eyes)
- Microscope
- Glucose Monitor
- Urine test strips and Hemoccult Test Strips
- Pregnancy test kits
- Sterile Drapes (lots)
- Portable Refrigerator A/C and D/C capacity
- Air Splints (arm/long-leg/short-leg)
- Plaster of Paris Cast Kits (to make casts for fractures) Adult and Pediatric
- Cast Removal Tools
- Crutches, Walking Canes, Wheelchair
- Drain and IV Sponges (dressings with a slit cutout) and Tegaderm film dressing
- IV Equipment, such as:
- Normal Saline (longest shelf life), Ringer's Lactate IV solutions
- IV Tubing sets - maxi-sets + standard sets
- Blood collection bags + filter transfusion sets
- Syringes 2/5/10/20 mL
- Needles 20/22/24 gauge
- IV Start Kits with Tegraderm Dressings
- Angiocath IV Needles: 16/18/20/24 gauge
- Paper Tape (1/2 or 1 inch) for IV lines
- IV Stands (to hang fluid bottles)
- Paracord (various uses)
- Assorted Clamps (curved and straight, small and large)
- Scalpel Handle with Blades (sizes 10, 11, 15) and/or disposable scalpels
- Triage Tags (for mass casualty incidents)
- Saline Solution for irrigation (can be made at home as well)
- Foley Catheters, Sterile Lubricant, Foley Insertion Trays and Urine Bags

- Nasogastric Tubes (to pump a stomach)
- Nasal Speculum (to look up the nose)
- Autoclave or Pressure Cooker (to sterilize instruments, etc.)
- Stainless Steel Tongs (to place inside sterilizer and use to pick out sterilized instruments)
- Self-sealing Sterilization Pouches with indicator strips
- Ultraviolet Sterilization Wand or Unit
- Vacuum Bags and Food Saver
- Cidex Solution or equivalent (for cleaning instruments)
- Dedicated Scrub Brushes for Cleaning Instruments only
- Surgical Trays and Bowls, stainless steel only
- Heavy Trash Bags and Biohazard Bags, various sizes
- Human Remains Pouch (HRP) with ID cards or tags
- Shovels and Hatchets
- Bucket, Scrub Brushes and Mop (to clean hospital surfaces and floors)
- Bleach and/or Pool Shock (to DIY bleach)
- Quick Lime Powder (sanitation of human waste)
- Toilet Paper, Tissues and Paper Towels
- Pill Bottles and Labels
- Books, Deck of Cards, Games, Music, Paper, pens, colored pencils/crayons and Activity books (for the sick patient)
- Poster Board, Permanent Markers and Red Duct Tape, for signage outside the Hospital

Surgery Tray items:

- Sterile Towels and Sterile Gloves
- Scrub Brushes in sterile single packages
- Hibiclens Antiseptic Surgical Scrub (to clean skin before invasive procedures)
- Mayo Scissors and Metzenbaum scissors
- Needle Holders, Sterile in various sizes
- Surgical Marking Pens
- Suction Pump with Internal 12V Rechargeable Battery
- Bulb and Large Syringes, Sterile (for irrigating wounds during procedures)
- Lap Sponges and large quantity of dressings and gauze

- Obstetric Forceps (for difficult deliveries)
- Vaginal Speculums, small to ex-large sizes
- Uterine Curettes (for miscarriages, various sizes)
- Uterine "Sound" (checks depth of uterine canal)
- Uterine Dilators (to open cervix; allows removal of dead tissue)
- Bone Saw Kit (for amputations)
- 1% or 2% Lidocaine (local anesthetic in injectable form-prescription medication)
- Chest Tube Set-up (connected to bedside suction)
- Penrose and Jackson-Pratt Drains (to allow blood and pus to drain from wounds)

Additional Prescription Medications

- Medrol Dose packs, oral steroids
- Epi Pens and Inhalers (Ventolin)
- Metformin 500mg, 1000mg or 750mg ER tablets
- Salbutamol Inhalers (for asthma/severe allergic reactions)
- Antibiotic and Anesthetic, Eye ointment/drops and Ear drops
- Oral Contraceptive Pills
- Metronidazole, oral antibiotic and anti-protozoal
- Amoxicillin, oral antibiotic
- Cephalexin, oral antibiotic
- Ciprofloxacin, oral antibiotic
- Doxycycline, oral antibiotic
- Clindamycin, oral antibiotic
- Trimethoprin/Sulfamethoxazole, oral antibiotic
- Ceftriaxone, IV antibiotic
- Diazepam IV sedative to treat seizures
- Diazepam in oral form, sedative
- Alprazolam, oral anti-anxiety agent
- Oxytocin (Pitocin) IV for post-delivery hemorrhage
- Percocet, (oxycodone with paracetamol/acetaminophen), strong oral pain medicine
- Morphine Sulfate or Demerol, strong injectable analgesic
- Tramadol (stronger pain medicine- prescription)

If you have any children in your family, or anticipated group, make sure you have pediatric versions of both supplies and medications. Also, if anyone in your family or group has specific medications they are currently taking, see the chapter on stockpiling medications for tips to accumulate a supply.

There are so many medical items that we're sure there is something that we might have missed, but the important thing is to accumulate supplies and equipment that you will feel competent using in the event of an illness or an injury.

Some of the above supplies, such as stretchers and tourniquets, can be improvised using common household items. Duct tape can be used as a butterfly dressing to close wounds and Paracord can be used to make a rope stretcher.

It should be noted that many of the advanced items are probably useful only in the hands of an experienced surgeon, and could be very dangerous otherwise. Why should you, perhaps, have medical or dental items that are beyond your pay grade? Because you never know when a medical professional experienced in their use might stumble across your threshold.

Some of the supplies listed would be more successful in their purpose with an intact power grid. These items just represent a wish list of what we would want if we were taking care of an entire community.

You should not feel that the more advanced supply lists are your responsibility to accumulate alone. Your entire group should contribute to stockpiling medical stores, under the medic's coordination. The same goes for all the medical skills that I've listed. To learn everything would take a lifetime of study; truthfully, more than even most formally-trained physicians can accomplish. Concentrate on the items that you are most likely to use regularly and be grateful of assistance from others in your group.

Medical Supplies As Barter Items

We recently received a communication from a paramedic who asked about the importance of silver and gold for barter purposes in a collapse.

Having some of this on hand would be very useful, but only in the early stages when people don't yet realize that "money" may be worthless in terms of your chances for long-term survival. Food, defensive items, and medical supplies will eventually become the most valuable surplus items you can have for successful trading.

Food will be in short supply, especially in urban environments once grocery stores are empty. Few have the knowledge of how to grow their own through gardening. Gardening has a learning curve and is subject to the whims of the weather such as the amount of rainfall, storms, and extremes in temperature. Soil conditions and pests will also be a factor. If you have food to barter, you have some real purchasing power.

Once people know you have surplus food to trade, items for defense will be important for protection. It's hard to believe you wouldn't be a target for the desperate or unscrupulous. Whatever materials you have for home defense, make sure that you know how to use them safely, and practice with them regularly. A gun, for example, in the hands of the inexperienced may be as dangerous to themselves as well as to those who wish them harm. Having said that, many survivalists believe that spare ammunition will be very valuable as a barter item.

So, why do medical supplies have barter value? These items and the knowledge of how to use them will become important materials and services both in the short and the long term. The reason is simple: You can easily make a wound with a weapon, but few will have the things necessary to heal a wound. Having bandages, antibiotics, blood clotting agents, and other medical materials are unique and irreplaceable goods in a world without ATMs, effective water treatment, or rule of law.

You can never have too many medical supplies in your survival storage. You'd be surprised how many dressings one major bleed will consume. If you have large quantities, they will become even more precious as time goes on and materials are consumed. Don't forget, however, that you'll be in charge of caring for wounds from beginning to end in a true survival scenario. That takes up supplies, so barter only what you can spare.

Let's take the value of your medical knowledge as a trade item: Not everyone knows how to stop bleeding, deal with orthopedic injuries, perform long-term wound care, or treat infection. If you are the medic, your services have a value. What do you think that value would be in circumstances where a family has a child that is sick or a loved one that is injured? To us, this is a compelling argument for taking the time and effort needed to learn these skills, even in normal times.

This doesn't mean that you should expect something in return every time you help someone in medical need. The value of good will in a survival community is not to be underestimated. Grateful parents, if they're able, will want to reward you in some way for saving a child's life. In this way, volunteering your services may increase the chances for your own family's survival. Indeed, your skills may be deemed so valuable that you become an asset that the community will make a priority to protect.

Even when the drugs and the equipment run out, your medical expertise will be valuable, especially if you studied some herbalism. An understanding of what plants in your area may have medicinal value will help cement your long term value to the group.

Food, water, and shelter are the most important things to have if things go South, but medical supplies and the knowledge of how to use them is a strong second. Keep this in mind as you put together your stockpile.

STERILE VS. CLEAN

Medical equipment is important to have, but that equipment must be clean enough to use on a patient. Some items are disposable in nature, but must be extended for survival situations. Other are meant to be reused, but shouldn't, unless they are returned to the condition they were in before they were utilized.

Thus, a significant factor in the quality of medical care given is the level of cleanliness of the equipment used. You may have heard of the terms "sterile" and "clean", but what's the difference?

When it comes to medical protection, "sterility" means the complete absence of microbes. Sterile technique involves hand washing with special solutions and the use of sterile instruments, towels, and dressings. When used on a patient, the area immediately around these items is referred to as a "sterile field". The sterile field is isolated and closely guarded to prevent contact with anything that could allow micro-organisms to invade it.

Of course, it may be very difficult to achieve a sterile field if you are in an extremely austere environment. In this case, we may only be able to keep things "clean". Clean techniques concentrate on prevention by reducing the number of microorganisms that could be transferred from one person to another by medical instruments or other supplies. Meticulous hand washing with soap and hot water is the cornerstone of a clean field.

In most survival settings, this may be as good as it gets, but is that so bad? With regards to wound care, there is very little research that compares clean vs. sterile technique. In one study, an experiment was conducted in which one group of patients had their wounds cleaned with sterile saline solution, the other group with tap water. Amazingly, the infection rate was 5.4% in the tap water group as opposed to 10.3% in the sterile saline group. Another study revealed no difference in infection rates in wounds treated in a sterile fashion as opposed to clean technique. Therefore, we usually recommend clean, drinkable water for most remote wound care.

Work surfaces must be clean or they will increase the risk of infection. To maintain a clean area, you should use "disinfectants". Disinfectants are substances that are applied to non-living objects to destroy microbes. This would include surfaces where you would treat patients or prepare food. Disinfection does not necessarily kill all bugs and, as such, is not as effective as sterilization, which goes through a more extreme process to reach its goal. An example of a disinfectant would be bleach. One part bleach to nine parts water would be a reasonable disinfectant solution.

Disinfection removes bacteria, viruses, and other bugs and is sometimes considered the same as "decontamination". Decontamination, however, may also pertain to the elimination of noxious chemicals or radiation. The removal of non-living toxins like radiation from a surface would, therefore, be decontamination but not disinfection.

It's useful to know the difference between a disinfectant, an "antibiotic", and an "antiseptic". While disinfectants kill bacteria and viruses on the surface of non-living tissue, antiseptics kill microbes on living tissue surfaces like skin. Examples of antiseptics include Povidone-Iodine (Betadine), Chlorhexidine (Hibiclens), and Benzalkonium Chloride (BZK).

Antibiotics are able to destroy microorganisms that live *inside* the human body. These include drugs such as Amoxicillin, Doxycycline, Metronidazole, and many others. We'll discuss these in detail later in the book.

How To Sterilize Medical Supplies

Many of your medical items, like instruments and some dressings, may come already sterile. In survival, dressings are consumed and the sterile instruments that you intend to reuse become dirty. This leads to the question of how to sterilize your medical "re-usables" and produce a store of sterile dressings. There are a number of ways that you can accomplish this goal:

- Simply placing them in gently boiling water for 30 minutes would be a reasonable strategy, but may not eliminate some bacterial "spores" and could cause issues with rusting over time, especially on sharp instruments like scissors or knives. Always sterilize scissors and clamps in the "open" position.

- Soaking in bleach (Sodium or Calcium Hypochlorite). 15-30 minutes in a 10% bleach solution will disinfect instruments but no longer or rusting will occur. Some recommend adding a teaspoon of baking soda to slow down deterioration. Instruments must be rinsed in sterilized water afterward.
- Soaking in 70% isopropyl alcohol for 30 minutes is another option. Some will even put instruments in a metal tray with alcohol and ignite them. The flame and alcohol, or even just fire itself (if evenly distributed) will do the job, but eventually causes damage to the instruments.
- Soaking in other chemical solutions that are specifically made for the purpose of high-level disinfection (not necessarily sterility) in the absence of heat, something very important if you have items that are made of plastic.

  A popular brand is Cidex OPA, a trade name for a solution with phthalaldehyde or glutaraldehyde as the active ingredient. Insert the instruments in a tray with the solution for 20 minutes for basic disinfection. Soaking overnight (10-12 hours) gives an acceptable level of "near-sterility" for survival purposes. There are test strips available which identify if contamination occurs. If not, the solution can be reused for up to 2 weeks.

  As an alternative, some have recommended using 6-7.5% hydrogen peroxide for 30 minutes (household hydrogen peroxide is only 3%, however).
- Ovens are an option if you have power. For a typical oven, metal instruments are wrapped in aluminum foil or placed in metal trays before putting them in the oven. The oven is then heated to 400 degrees Fahrenheit for 30 minutes or, alternatively, 325 degrees Fahrenheit for 2 hours.
- Although ovens and microwaves have been used to sterilize instruments, probably the best way to guarantee sterility in an austere setting is a pressure cooker. Hospitals use a type of pressure cooker called an "autoclave" that uses steam to clean instruments, surgical towels, bandages, and other items. All modern medical facilities clean their equipment with this type of device.

> Having a pressure cooker/canner as part of your supplies will allow you to approach the level of sterility required for minor surgical procedures. You'll need to reach 15-20 psi for 20-30 minutes and then allow everything to cool gradually. As you can imagine, pressure cookers aren't easy to lug from place to place, so it's best for those who plan to stay in place in a disaster scenario.

A significant development in the quest to put together a portable and reliable method to sterilize instruments comes from a recent study commissioned by the military. The study, published in the journal *Wilderness and Environmental Medicine*, explored the use of UVC light as a survival medical tool.

In this study, instruments laden with MRSA and other bacteria were first scrubbed with Chlorhexidine (Hibiclens) for 30 seconds, and dried with a sterile gauze 4 x 4. Then, an ultraviolet C (UVC) wand was passed within 4 inches over the instruments for 45 seconds. Evaluation afterwards revealed a 100% reduction of bacteria and achieved levels of sterilization acceptable for use in the field. If the instruments were not used right away, rapid vacuum sealing extended the life of sterility.

INTRODUCTION TO NATURAL REMEDIES

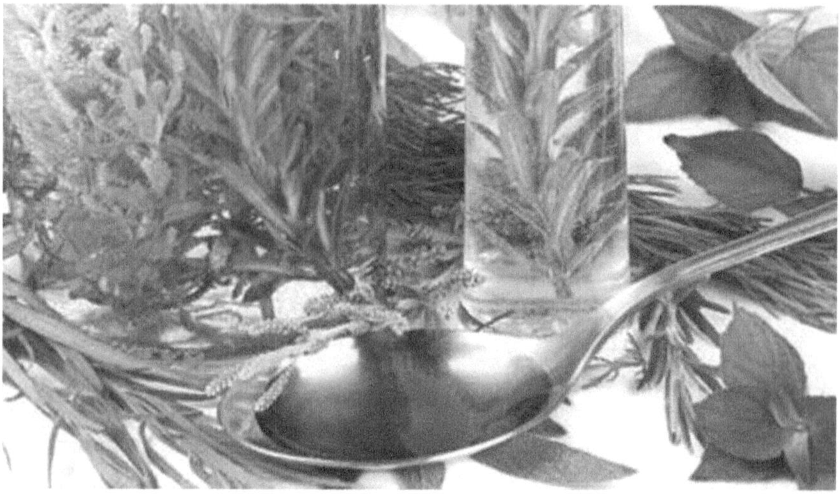

There are many issues that you, the medic, would best handle with the support of the latest technology and modern equipment and facilities. Sure enough, we've just spent the entire last chapter telling you to stock up on all sorts of high-tech items (even defibrillators) and, indeed, many of these are indispensable when it comes to dealing with certain medical conditions.

Unfortunately, you probably will not have the resources needed to stockpile a massive medical arsenal. Even if you are able to do so, your supplies will last only a certain amount of time. Depending on the number of people you are medically responsible for, you'll be shocked at how quickly precious medications and other items are used up. Tough decisions are ahead when you're down to that last box of gauze or bottle of pain meds.

One solution is to grossly overstock on commonly used medical supplies. This isn't a bad idea, but costly and doesn't really give you a sustainable solution. Even large stockpiles will eventually dry up when you're dealing with common injuries and illnesses on a daily basis. Let's face it: in a true long term survival scenario, no one is manufacturing medical supplies. There is no way to replace what you have used up.

Therefore, you must devise a strategy that will allow you to provide medical care for the long run. You will need a way to produce substances that have medical benefits without having a pharmaceutical factory at your disposal.

You might be surprised to know that there is, indeed, another option: The plants in your own backyard or nearby woods.

You might ask yourself, "I thought this was a book by medical types that worked in hospitals. What's all this plant stuff?" Good question. It's true that we were trained conventionally at large inner-city hospitals with little exposure to natural remedies. We're not herbalists and this isn't an herbalism book. However, one thing that we have realized is that the pharmaceuticals will eventually run out in a true long term survival scenario. We have to examine alternatives that might have medicinal benefits.

Let's look at the history of medicine. Physicians have occupied different niches in society over the ages, from priests during the time of the pharaohs, slaves in imperial Rome, and barber-surgeons in medieval times. All of these ancient healers used different methods but there was one thing they had in common: They knew the use of natural products for medicinal purposes. If modern medical care is no longer available one day, we'll have to take advantage of time-honored remedies.

If the medicine man needed more of a particular plant than occurred in their native environment, they cultivated it. They learned to make teas, tinctures and salves containing these products and how best to use them to treat illness.

A little more history: Salicin is a natural pain reliever found in the under bark of Willows, Poplar, and Aspen trees. In the 19th century, we first developed a process to commercially produce Aspirin (Salicylic acid) from trees commonly found in our environment.

That's right: Many conventional therapies are rooted in what is now considered alternative "herbal" medicine. Look at any standard medical text from the 19th century and you'll see that's about all they had.

Today, most artificially produced drugs involve many different chemicals in their manufacture. To make Insulin or Penicillin, for example, so many chemicals are used that it would be nigh impossible to reproduce the process in any type of austere scenario.

We have gone so far in our ability to synthesize medications that we use them far too often in our treatment of patients. This is a detriment to the survival medic for two reasons:

- We can't reproduce any of these drugs with limited supplies in an austere environment.
- We've lost the knowledge of how to use natural substances as a medical tool.

Physicians are realizing that we are too fast in reaching for the prescription pad. Medical journals now call for physicians to focus on prevention instead of intervention. Additionally, when doctors use pharmaceuticals, they are now being asked to prescribe one drug at a time when possible. Multiple medications lead to unpredictable interactions. The conventional medical wisdom is being challenged, and it just might be good for your health.

Having said this, not all pharmaceuticals are bad. Indeed, some of them can save your life. Natural remedies, however, should be integrated into the medical toolbox of anyone willing to take responsibility for the well-being of others. Why not use all the tools that are available to you? At one point or another, the medicinal herbs and plants you grow in your garden may be all you have.

Natural substances can be used in "home remedies" via several methods, including:

Teas: A hot drink made by infusing the dried, crushed leaves of a plant in boiling water.

Tinctures: Plant extracts made by soaking herbs in a liquid (such as water, grain alcohol, or vinegar) for a specified length of time, then straining and discarding the plant material. (also known as a "decoction").

Essential Oils: Liquids comprised of highly concentrated aromatic mixtures of natural compounds obtained from plants. These are typically made by a process called "distillation". Most have long shelf lives.

Salves: Highly viscous or semisolid substances used on the skin (also known as an ointment, unguent, or balm).

Some of these products may also be ingested directly or diluted in solutions. A major benefit of home remedies is that they usually have fewer side effects than commercially produced drugs.

It is the obligation of the group medic to obtain a working knowledge of how to use and, yes, grow these plants. You should also consider learning how to produce tinctures, salves, and oils so as to keep your survival medicine cabinet stocked. A number of reference books are available on the subject of natural remedies, and are listed in the appendix of this book.

Another alternative therapy thought by some to boost immune systems and treat illness is **colloidal silver**. A colloid is a substance in which one microscopic substance is suspended throughout another. Colloidal silver, therefore, is made of tiny silver particles, silver ions, or silver proteins, all suspended in a liquid. Various silver compounds were used in the past to treat infection before the development of antibiotics.

Colloidal silver products are commonly ingested in liquid form as dietary supplements. They also come as balms or ointments that can be applied to the skin, where they are thought to improve healing by preventing infection.

Many traditional institutions agree that silver ions may have medicinal uses. For example, laboratory studies at the department of Biochemistry at Jiaxing College, China, have shown that "silver-containing alginate fibers" provide a sustained release of silver ions when in contact with samples of wound drainage, and are "highly effective against bacteria".

Ionic silver (Ag^{+}) and silver particles in concentration has been shown to have an antimicrobial effect in certain laboratory studies. In the face of rising bacterial resistance to antibiotics, wound dressings containing silver are being used more and more often. A study at the Hull York Medical School found that a dressing containing silver was "a highly effective and reliable barrier to the spread of MRSA (an antibiotic-resistant bacteria) into the wider hospital." Physicians use wound dressings containing silver sulfadiazine (Silvadene) to help treat bedsores and burns.

Silver use is, luckily, only rarely associated with ill effects. Silver is not an essential mineral in humans, and continuous ingestion of silver may result in a condition known as Argyria. This condition causes your skin to turn blue. Although certainly a strange effect, it's mostly a cosmetic concern.

Although the benefits of silver applied to skin wounds are well-accepted, less evidence is available for the effectiveness of ionic silver solutions for internal use.

The reasoning goes as follows: Ions are charged particles. Silver ions are bioactive, but they are like members of the "lonely hearts club": Positively charged particles that are desperately looking to bond with negatively charged ones. Once inside our body, they have a willing partner in the form of the chloride from the salt (sodium chloride) in our cells. Once bonded, it becomes Silver Chloride, a compound that is essentially inactive in the body. As such, the amount of benefit that internal use of silver will give you is uncertain.

Despite this, there are many prominent naturopaths who strongly support its use. Home ionic silver generators are available for sale at a multitude of online sites.

Silver proteins are another form of therapy. In this process, organic materials bind to silver to form a compound. In this way, silver proteins are a different product than ionic silver.

The issue with silver proteins is that, unless suspended in gelatin, they have a tendency to drop to the bottom of the solution (this is called "precipitation") and lose their antimicrobial effect. The larger the silver particle, the more likely this will occur. Also, the presence of organic matter in the compound could lead to rare cases of contamination.

It is important to understand that colloidal effectiveness is determined by particle surface area. Large silver particles tend to precipitate and become inactive. Since the smallest silver particles stay suspended in the solution, more will be available for antimicrobial effects. If you pursue this option, seek out products that will produce the smallest silver particles in their solutions.

We have to mention that the FDA remains dubious as to the medical benefits of colloidal silver and has banned sellers from claiming any therapeutic or preventive value. As a result, the product cannot be marketed as preventing or curing any illness. More evidence is needed before colloidal silver becomes a standard part of your medical arsenal.

ESSENTIAL OILS AND HERBAL TEAS

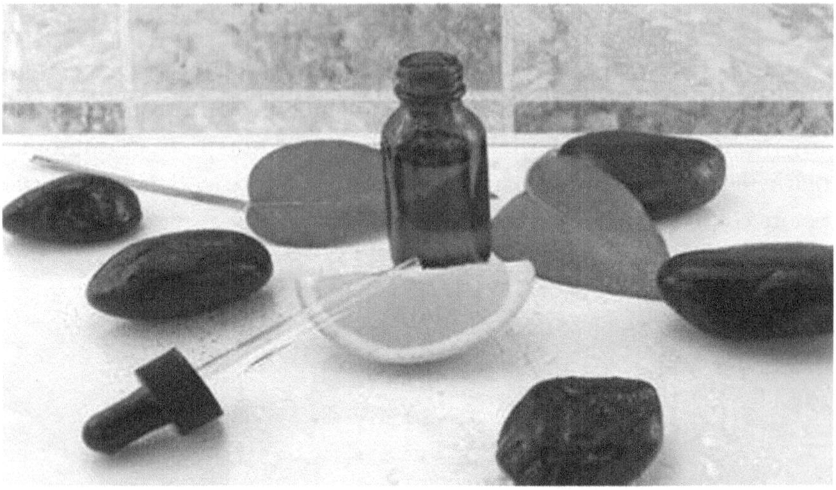

As a medical doctor and a nurse practitioner, we received conventional medical training at university hospitals while getting our degrees. Since that time, however, we have explored various alternative methods of healing. We did this not to replace our education, but as an additional tool in the medical woodshed.

The truth is that, in a long term survival scenario, nature may be your only pharmacy. Over time, your stockpile of medicine will run out, and you'll be thrown back to an earlier era, at least medically. In a situation where regular medications are no longer produced, it is imperative to learn the medicinal benefits of plants that you can grow in your own garden. It worked to sustain our ancestors, and in a disaster, it might again be necessary to keep your family healthy.

Many popular alternative remedies use substances that are called Essential Oils. These liquids are called "essential" because they capture the "essence" of the plant. Essential oils are produced by plants to serve as either an attractant to pollinator insects (hence their strong fragrance) or as a repellant against anything from bacterial to animal invaders.

Unlike cooking oils such as olive or corn, essential oils are less fixed and more volatile. That means that they tend to evaporate easily, making them a favorite component of aromatherapy and inhalation therapy.

An essential oil is distilled from whole plant material, not a single ingredient; therefore, each one has multiple compounds that might be medically useful. To take an example, English lavender has about 20 different chemicals, including esters, ketones, and terpenes. These combinations make each oil unique. Oils may be produced by leaves, bark, flowers, resin, fruit or roots. For example, Lemon oil comes from the peel, Lavender oil from flowers, and Cinnamon oil from bark.

Although you might not realize it, you've been using essential oils all your life in soaps, furniture polishes, perfumes, and ointments. Previous generations of conventional physicians commonly included them in their medical bags. Indeed, many standard medical texts of the past were really instruction manuals on how to use these products.

Essential oils aren't easy to produce without distillery equipment. Although it only takes a few leaves of peppermint to make a tea, you would need 5 pounds of leaves to make 1 ounce of essential oil. One source states that it takes an entire acre of peppermint to produce just 12 pounds. The same source says that 12,000 rose blossoms are required to produce a tablespoon of rose oil. These concentrated versions are the ones you see marketed in small, dark bottles. Unless you intend to buy distilling materials, you should accumulate essential oils early and use them sparingly.

Some plant materials produce a great deal of oil; others produce very little. The strength or quality of the oil is dependent on multiple factors, including soil conditions, time of year, subspecies of plant, rainfall, and even the time of day the plant is harvested. This is akin to the conditions that determine the quality of a particular vintage of wine. It also explains the significant variance you'll see in the effects of the same oil from year to year.

You might be surprised to learn that the Food and Drug Administration only requires 10% essential oil in the bottle to be marketed as "Pure Essential Oil". Beware of claims of FDA certification; the FDA has no certification or approval process for these products.

Essential Oils

The manufacture of essential oils, known as "extraction", can be achieved by various methods:

- **Distillation Method**: Using a "still" like old-time moonshiners, water is boiled through an amount of plant material to produce a steam that travels through cooled coils. This steam condenses into a "mixture" of oil and water from which the oil can be extracted.
- **Pressing Method:** The oils of citrus fruit can be isolated by a technique which involves putting the peels through a "press". This works well only with the oiliest of plant materials, such as orange skins.
- **Maceration Method**: a fixed oil (sometimes called "carrier" oil) or lard may be combined with the plant part and exposed to the sun over time, causing the fixed oil to become infused with the plant "essence". Oftentimes, a heat source is used to move the process along. The plant material may be added several times during the process to manufacture stronger oil. This is the method by which you obtain products such as "garlic-infused olive oil". A similar process using flowers is referred to as "Enfleurage".
- **Solvent Method:** Alcohol and other solvents may be used on some plant parts, usually flowers, to release the essential oil in a multi-step process.

As each essential oil has different chemical compounds in it, it stands to reason that the medicinal benefits are also different. An entire alternative medical discipline has developed to find the appropriate oil for the condition that needs treatment. The method of treatment may differ, as well. Common methods are:

1) **Inhalation Therapy:** This method is also known as "aromatherapy". Direct inhalation therapy simply involves putting 2 or 3 drops of essential oil on your hands, rubbing them together, and inhaling.

   Steam inhalation therapy utilizes the addition of a few drops of the essential oil in a bowl of steaming water (distilled or sterilized), which is then inhaled. This method is most effective when placing a towel over your head to catch the vapors.

   Many people will place essential oils in potpourri or use a "diffuser" to spread the aroma throughout the room. This technique probably dilutes any medicinal effects, however.

2) **Topical Application:** The skin is an amazing absorbent surface, and using essential oils by direct application is a popular method of administration. The oil may be used as part of a massage, or directly placed on the skin to achieve a therapeutic effect on a rash or muscle. Always test for allergic reactions before using an essential oil in this manner: Even though the chemical compounds in the oil are natural, you could exhibit an allergy to it or react against an irritant (case in point: poison ivy).

   A simple test involves placing a couple of drops on the inside of your forearm with a cotton applicator. Within 12-24 hours, you'll notice redness and itch if you're allergic. Mixing some of the essential oil with "carrier" oil such as olive oil before use is a safer option for topical use. Another concern, mostly with citrus oils applied to the skin, is "phototoxicity" (an exaggerated burn response to sun exposure).

   Although we have seen many sources recommend applying essential oil over the location of an internal organ, some reservations exist about whether such an application will really have an effect on that organ. It is much more likely to work on skin issues or, perhaps, underlying muscle tissue.
3) **Ingestion:** Direct ingestion is unwise for many essential oils, and this method should be used with caution. Professional guidance is imperative when considering this method, except for a very few instances. A reasonable alternative to consider is a tea made with the dried herb. This is a safer mode of internal use, but the effect may not be as strong.

Essential oils have been used as medical treatment for a very long time, but it's difficult to provide definitive evidence of their effectiveness for several reasons. Essential oils are difficult to standardize, due to variance in the quality of the product based on soil conditions, time of year, and other factors that we mentioned above.

In addition, there are many subspecies of plants that may differ in their effects. An essential oil of Eucalyptus, for example, may be obtained from Eucalyptus Globulus or Eucalyptus Radiata; these plants may have their own unique properties. These factors combine to make scientific study problematic.

In most university experiments, a major effort is made to be certain that the substance tested caused the results obtained. As essential oils have a number of different compounds and are often marketed as blends, which ingredient was the cause of the effect? If the oil is applied with massage, was the effect related to the oil itself or from the physical therapy?

The majority of studies on essential oils have been conducted by the cosmetics and food industries. Some have been conducted by individuals or small companies with a vested interest in the product. Definitive studies for medicinal benefit are usually performed in universities sponsored by the pharmaceutical industry. Unfortunately, they generally have little interest in herbal products because they have few ways to patent them.

Therefore, serious funding is hard to find because of the limited profit potential. Despite this, essential oils have various reported beneficial effects, mainly based on their historical use on thousands of patients by generations of healers. Although there are many essential oils, a number of them are considered mainstays of any herbal medicine cabinet. Here are just some:

Lavender Oil: An analgesic (pain reliever), antiseptic, and immune stimulant. It is thought to be good for skin care and to promote healing, especially in burns, bruises, scrapes, acne, rashes and bug bites. Lavender has a calming effect and is used for insomnia, stress and depression. It has been reported effective as a decongestant through steam inhalation. Lavender oil may have benefit as an antifungal agent, and has been used for athlete's foot or other related conditions.

Eucalyptus Oil: An antiseptic, antiviral, and decongestant (also an excellent insect repellent), Eucalyptus oil has a "cooling" effect on skin. It also aids with respiratory issues and is thought to boost the immune system. Consider its use for flus, colds, sore throats, coughs, sinusitis, bronchitis, and hay fever. Eucalyptus may be used in massages, steam inhalation, and as a bath additive. Although eucalyptus oil has been used in cough medicine, it is likely greatly diluted and should not be otherwise ingested in pure form.

Melaleuca (Tea Tree) Oil: Diluted in a carrier oil such as coconut, Tea Tree oil may be good for athlete's foot, acne, skin wounds, and even insect bites. In the garden, Tea Tree oil is a reasonable organic method of pest control. In inhalation therapy, it is reported to help relieve respiratory congestion. Studies have been performed which find it effective against both Staphylococcus and fungal infections. Some even recommend a few drops in a pint of water for use as a vaginal douche to treat yeast. Tea Tree oil may be toxic if used in high concentrations, around sensitive areas like the eyes, or ingested.

Peppermint Oil: This oil is said to have various therapeutic effects: antiseptic, antibacterial, decongestant, and anti-emetic (stops vomiting). Peppermint oil is applied directly to the abdomen when used for digestive disorders such as irritable bowel syndrome, heartburn, and abdominal cramping. Some herbalists prescribe Peppermint for headache; massage a drop or two to the temples as needed. For achy muscles or painful joints, massage the diluted oil externally onto the affected area. As mentioned previously, definitive proof of topical application effects on deep organs is difficult to find.

Lemon Oil: Used for many years as a surface disinfectant, it is often found in furniture cleaners. Many seem to think that this disinfecting action makes it good for sterilizing water, but there is no evidence that it is as effective as any of the standard methods of doing so, such as boiling. Lemon oil is thought to have a calming effect; some businesses claim to have better results from their employees when they use it as aromatherapy. Don't apply this oil on the skin if you will be exposed to the sun that day, due to increased likelihood of burns.

Clove Oil: Although thought to have multiple uses as an anti-fungal, antiseptic, antiviral, analgesic, and sedative, Clove oil particularly shines as an anesthetic and antimicrobial. It is marketed as "Eugenol" to dentists throughout the world as a natural painkiller for toothaches. A toothpaste can be made by combining clove oil and baking soda. When mixed with zinc oxide powder, it makes an excellent temporary cement for lost fillings and loose crowns. Use Clove oil with caution, as it may have an irritant effect on the gums if too much is applied.

Arnica Oil: Arnica oil is used as a topical agent for muscle injuries and aches. Thought to be analgesic and anti-inflammatory, it is found in a number of sports ointments. As a personal aside, we have tested this oil on ourselves and found it to be effective, though not very long lasting. Frequent application would be needed for long term relief. Although some essential oils are used as aromatherapy, Arnica oil is toxic if inhaled.

Chamomile Oil: There are at least two versions of Chamomile oil, Roman and German. Roman Chamomile is a watery oil, while German Chamomile seems more viscous. Both are used to treat skin conditions such as eczema as well as irritations due to allergies. Chamomile oil is thought to decrease gastrointestinal inflammation and irritation, and is thought have a calming effect as aromatherapy, especially in children.

Geranium Oil: Although variable in its effects based on the species of plant used, Geranium oil is reported to inhibit the production of sebum in the skin, and may be helpful in controlling acne. Some believe that it also may have hemostatic (blood-clotting) properties, and is often recommended for bleeding from small cuts and bruising. When a small amount of oil is diluted in shampoo, it may be considered a treatment for head lice.

Helichrysum Oil: Thought to be a strong analgesic and anti-inflammatory, Helichrysum is used to treat arthritis, tendonitis, carpal tunnel syndrome, and fibromyalgia as part of massage therapy. It has also been offered as a treatment for chronic skin irritation.

Rosemary Oil: Represented as having multiple uses as an antibacterial, anti-fungal, and anti-parasitic, Rosemary oil is proven to control spider mites in gardens. Use a few drops with water for a disinfectant mouthwash. Inhalation, either cold or steamed, may relieve congested or constricted respiration. Mixed with a carrier oil, it is used to treat tension headaches and muscle aches.

Clary Sage Oil: One of the various chemical constituents of Clary Sage has a composition similar to estrogen. It has been used to treat menstrual irregularities, premenstrual syndrome, and other hormonal issues. Sage is also believed to have a mild anticoagulant effect, and may have some use as a blood thinner. Clary Sage also is thought to have some sedative effect, and has been used as a sleep aid.

Neem Oil: With over 150 chemical ingredients, the Neem tree is called "the village pharmacy" in its native India. The majority of Ayurvedic alternative remedies have some form of Neem oil in them.

Proven as a natural organic pesticide, we personally use Neem Oil in our garden. Reported medicinal benefits are too numerous to list here and seem to cover just about every organ system. It should be noted, however, that it may be toxic when the oil is taken internally.

Wintergreen Oil: A source of natural salicylates, Wintergreen oil is a proven anticoagulant and analgesic. About 1 fluid ounce of Wintergreen Oil is the equivalent of 171 aspirin tablets if ingested, so use extreme caution. It may also have beneficial effects on intestinal spasms and might reduce elevated blood pressures.

Frankincense Oil: One of the earliest documented essential oils, evidence of its use goes back 5000 years to ancient Egypt. Catholics will recognize it as the incense used during religious ceremonies. Studies from Johns Hopkins and Hebrew Universities state that Frankincense relieves anxiety and depression in mice (we're unsure how, exactly, this was determined, but it probably involved a cat). Direct application of the oil may have antibacterial and antifungal properties, and is thought to be helpful for wound healing. As a cold or steam inhalant, it is sometimes used for lung and nasal congestion.

Blue Tansy Oil: Helpful as a companion plant for organic pest control, Blue Tansy is sometimes planted along with potatoes and other vegetables. The oil has been used for years to treat intestinal worms and other parasites. One of its constituents, Camphor, is used in medicinal chest rubs and ointments. In the past, it has been used in certain dental procedures as an antibacterial.

Oregano Oil: An antiseptic, oregano oil has been used in the past as an antibacterial agent. It should be noted that Oregano oil is derived from a different species of the plant than the Oregano used in cooking. One of the minority of essential oils that are safe to ingest, it is thought to be helpful in calming stomach upset, and may help relieve sore throats. Its antibacterial action leads some to use the oil in topical applications on skin infections when diluted with a carrier oil. Oregano Oil may reduce the body's ability to absorb iron, so consider an iron supplement if you use this regularly.

Thyme Oil: Reported to have significant antimicrobial action, diluted Thyme oil is used to cure skin infections, and may be helpful for ringworm and athlete's foot. Thyme is sometimes used to reduce intestinal cramps in massage therapy. As inhalation therapy, it may loosen congestion from upper respiratory infections.

"Thieves' Oil": Many essential oils are marketed as blends, such as "Thieves' Oil". This is a combination of clove, lemon, cinnamon bark, eucalyptus, and rosemary essential oils. Touted to treat a broad variety of ailments, studies at Weber State University indicate a good success rate in killing airborne viruses and bacteria. Of course, the more elements in the mixture, the higher chance for adverse reactions, such as phototoxicity.

Some important caveats to the above list should be stated here. Most of the essential oils listed are unsafe to use in pregnancy, and some may even cause miscarriage. Also, allergic reactions to essential oils, especially on the skin, are not uncommon; use the allergy test we described earlier before starting regular topical applications.

Even though essential oils are natural substances, they may interact with medicines that you may regularly take or have adverse effects on chronic illness such as liver disease, epilepsy or high blood pressure. Thorough research is required to determine whether a particular essential oil is safe to use.

Having said that, essential oils are a viable option for many conditions. Anyone interested in maintaining their family's well-being should regard them as just another weapon in the medical arsenal. Learn about them with an open mind, but maintain a healthy skepticism about "cure-all" claims.

Herbal Teas

For long term storage, essential oils are probably some of the best natural products the medic can stockpile. Producing new supplies of them, however, is another story. Without distilling equipment and a large amount of plant material, you will not be able to replenish oils in any significant quantity.

A more realistic option for sustainable herbal medicines is using fresh or dried plant materials in teas. These require little more than a garden and some knowledge regarding each herb.

It should be noted that the term "tea" is incorrect: The word actually refers to various drinks made from the leaves of one species, *Camellia sinensis.* Indeed, green, black, white, and oolong teas are made from the same plant; only the processing differs. The proper term for a drink made by steeping herbs in hot water would be an "herbal infusion" or "tisane". For simplicity's sake, though, we'll call them teas.

Standard teas from Camellia Sinensis, like green, black, white, and oolong, are high in antioxidants with many health benefits ascribed to them. These include heart disease, type 2 diabetes, liver dysfunction, and more.

Making a tea is one of the simplest ways to prepare medicinal herbs. If you can boil water, you can brew tea. You just:

- Bring some water to a roiling boil in a pot or other container.
- Crush herb leaves and/or flowers.
- Pour the boiled water over 1 teaspoon of herbs and let steep for about five or ten minutes.
- Keep a cover on while steeping.
- Unless using a tea bag or "bob", place a strainer over a cup, and pour.
- Use honey or lemon to add flavor if desired.

A tea doesn't have to be ingested to be of benefit: Some may be used as an eye wash, an irrigation solution for wounds, or in cold or warm compresses.

There are many herbs that can be made into a tea. Although some of the information below lacks hard scientific data, these are some of the teas made by your ancestors for their medicinal benefits.

Alfalfa: The seeds and leaves contain vitamins A, C, E, and K, as well as calcium, phosphorous, iron, and potassium. It has been used as a diuretic to help urine flow and for upset stomachs. There are claims that it helps arthritis pain and may lower cholesterol. Use 1 to 2 teaspoons of dried leaves, steeped in 1 cup of boiling water, for 10-20 minutes.

Burdock: The dried root has been used in teas to help clear acne and to treat psoriasis. Use 2 tablespoons of fresh grated root or 1 tablespoon of well-dried root in 3 cups of boiling water.

Catnip: Leaves and flowers are used to treat intestinal cramping, indigestion, diarrhea, and other stomach ailments. Also thought to treat respiratory infections like the common cold. A substance in catnip called nepetalactone is thought to produce a mild sedative effect. Use 1 teaspoon of dried leaves or 1 tablespoon of fresh leaves per cup.

Chamomile: A favorite tea of many, it contains the amino acid Tryptophan, which gives it a sedative and relaxing effect. As such, it may help treat anxiety and insomnia. Antioxidants in chamomile may help slow down progression of visual, kidney, and nerve damage in diabetics. Use 2-3 teaspoons of dried flowers per cup.

Chicory: When supplies of coffee ran out, soldiers in the Civil War used the root of this common plant as a substitute. It doesn't have caffeine, though, and has more of a sedative than stimulant effect in large amounts. Chicory root has an effect against intestinal worms, and has been shown in animal studies to improve calcium absorption and bone mineral density. Scrape the "bark" off the root before drying; use 1 teaspoon to 1 cup of water. Tea made from leaves has a laxative effect.

Dandelion: You might be surprised to know that the common dandelion contains vitamins and minerals. Indeed, it's thought to have more beta-carotene than a similar serving of carrots. Young flowers and leaves make a good tea for constipation (steep for 20 minutes). Roasting the roots produces a coffee-like drink; use 2 teaspoons dried chopped root in 1 cup of water.

Echinacea: Well-known to decrease the duration of colds and flus, Echinacea boosts the immune system and may have some antiviral activity. Steep 1-2 teaspoons of leaf, flower, or ½ teaspoon of root to 1 cup of boiling water

Elder: Elderberry flowers make a tea that is used for many upper respiratory infections such as sinusitis, colds, flus, and laryngitis. Applied in a compress, the tea may be helpful for wound healing and some skin conditions.

The blue or purple berries are high in antioxidants and may be made into a juice or syrup: Put two pounds of elderberries and four cups of water and bring to a boil, then simmer for a half hour. Use a fine mesh strainer to press out the juice. Sugar may be added under medium heat to make a syrup.

Eucalyptus: Tea made from eucalyptus leaves offer relief from asthma as well as respiratory infections, mostly by opening airways and loosening thick mucus. It may have antibacterial and antiviral effects. Steep ½ teaspoon of dried or fresh leaves in 1-2 cups of water.

Ginger: The underground stems, or rhizomes, of Ginger are used to treat nausea of all types from morning sickness to motion sickness. Slice one inch of the rhizome into small pieces and simmer in two cups of water on low heat for 15 minutes. Then strain. ¼ - ½ teaspoon of ginger powder is another option.

Ginseng: Both Asian and American Ginseng root can be made into herbal teas that are thought to lower blood sugar levels, a useful benefit for those with diabetes. Simmer three to six teaspoons of the root for 45 minutes in three or four cups of water, then strain.

Lavender: Used in aromatherapy, lavender may improve nausea and other digestive symptoms when drunk as a tea. It's thought to decrease migraine headaches and possibly limit convulsions and muscle spasms. Use 1 tablespoon of dried herb in 1 cup of water.

Lemon Balm: An herb with antiviral effects, it's a member of the mint family. A tea made from lemon balm leaves and flowers was used in the past to treat mouth, throat, and dental infections like gingivitis and herpes sores. Also thought to decrease anxiety and aid sleep. Lemon balm may help improve intestinal spasms and nausea. 1 teaspoon of dried herb or 5-6 fresh leaves to one cup of boiling water makes a fine tea.

Licorice: Better known as an ingredient in candy, its coating properties may help with sore throats, coughs, and heartburn. Licorice can, however, raise blood pressure and should be avoided during pregnancy. Add 1-2 teaspoons of chopped root to 2 cups of boiling water to make a decoction. Drink ½ cup at a time.

Passionflower: Tea made from passionflower has a beneficial effect on anxiety and may serve as a sleep aid if taken regularly. Boil 1-2 teaspoons of herb (avoid the root) in 2 cups of water for 5-10 minutes.

Peppermint: A long-standing herbal remedy, tea made from peppermint calms the stomach and helps Irritable Bowel Syndrome (IBS), but can worsen heartburn. The tea helps thin respiratory mucus and relieves nasal congestion. Put 1 teaspoon of dried herb or 6-8 fresh leaves over 1 cup of boiling water.

Rose: Rose "hips" make a tea with vitamin C, as well as calcium, selenium, zinc, manganese, and others. It boosts the immune system and is thought to be beneficial for the adrenal gland, responsible for the stress hormone cortisol. Boil 1 teaspoon of dried rose hips in water and steep for 20 minutes.

Sage: Sage leaf tea is a time-honored remedy for sore throat as well as the common cold as a tea or gargle. It may also aid digestion and decrease cramping, and may even improve memory. Steep 1 teaspoon of dried leaves in one cup of water.

Stinging Nettle: Stinging nettle root is thought to have benefits as a diuretic to improve urine flow, even in those with enlarged prostates. The leaves may decrease the pain of arthritis in joints. Use 1 teaspoon dried leaves in 1 cup boiling water or boil 5 grams of dried root in 2 cups of water for 5-10 minutes.

St. John's Wort: One of the few herbs that has known activity against minor depression, leading it to be called "herbal Prozac". Beware of interactions with prescription drugs, however. Pour 1 cup of boiling water over 1 teaspoon herb.

Thyme: Teas made from thyme will loosen thick phlegm and may help coughs. It's known to inhibit bacteria, viruses, and fungi, including many that cause respiratory infections. Steep 1 to 2 teaspoons of fresh or dried leaves in 1 cup of water.

Turmeric: This herb contains curcumin, an anti-inflammatory compound that may treat Crohn's disease and other digestive tract issues. As well, it may have beneficial effects on joint pain due to rheumatoid arthritis and other disorders.

Valerian: The dried roots of this plant have been utilized for centuries to deal with anxiety and insomnia. It may even decrease the frequency of seizures in patients with epilepsy. Its mild sedative effect eases pain and promotes sleep. Avoid alcohol or sedative drugs.

Willow Bark: The green underbark of willow trees contain salicin, the original ingredient used to produce aspirin in the 19th century. It is especially useful for muscle aches and joint pain. Simmer 1 teaspoon of bark in 1 cup of water for 10 minutes.

There is much research to be done to confirm all of the effects of these plants, and there may be other benefits not mentioned. Many other plants have medicinal effects other than the ones in the list above. These, however, are easily made into easily-made teas that can be produced even while on the move.

Medicinal Gardens

Planting your own medicinal garden is a prudent way to provide alternatives to modern medicine. Until pharmaceuticals were produced in factories, people had to grow their own "medicine". This common practice was a natural part of the landscape and provided needed remedies for many medical issues. Oftentimes, a community would have a person that served as an herbalist and supervised the cultivation and processing.

Growing your own medicinal garden is both rewarding and beneficial; in times of trouble, you will likely have limited access to pharmaceuticals. The gardening learning curve when gardening can be steep, so don't wait until the situation is critical to get started.

Select a well-drained, sunny area with healthy soil. Although some herbs grow well in shade, most plants need at least 6-8 hours of full sun for proper growth and development. Potting is appropriate for medicinal plants that will need to be transported inside during a cold winter. Water should be provided on a regular basis to allow the soil to stay moist, but not muddy or waterlogged. A small amount of natural mulch is perfect for maintaining even moisture levels in very dry conditions.

Use only organic pest and disease control. A soapy mixture of 1 tablespoon of neem oil, 1 teaspoon of Dr. Bronner's lavender, peppermint Castile soap and, perhaps, a few drops of tea tree essential oil to

4-8 cups of water makes a great disease and natural pest control. Spray foliage in the late afternoon every 5-7 days or after a heavy rain.

The medicinal plants you select should match the climate as best as possible. For some, that means that the herbs must survive the winter; for others, the summer heat. The Department of Agriculture publishes both "Plant Hardiness" maps for cold weather and "Heat Zone" maps to help you choose what to grow.

You may be able to grow warmer climate plants by protecting them from the cold with greenhouses or using row covers. This will expand the range of medicinal plants you may choose to grow either in pots or around your homestead.

Harvest mature herbs in dry weather after the dew has evaporated. The different parts of the plant may require specific times of the year or other conditions for collection:

- **Leaves**: Usually best when collected soon after they open in spring and summer.
- **Flowers**: Harvest just as they start to bloom.
- **Roots**: Harvest in the fall.
- **Bark**: Collect in the spring or fall in small amounts.
- **Berries, Fruits, and Seeds**: As you might imagine, best harvested when ripe but before they drop.

It's preferable to take just the amount of plant material that you are ready to process for use or storage. Otherwise, rapid deterioration could occur and degrade the medicinal benefit of the herbs. Herbs can be preserved by air- or oven-drying, and then stored in a sterile dark glass jar with airtight lids. For the longest shelf life of about 12 months, make sure conditions are cool, dry, and dark.

Here is a short list of medicinal plants you may consider growing, as well as their benefits and the most commonly used part of the plant:

Aloe Vera- the slimy gel from the leaf is used to heal and soothe rashes, burns, and cuts.

Angelica- rhizomes (similar to a root but actually an underground stem) are used to make tinctures and infusions to treat menstrual cramps.

Arnica- flowers and rhizomes (underground stems) are utilized to produce very dilute concentrations in an ointment or salve. Used only externally on unbroken skin for bruises or joint/muscle pain.

Calendula- the flowers are used fresh or dried and made into teas, tinctures, creams and salves. Calendula tea or tincture may relieve menstrual and intestinal cramps and decrease the severity of a viral infection. Rich in antioxidants, Calendula can be applied externally as a cream, salve, infused oil, or as a compress. Calendula reduces pain and heals minor burns, cuts, rashes, ringworm and athlete's foot. Cool, weak tea compresses may heal an eye infection; apply to the affected eye three times daily.

Cayenne Pepper-the pepper itself is used dried and powdered, infused in oil, as a tincture, or mixed in a salve or cream. Good externally for arthritic pain as a salve. Applied directly to a wound, it may be useful to stop mild to moderate bleeding. Cayenne can be taken internally as a tincture or as a pinch of powder in a tea for to treat intestinal infections, sore throat pain, or gas. Some consider it a broad spectrum antibacterial. It has even been used as a tea or tincture in cases of heart attack.

Chamomile, German-the flowers are used in teas, salves, and creams. Internally taken, the tea is known to be relaxing and is used as an antispasmodic (relaxes muscle tension and cramps). It also helps with insomnia, calms an upset stomach, and may also reduce the inflammation of joints. Externally used, cooled tea compresses or eyewash may treat eye infections. Applied to painful rashes, itchy skin, or sore nipples, a poultice (a mass of warmed crushed flowers), cream, or salve may relieve and heal skin conditions.

Comfrey-the leaves, aerial parts, and root are used in creams, salves, infused oils, ointments, poultices, and tinctures. Use externally and only on unbroken skin. Common uses for comfrey are to help heal broken bones, sprains, strains and bruises. Comfrey may help with acne by reducing scar formation.

Echinacea-the flowers and roots are used to produce tinctures, teas, capsules, and pills. It is known to have immune stimulating effects. Some use it to help reduce allergies, such as hay fever.

Elder- this tree produces two parts used medicinally: the fresh or dried flowering tops and blue or purple berries (red are poisonous). A tea, tincture or syrup made of the flowering tops are good for coughs, colds, flu and reducing allergies. Cooking is preferred to prevent poisoning from elderberries and makes a reasonable syrup. Syrup made from berries can be used for the same ailments as the flowering tops.

Witch Hazel-tincture of the bark is used as an astringent to reduce hemorrhoids. It can also stop itching from insect stings.

Feverfew-the fresh or dried aerial parts (stems, leaves and flowers) are used to produce a tea, tincture, capsules, or pills. As a tea or tincture, the leaves may help treat or prevent migraine headaches and also reduce fevers. This herb may also help with arthritic conditions. Do not use in combination with blood-thinning medications.

Garlic- the fresh cloves are used (crushed) to make a tea, tincture, syrup, or capsules. Garlic may help lower blood pressure, reduce cholesterol, thin the blood to help protect against blood clots, and lower blood sugar levels. It has antibacterial and antiviral properties, which makes it useful for treating both digestive and respiratory infections. It can be applied externally to dress wounds to reduce infection rates. Use with caution if taking blood thinners or antihypertensive medications.

Ginger-the rhizomes are used to make a tea, essential oil, capsule or tincture. Ginger is excellent for use in digestive disorders. It can help relieve both morning sickness and motion sickness. Some types of food poisoning may be treated effectively with ginger. Ginger may also lower blood pressure. It is thought to increase sweating, which is beneficial to reduce a fever.

Ginkgo-the leaves are used, fresh or dried, in a tea, tincture, or extract to help improve circulation and memory. Gingko also has anti-allergenic properties, which makes it helpful to relieve wheezing in asthmatics.

Ginseng- the roots are used to make a tea, tincture or incorporated into capsules. It is used to reduce the effects of physical and mental stress. It stimulates the immune system to help the body fight viruses and bacterial infections.

Goldenseal-the rhizomes are used to produce a tincture, tea, powder, or infusion. It is said to be a mild laxative. It also may reduce heavy menstrual bleeding. A dilute infusion can be used as eyewash for infections, as a mouthwash for swollen or infected gums, or as an external treatment for psoriasis. Goldenseal is not appropriate for use in pregnancy.

Lavender-the fresh or dried flowers are used to produce a tea, tincture, infusion or essential oil. It enhances relaxation and calms nervous conditions, including muscle or intestinal cramps, and loosens tight airways in asthmatics. Applied externally, it is an antiseptic for open wounds and mild burns. It relieves itching and inflammation, and can be used to relieve bug bites and rashes.

Lemon Balm- the fresh or dried aerial parts are used to produce a juice, tea, tincture, infusion, lotion and salve/cream. It can alleviate nervous conditions and cramps, and is useful for anxiety and muscle aches. Lemon balm can relieve cold sores and reduce future outbreaks.

Licorice-the dried or fresh root is used to create a tea, fluid extract, tincture, dried juice stick or powder. It is a gentle laxative. It is also considered to have anti-inflammatory effects. It helps with canker sores, upset stomach, and acid reflux. This same action also helps it reduce arthritic pain and inflamed joints. Do not take if anemic, have high blood pressure, or during a pregnancy.

Peppermint-the fresh or dried aerial parts are used to make a tea, tincture, lotion, capsules and essential oil. The tea or tincture is helpful for digestive problems and may reduce gas, cramps, and diarrhea. As a lotion or diluted essential oil, it helps relieve headaches and migraines when a small amount is applied to the temples in a gentle massage.

Rosemary-the fresh or dried leaves are used to produce a tea, tincture, or essential oil. The tea or tincture can help reduce stress and relieve headaches. Applied as a diluted essential oil or lotion, it may relieve sore muscles or joint pain. Do not take the essential oil internally.

Sage-the fresh or dried leaves are used to make a tea or tincture. Fresh leaves are sometimes crushed and applied directly to the skin for the relief of stings and bug bite irritation. The tea is good to relieve a sore throat, canker sores, or sore gums when used as a gargle. Drinking the tea can help reduce menopausal symptoms.

Skullcap-the fresh or dried aerial parts are used to create an infusion, tincture or capsules. It is said to calm and relax nervous conditions, including insomnia and menstrual pain. The tincture may help relieve headaches.

Senna-the fresh or dried pods are used commonly to make a tea. It is a laxative, with a number of over-the-counter preparations available to treat constipation. Senna should be used only in dilute, small dosages. Do not take for more than 10 days.

St. John's Wort-the fresh or dried flowering tops are used to make a tea, tincture, cream, or infused oil.. Most commonly said to be a relaxant and helpful to treat depression, PMS and menopausal symptoms. The infused oil is useful when applied externally to help with stimulating tissue repair on wounds and burns; it may also may reduce joint and muscle pains. This herb may cause sensitivity to sunlight and is known to interact with some prescription drugs.

Thyme-the fresh or dried aerial parts are used to produce a tea, tincture, syrup, and essential oil. A tea may be helpful for use in treating colds and flu. Syrup made from thyme is a traditional cough remedy. A tincture applied externally may help with vaginal fungal infections. Thyme has been used as a treatment for intestinal worms. Do not use the essential oil during pregnancy.

Turmeric-the fresh or dried rhizome is used in a tea, tincture, poultice, or powder. It is said to have a strong anti-inflammatory action, and may help with asthma, arthritis and eczema. A beneficial effect on stomach and intestinal cramps is also attributed to this herb. Externally, it is useful in treating fungal infections, psoriasis, and other itchy rashes; as a result, it could be utilized as a replacement for hydrocortisone if modern medicines are unavailable. Turmeric may cause stomach upset, heartburn, and sensitivity to sunlight if taken regularly. Turmeric has blood thinning properties and should be avoided if taking anti-coagulants like Coumadin.

Valerian-the roots and rhizome are used to produce a tea, tincture, or powder. It has a sedative effect and, thus, is commonly used to reduce stress, induce relaxation, and treat insomnia. It can help relax muscle tension, intestinal cramps, and menstrual pain. Do not take with alcohol or if using sleep-inducing medications.

Yarrow-fresh or dried aerial parts are used to make a tea, tincture, essential oil, or a poultice. Yarrow is used externally to heal wounds as a poultice. Traditionally mixed with other herbs in a tea, it may help with colds and flus. Some claim that it reduces menstrual bleeding. There are reports of allergic reactions to Yarrow by some; do not use it during pregnancy.

Note that some of the above are also mentioned in the chapters on teas and oils. The ones here, however, are especially amenable to cultivation in the average garden.

The same issues regarding proof of effectiveness and uncertainty of dosage that we relate in previous chapters are relevant for the herbs on this list. Perform your own research into these alternatives and come to your own conclusions. For useful books on herbalism and other medical subjects, go to the reference section at the end of this book.

THE HISTORY AND PHYSICAL

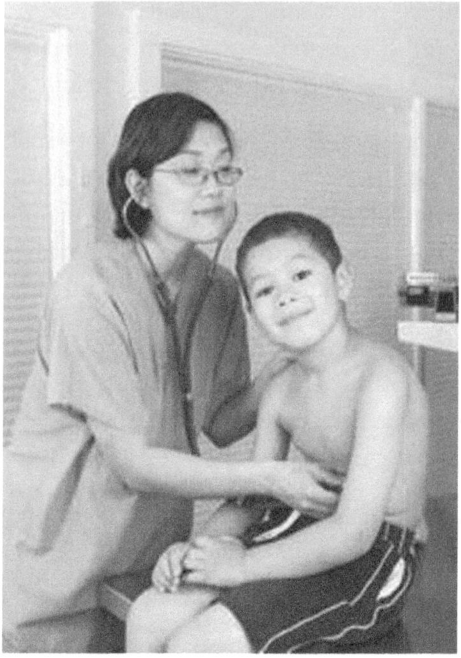

For those willing to take responsibility for the medical care of others in the aftermath of a disaster, success involves familiarity with the patient's past and present medical issues as much as knowledge of the reason for the current visit.

It's important for you to compile as complete a medical history as possible for every person in your group before a disaster occurs. In this way, you can help them plan to stay healthy in harder times.

The patient should be interviewed when there isn't an emergency ongoing, or else you may have to rely on family members or even bystanders to give you (possibly erroneous) information.

Past surgeries, chronic illnesses, allergies, risk factors, and current medications will factor into your evaluation. Even things you might not think would matter in a survival setting, like smoking history, might help you make sense of strange respiratory complaints later on. You'll have to keep a written record of this information. Don't depend on your memory; it isn't perfect and it won't help other medics if you're not around.

In addition to taking a history, you must learn how to physically evaluate a patient and make a diagnosis. This means putting your (gloved) hands on them and looking for physical signs of illness or checking out a wound. Sometimes the problem is obvious in seconds; other times, you will have to examine the entire body to determine the problem. This can be done efficiently and in an organized manner.

The most basic information is obtained by simply observing the appearance of the patient. Are they well-nourished or sickly? Are they calm or in distress? Does one side of the patient match the other? What is their chief complaint (CC)? This takes no medical skill to ascertain and a general impression can be reached while the patient tells you the reason for their visit.

Vital Signs

Once you have heard the history of the patient and their current medical problem, you can begin the physical portion of the exam by checking the vital signs. These are a set of measurements that give an idea of the general condition of the patient. Vital signs include the following;

- **Pulse rate** – Take a pulse by using 2 fingers to press on the side of the neck to feel the carotid artery. This action is called "**palpation**". A more common alternative is to feel the radial artery on the inside of the patient's wrist by the base of the thumb. Speaking of thumbs, don't use that finger to take a pulse as it has a pulse of its own. You may wind up counting your own pulse instead of the patient's.

  A normal pulse rate at rest is 60-100 beats per minute. You may choose to feel the pulse for, say, 15 seconds and multiply the number you get by 4 to get beats per minute. A full minute would be more accurate, however.

  You will find that most people who are agitated from having suffered an injury will have a high pulse rate over 100. This is called "**tachycardia**". A low pulse rate below 60 is called "**bradycardia**" and might be seen in patients with heart problems. It's also sometimes seen in highly athletic patients as a normal finding.

- **Respiration rate** – Simple observation of a patient breathing will give you a rate per minute. You can, as an alternative, place hands on their back to feel the raising and lowering of the chest wall. Respiration rate is best evaluated for an entire minute to get an accurate reading.

  The normal adult rate at rest is 12-18 breaths per minute, somewhat more for children. Note any unusual aspects, such as wheezing or gurgling noises during inhalation or exhalation. A respiration rate over 20 per minute is usually a sign of a person in distress, and is known as "**tachypnea**".

- **Blood pressure** – blood pressure is a measure of the work the heart has to do to pump blood throughout the body. This is determined partially by the elasticity of the walls of the arteries. The less elastic the wall, the more pressure is required to force blood through it.

  Your blood pressure is at its highest when the heart beats. This is called the **systolic pressure**. Pressure is at its lowest when the heart is between beats. This is called the **diastolic pressure**. These readings are taken with an instrument called a **sphygmomanometer**, but we'll call it a blood pressure cuff. It's an item that should be part of every medic's kit.

  You're looking for a reading less than 140/90 at rest. Blood pressure may be temporarily high after extreme physical exertion and a number of other causes. As such, it should be taken more than once, especially if an abnormal result is noted.

  Of course, some people have chronically high blood pressure as a medical condition. A very low blood pressure may be seen naturally in very thin persons and athletes, but is also seen in major hemorrhages and shock. Step-by-step instructions on how to take a blood pressure can be found in the chapter on high blood pressure, also called "**hypertension**".

- **Mental status** – You want to know that your patient is alert and can respond appropriately to questions and commands. If they seem disoriented, ask simple questions like their name, where they are, or what year it is. Note whether the patient is lethargic, alert, or agitated.

Some patients may appear unconscious, but may respond to a spoken command. For example: "Hey! Open your eyes!" If no result, determine if they respond to a stimulus, such as pressure on their breastbone with your knuckles. If they don't, they are termed "unresponsive to pain". This occurs for a number of reasons, including brain injuries, lack of oxygen, and uncontrolled diabetes, discussed elsewhere in this book. Prolonged unconsciousness is called a "**coma**".

- **Body Temperature** - Take the person's temperature to verify that they don't have a fever. A person with a fever is referred to as being "febrile".

  A normal temperature will range from 97.5 to 99.0 degrees Fahrenheit or about 37 degrees Celsius. A significant fever is defined as a temperature above 100.4 degrees Fahrenheit (38 degrees Celsius). Very low temperatures (less than 95 degrees Fahrenheit (35 degrees Celsius) may indicate cold-related illness, also known as **hypothermia**. On the opposite hand is heat stroke (**hyperthermia**), where the temperature may rise above 105 degrees Fahrenheit (40.5 degrees Celsius). These issues are discussed in detail later in this book.

Once you've taken the vital signs and determined that there is no obvious injury, perform a general exam from head to toe in an organized fashion. This can be done with limited equipment.

Before an exam, always communicate to your patient in a calm manner who you are, what you will be doing, and why. During the process, be very careful to avoid forcing them to perform any action that is beyond their capability. Explain each part of the exam as you get to it, and keep body parts covered unless they must be exposed for evaluation.

To begin, touch the patient's skin; is it hot or cold, moist or dry? Is there redness? Is the patient pale? Do you see any skin abnormalities, also known as "lesions"?

Once you've made general observations, examine the head area and work your way down. Look for bumps, bleeding, cuts, abrasions, or other evidence of trauma to each part of the body you examine. Later chapters of this book will go deeper into the significance of abnormal findings.

HEENT: Head, Ears, Eyes, Nose, Throat

Head, Ears, and Nose: You've probably already looked at the patient's head for evidence of trauma like cuts and bruises. Rub your fingers together by each ear to test hearing. If you have an instrument to see inside the ear canal (an "otoscope"), evaluate the eardrum; it should be a shiny grey. If dull, it could represent an ear infection. Are there any foreign objects? The otoscope could also be used to look up the nose.

Eyes: Pull just below the eye to see under the eyelid. If pale, it could represent someone that has a low red blood cell count, otherwise known as "anemia". Are the whites of the eyes yellowed or reddened? These could represent liver dysfunction or infections like "pink eye", respectively. Use a light to see if pupils retract similarly in both eyes. Have the patient follow your finger as it outlines a square to verify that the eyes move appropriately and in concert with each other.

You might design a chart to test the vision in each eye. Normal vision is called "20/20". This means that your patient can read the same letters at 20 feet as a person without visual impairment. Further, 20/40 vision means that the subject can only read at 20 feet what a normal person can read at 40 feet. On the other hand, someone with 20/10 vision can read at 20 feet what a normal person can only read if the chart is moved to 10 feet.

Oral Cavity: Have the patient open their mouth and check for redness, sores, or other dental issues with a light source and a tongue depressor. Swollen, red gums would be seen in those with poor dental hygiene. Decay appears as brown or black indentations on teeth, and an abscess appears as a shiny red swelling, often with a white pimple-like head. Sore throats present as redness and swelling in back and, often, on the tonsils on each side.

Neck: Feel ("palpate") the neck to feel the pulse bilaterally (on both sides) in front of the neck muscle or for any unusual lumps down to the collarbone. The thyroid gland is usually very small and is located over the windpipe a couple of inches below the Adam's apple. Lightly touch each side of the windpipe in that area and have the patient swallow; the thyroid should move up and down. This is easiest done if you are positioned behind the patient.

Chest And Abdomen

Take your stethoscope and listen to the chest. This is called "**auscultation**". Starting with the back, have the patient breathe in deeply through their open mouth. Listen over the lower, middle, and upper left lung and compare to the same area on the right and work your way to the front of the chest. Lung sounds over the major airways in the center of the chest are called "bronchial"; sounds over the periphery are called "vesicular".

Do you hear the patient's breathing as you place the instrument over different areas of each lung? Are there areas where much less or no breathing is heard on one side? Do they differ during inhalation and exhalation (breathing in and out)? Are there rough or bubbling noises that shouldn't be there? Noises get louder and coarser as you approach the windpipe. Practice listening to healthy people to get a good idea of what clear lungs should sound like.

Abnormal sounds would include wheezing, gurgles, coarse sounds, and crackles. Depending on the sound, these could represent pneumonia, an asthma attack, a foreign object in the airways, or a number of other issues. We have included some references to videos at the end of the book that allow you to hear these sounds and compare them to normal "clear" lungs.

Listen to the heart and see if the heartbeat is regular or irregular in rhythm. Check along the ribs for rough, bruised, or painful areas that might signify a fracture. Check the armpits (also known as the "axilla") for masses. Perform a breast exam in women by moving your fingers in a circular motion over the breast tissue, starting from the periphery near the axilla and ending at the nipple.

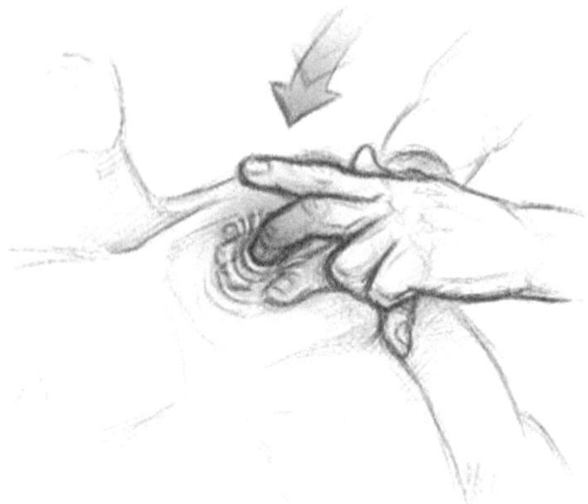

PERCUSSION

Palpate the abdomen with your open hand. Is there pain? Is the belly soft or is it rigid and swollen? Do you feel any masses? Use your stethoscope to listen to the gurgling of bowel sounds. Lack of bowel sounds may indicate lack of intestinal movement; excessive bowel sounds may be seen in some diarrheal disease. Place your open hand on the different quadrants of the abdomen and tap on your middle finger, as in the image above. This is called "**percussion**". The abdomen will sound "hollow" normally, but dull where there might be a mass or enlarged liver. An enlarged liver can also be found by pressing down on the upper right side below the rib cage and feeling firmness (it's normally soft if the liver isn't enlarged).. An enlarged spleen will be felt as a mass on the left side under the bottom of the rib cage.

Check along the patient's spine for evidence of pain or injury. Pound lightly with a closed hand on each flank below the last rib. The kidneys are in this location, and injury or infection would cause this action to be very painful to the patient. Pain on either side of the spine might indicate a muscle strain.

Extremities

Check each limb for painful muscles or joints. Determine if an arm or leg has decreased range of motion. Make sure that there is good circulation by checking the color on the tips of the fingers and toes.

Poor circulation will make these areas white or blue in color. Check for sensation by lightly tapping with a safety pin or pen tip, especially at the ends of extremities.

It's important to identify areas of weakness. Place your hands on the patient's thighs and ask them to lift up against light resistance. Ask them to grasp your fingers with each hand; then, try to pull your hand away. Check to see if you can block motion easily with your hands, as in the image below. You're trying to see not only if they have good strength but that the strength on each side is about equal.

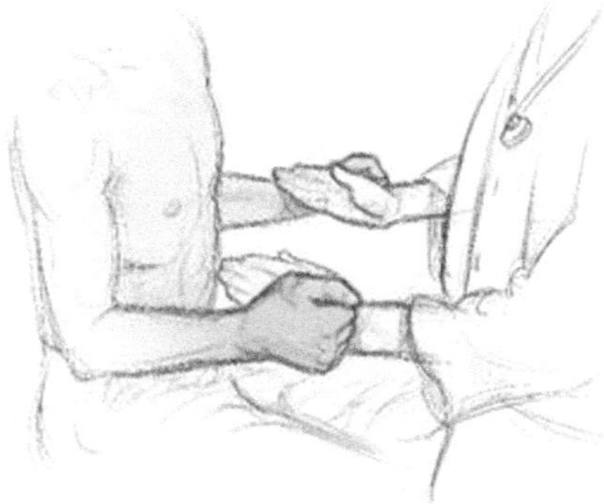

STRENGTH TESTING

Human beings are what we call "bilaterally symmetrical". If you draw a line vertically down the length of their body, each side is essentially the same. This means that, if you are uncertain whether a limb is injured or deformed, you can compare it to the other side.

These are just some basics. Certainly, there's a lot more to a physical exam than what you've just read, but practicing exams on others will give you experience. As time goes by, you'll get the feel of what is normal and what isn't. Once you get the hang of it, your efforts will prepare you for making a diagnosis if we find ourselves without access to modern medical care.

THE MASS CASUALTY INCIDENT

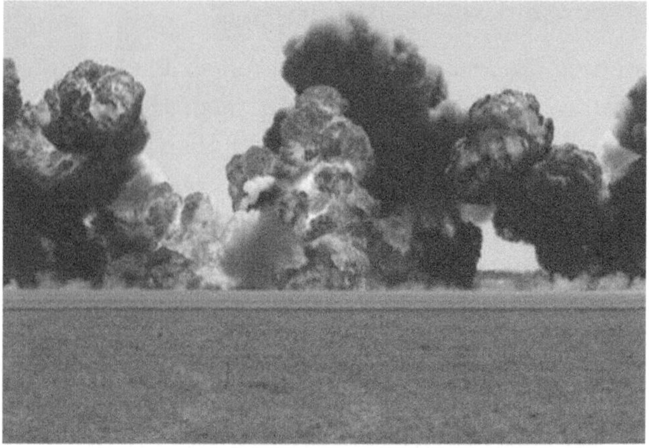

The last section discussed performing a general physical exam. Although most patient encounters will be unhurried and routine, occasionally you will have to make quick decisions. For major trauma, it is important to take note of the "Golden Hour". A victim's chance of survival decreases significantly if not treated within 1 hour of the injury. For severe bleeding, it might be more accurately described as the "Platinum Five Minutes". If bleeding isn't stopped quickly, your patient will likely succumb to their wound.

Your responsibilities in times of trouble will usually be one-on-one; that is, the healthcare provider will be dealing with one ill or injured individual at a time. If you have trained and accumulated supplies, your encounter with any one patient should be, with any luck, within your expertise and resources. There may be a day, however, when you find yourself confronted with a scenario in which multiple people are injured. This is referred to as a **Mass Casualty Incident** (MCI).

A mass casualty incident is any event in which your medical resources are inadequate for the number and severity of injuries incurred. Mass Casualty Incidents (we'll call them "MCIs") can be quite variable in their presentation. They might be:

- Doomsday scenario events, such as nuclear weapon detonations
- Terrorist bombings, such as occurred on 9/11

- Active shooter events
- Consequences of a storm, such as a tornado or hurricane
- Consequences of civil unrest
- Mass transit mishap (train derailment, plane crash, etc.)
- A car accident with, say, three people significantly injured (and only one ambulance)
- Many others

The effective medical management of any of the above events requires rapid and accurate triage. **Triage** comes from the French word "trier" (to sort) and is the process by which medical personnel rapidly assess and prioritize injured individuals at the scene. In this way, you do the most good for the most people. Note that we didn't say: "the best possible care for *each* individual".

Let's assume that you are in a marketplace somewhere in the Middle East or perhaps in your survival village near the border with a hostile group. You hear an explosion. You are the first one to arrive at the scene. There are twenty people on the ground, some moaning in pain. There were probably more, but only twenty are in one piece. The scene is horrific.

S.T.A.R.T.

As the first to respond to the scene, you are Incident Commander until someone with more medical expertise arrives. What do you do? Your initial actions comprise what we call the "5 S's" of evaluating a mass casualty scene:

- Safety
- Size up
- Send for help
- Set-up of areas for care of the injured
- **START** – Simple Triage And Rapid Treatment

1. **Safety Assessment**: Many terrorists employ an insidious strategy using primary and secondary bombs. The main bomb causes the most casualties, and the second bomb is triggered as rescue personnel arrive.

Many wince when we advise not approaching the injured in a hostile setting. Yet, your primary goal as medic is your own self-preservation. Keeping the medical personnel alive is likely to save more lives down the road. You do your family and community a disservice by becoming the next casualty.

In the immediate aftermath of the Oklahoma City bombing, various medical personnel rushed in to aid the victims. One of them was a heroic 37 year old Licensed Practical Nurse who, as she entered the area, was struck by a falling piece of concrete. She sustained a head injury and died five 5 days later.

As you arrive, be as certain as possible that there is no ongoing threat. Do not rush in there until it is safe to enter the area.

2. **Size up the Scene:** Ask yourself the following questions:
   - What's the situation? Is this a mass transit crash? Did a building on fire collapse? Was there a shooting or explosion?
   - How many injuries and how severe? Are there a few victims or dozens? Are there any uninjured that could assist you?
   - Are the victims all together or spread out over a wide area?
   - Are there lanes open enough for vehicles to come through to help transport victims?
3. **Send for Help:** If modern medical care is available, call 911 and say (for example): "I am calling to report a mass casualty incident involving a multi-vehicle auto accident at the intersection of Hollywood and Vine (location). At least 7 people are injured and will require medical attention. There may be people trapped in their cars and one vehicle is on fire."

   In three sentences, you have informed the authorities that a mass casualty event has occurred, what type of event it was, where it occurred, an approximate numbers of patients that need help, and the types of care or equipment that may be required.

   In survival settings, use your walkie-talkie or other communication device to notify base camp of the situation. Let them know what you'll need in terms of personnel and supplies. If you are not medically trained, contact the person who is the group medic. The most experienced medical person who arrives becomes the new Incident Commander.

4. **Set-Up:** Determine likely areas for various triage levels (see below) to be further evaluated and treated. Also, determine the appropriate entry and exit points for victims that need immediate transport to medical facilities, if they exist. If you are blessed with lots of help at the scene, assign triage, treatment, and transport team duties.
5. **S.T.A.R.T.:** Triage uses the acronym S.T.A.R.T., which stands for **S**imple **T**riage **A**nd **R**apid **T**reatment. The first round of triage, known as "primary triage", should be fast (30 seconds per patient if possible) and does not involve extensive treatment of injuries. It should be focused on identifying the triage level of each patient.

Evaluation in primary triage consists mostly of quick evaluation of respirations (or the lack thereof), perfusion (adequacy of circulation), and mental status. Other than controlling massive bleeding and clearing airways, very little treatment is performed in primary triage.

Although there is no international standard, triage levels are usually determined by color:

Immediate (Red tag): The victim needs immediate medical care and will not survive if not treated quickly (for example, a major hemorrhagic wound/internal bleeding). This person has top priority for treatment.

Delayed (Yellow tag): The victim needs medical care within 2-4 hours. Injuries may become life-threatening if ignored, but can wait until Red tags are treated (for example, an open fracture without major bleeding).

Minimal (Green tag): Generally stable and ambulatory ("walking wounded") but may need some medical care (for example, broken fingers or a sprained wrist).

Expectant (Black tag): The victim is either deceased or is not expected to live (for example, open fracture of skull with brain damage, multiple penetrating chest wounds).

Knowledge of this system allows a caregiver to understand the urgency of a patient's situation. You should know that, without modern medical care, a lot of red tags and even some yellow tags will become black tags. It will be difficult to save someone with major internal bleeding without surgical intervention.

Let's go through an example of a mass casualty incident and discuss how you would perform primary triage.

Primary Triage: MCI scenario

Here's our hypothetical scenario: you are in your village near the border with another (hostile) group. You hear an explosion. You are the first one to arrive at the scene, and you are alone. There are about twenty people down, and there is blood everywhere. What do you do?

Referring back to the 5 S's, let's say that you have already determined the SAFETY of the current situation and SIZED UP the scene. It appears that a bomb has exploded. There are no hostiles nearby, as far as you can tell. Therefore, you believe that you aren't currently in danger. The injuries are significant (there are body parts) and the victims are all in an area no larger than, say, 30 yards.

The incident occurred on a main thoroughfare in the village, so there are ways in and ways out. You have SENT FOR HELP on your handie-talkie and described the scene. Several group members have replied, including a former ICU nurse. The area is relatively open, so you can SET UP different areas for various triage categories. Now you can START (Simple Triage And Rapid Treatment).

You will call out as loudly as possible: "I'm here to help, everyone who can get up and walk and needs medical attention, get up and move to the sound of my voice. If you are uninjured and can help, follow me."

You're lucky, 13 of the 20, mostly from the periphery of the blast, sit up, or at least try to. 10 can stand, and 8 go to the area you designated for walking wounded. These people have cuts and scrapes, and a couple of them are limping; one has obviously broken an arm. 2 bruised but sturdy individuals join you. By communicating, you have made your job as temporary Incident Commander easier by identifying the walking wounded (Green Tags) and getting some immediate help. You still have 10 victims down.

You then go to the *closest* victim on the ground and proceed in an organized manner to the next nearest victim in turn. In this way, you will triage faster and more effectively than trying to figure out who needs help the most from a distance.

Let's cheat just a little and say that you happen to have SMART tags in your pack. SMART tags are handy tickets which allow you to mark a particular triage level on a patient. Once you identify a victim's triage level, you remove a portion of the end of the tag until you reach the appropriate color and place it around the patient's wrist.

You could, instead, use colored adhesive tape, colored markers, or numbers placed on the forehead. If you use numbers:

- Priority 1 is immediate/red (top priority)
- Priority 2 is delayed/yellow
- Priority 3 is minimal/green
- Priority 4 is dead/expectant/black

The number method is used in some other countries; it is also useful if you're color blind.

It is important to remember that you are triaging, not treating. The only treatments in START will be the control of heavy bleeding, opening airways, and elevating the legs in case of shock.

As you go from patient to patient, stay calm, identify who you are and that you're here to help. Your goal is to find out who will need help most urgently (red tags). You will be assessing **RPMs** (**R**espirations, **P**erfusion, and **M**ental Status):

Respirations: Is your patient breathing? If not, tilt the head back or, if you have them, insert an oral airway (Note: in a MCI triage situation, the rule against moving the neck of a victim due to risk of cervical spine injury is, for the time being, suspended) If you have an open airway and no breathing, that victim is tagged black. If the victim breathes once an airway is restored or is breathing more than 30 times a minute, tag red. If the victim is breathing normally, move to perfusion.

Perfusion: Perfusion is an evaluation of how normal the blood flow or circulation is. Check for a (wrist or neck) pulse, then press on a nail bed or finger pad firmly and quickly remove. The color will go from white back to normal color in less than 2 seconds if circulation is good. This is referred to as the **Capillary Refill Time (CRT)**. If you have trouble feeling a weak pulse or it takes longer than 2 seconds for nail bed color to return, tag red. If a pulse is present and CRT is normal, move to mental status.

Mental Status: Can the victim follow simple commands ("open your eyes", "what's your name")? If the patient isn't breathing excessively fast and has normal perfusion, but is unconscious or disoriented: Tag red. If they can understand you and follow commands, tag yellow if they can't get up or green if they can. Remember that, as a consequence of the explosion, some victims may not be able to hear you well.

It might be easier to remember all this by just thinking 30 -2- Can Do:

30 (respirations)
2 (CRT)
Can Do (Commands)

If there is any doubt as to the category, always tag the highest priority triage level. Not sure between yellow and red? Tag red. Once you have identified someone's triage level, tag them and move immediately to the next patient unless you have major bleeding to stop. Any one RPM check that results in a red result tags the victim as red. Elevate the legs if you suspect shock.

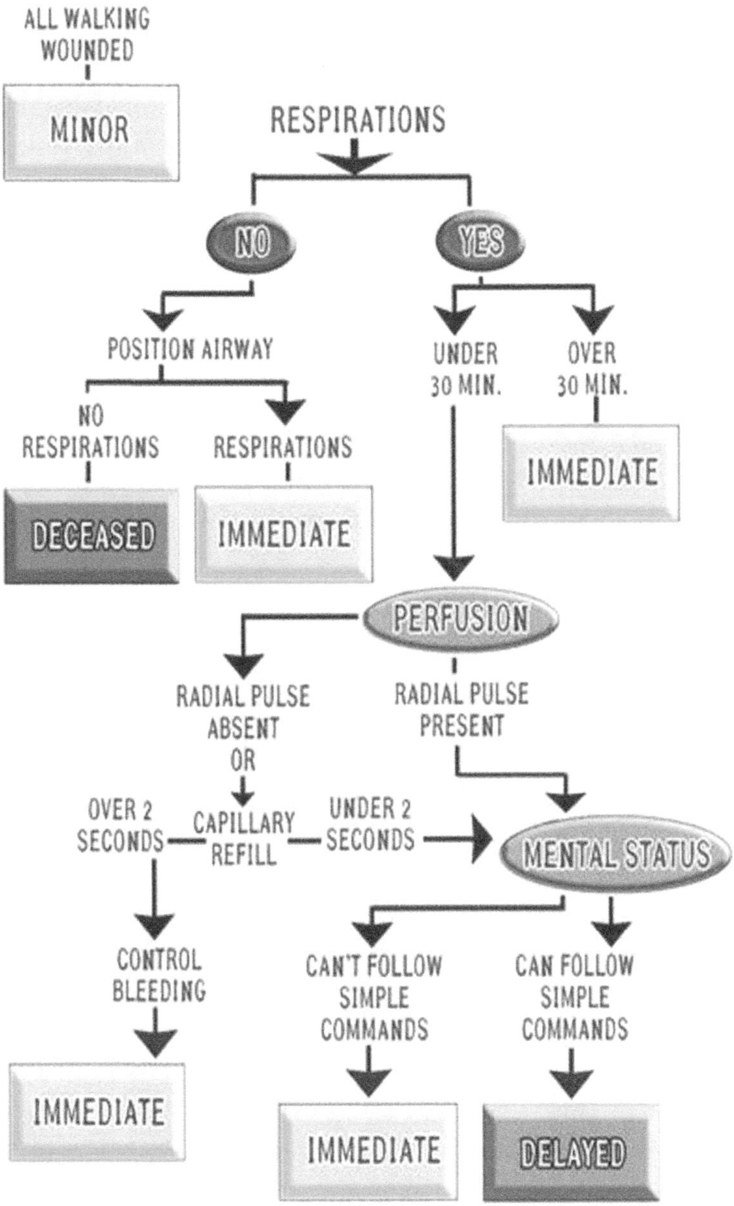

TRIAGE CASCADE

Now, let's return to our mass casualty event. You have identified 8 walking wounded and moved them to a designated area. You have 2 relatively unhurt victims who will assist your triage efforts. Finally, the list below contains your 10 patients on the ground, in order. Read the descriptions and decide the primary triage level; utilize your helpers wisely. We'll discuss how we triaged them in detail in the next section:

1. Male in his 30s, complains of pain in his left leg (obviously fractured), Respirations 24, pulse strong, CRT 1 second, no excessive bleeding.
2. Female in her 50s, bleeding from nose, ears, and mouth. Trying to sit up but can't, respirations 20, pulse present, CRT 1 second, not responding to your commands.
3. Teenage girl bleeding heavily from her right thigh, respirations 32, pulse thready, CRT 2.5 seconds, follows commands.
4. Another teenage girl, small laceration on forehead, says she can't move her legs. Respirations 20, pulse strong, CRT 1 second.
5. Male in his 20s, head wound, respirations absent. Airway repositioned, still no breathing.
6. Male in his 40s, burns on face, chest, and arms. Respirations 22, pulse 100, CRT 1.5 seconds, follows commands.
7. Teenage boy, multiple cuts and abrasions but not hemorrhaging, says he can't breathe, respirations 34, radial pulse present, CRT 2.5 seconds.
8. Female in her 20s, burns on neck and face, respirations 22, pulse present, CRT 1 second, asks to get up and can walk, although with a limp.
9. Elderly woman, bleeding profusely from an amputated right arm (level of forearm), respirations 36, pulse on other wrist absent, CRT 3 seconds, unresponsive.
10. Male child, multiple penetrating injuries, respirations absent. Airway repositioned, starts breathing. Radial pulse absent, CRT 2 seconds, unresponsive.

MCI Scenario Results

On the previous pages, we described a mass casualty incident scene with 20 victims. We told you about initial considerations before beginning

START (Simple Triage and Rapid Treatment) and the RPM system for determining triage level. You ended up with 10 victims on the ground, 8 walking wounded, and 2 uninjured but unskilled helpers. You moved the walking wounded to a separate area and are now ready to quickly triage the remaining 10 victims.

To review the primary triage categories:

Immediate (Red tag): The victim needs immediate medical care and will not survive if not treated quickly (for example, a major hemorrhagic wound/internal bleeding) Top priority for treatment.

Delayed (Yellow tag): The victim needs medical care within 2-4 hours. Injuries may become life-threatening if ignored, but can wait until Red tags are treated (for example, open fracture of femur without major hemorrhage).

Minimal (Green tag): Generally stable and ambulatory ("walking wounded") but may need some medical care (for example, 2 broken fingers, sprained wrist).

Expectant (Black tag): The victim is either deceased or is not expected to live (for example, open fracture of cranium with brain damage, multiple penetrating chest wounds).

And here are your previously-described triage evaluation parameters (**RPMs**):

- Respirations
- Perfusion
- Mental Status

Remember this: **30** (respirations) – **2** (CRT) – **Can Do** (follows commands)

Your 2 uninjured helpers are an able-bodied man and woman. The woman knows how to take a pulse. You have no medical equipment with you other than some oral airways and triage tags to work with.

Begin with the nearest victim (#1 on the list in the previous section):

1. Male in his 30s, complains of pain in his left leg (obviously fractured), Respirations 24, pulse strong, CRT 1 second, no excessive bleeding.

Respirations are within acceptable range (less than 30), pulse and CRT normal. Complains of pain, and is communicating where it hurts, so mental status probably normal. This patient is tagged YELLOW: needs care but will not die if there is a reasonable (2-4 hour) delay. Move on.

2. Female in her 50s, bleeding from nose, ears, and mouth. Trying to sit up but can't, respirations 20, pulse present, CRT 1 second, not responding to your commands.

   This victim has a significant head injury, but is stable from the standpoint of respirations and perfusion. As her mental status is impaired, tag RED (immediate). Move on.

3. Teenage girl bleeding heavily from her right thigh, respirations 32, pulse thready, CRT 2.5 seconds, follows commands.

   This victim is seriously hemorrhaging, one of the reasons to treat during triage. Respirations elevated and perfusion impaired. You use your unskilled male helper to apply pressure by placing his hands on the bleeding and applying pressure, preferably using his shirt or bandanna as a "dressing". Tag RED. As the patient is already RED, you don't really have to assess mental status. You and your female helper move on.

4. Another teenage girl, small laceration on forehead, says she can't move her legs. Respirations 20, pulse strong, CRT 1 second.

   Probable spinal injury but otherwise stable and can communicate. Tag YELLOW. Move on.

5. Male in his 20s, head wound, respirations absent. Airway repositioned, still no breathing.

   If not breathing, you will reposition his head and place an airway. This fails to restart breathing. This patient is deceased for all intents and purposes. Tag BLACK, move on.

6. Male in his 40s, burns on face, chest, and arms. Respirations 22, pulse 100, CRT 1.5 seconds, follows commands.

   This victim has significant burns on large areas, but is breathing well and has normal perfusion. Mental status is unimpaired, so you tag YELLOW and move on.

7. Teenage boy, multiple cuts and abrasions but not hemorrhaging, says he can't breathe, respirations 34, radial pulse present, CRT 2.5 seconds.

This victim doesn't look so bad but is having trouble breathing and has questionable perfusion. Mental status is unimpaired, but he likely has other issues, perhaps internal bleeding. You tag RED (respirations over 30, impaired perfusion) and move on.

8. Female in her 20s, burns on neck and face, respirations 22, pulse present, CRT 1 second, asks to get up and can walk, although with a limp.

   Obviously injured, this young woman is otherwise stable and communicating. With assistance, she is able to stand up, and can walk by herself. She becomes another of the walking wounded, tag GREEN. Point her to the other GREEN victims and move on.

9. Elderly woman, bleeding profusely from an amputated right arm (level of forearm), respirations 36, pulse on other wrist absent, CRT 3 seconds, unresponsive.

   Obviously in dire straits, you use your shirt as a tourniquet and sacrifice your remaining helper to apply pressure on the bleeding area. Tag RED, move on.

10. Male child, multiple penetrating injuries, respirations absent. Airway repositioned, starts breathing. Radial pulse absent, CRT 2 seconds, unresponsive.

You initially think this child is deceased, but you follow protocol and reposition his airway by tilting his head back. He starts breathing even without an oral airway, to your surprise, so you tag him RED. If he is bleeding heavily from his injuries, you apply pressure and wait for the additional help you originally requested to arrive.

You have just performed triage on 20 victims, including the walking wounded, in 10 minutes or less. Help begins to arrive, including the ICU nurse that you contacted initially. You are no longer the most experienced medical resource at the scene, and you are relieved of Incident Command. The nurse begins the process of assigning areas for where secondary triage and treatment can occur.

There is still much to do, but you have performed your duty to identify those victims who need the most urgent care. In a normal situation, your modern medical facilities will already have ambulances and trained personnel with lots of equipment on the scene. In a collapse situation, however, the prognosis for many of your victims is grave. Go over our list of victims and see who you think would survive if modern medical care is not available. Many of the RED tags and even some of the YELLOW tags would be in serious danger of dying from their injuries.

THE ACTIVE SHOOTER EVENT

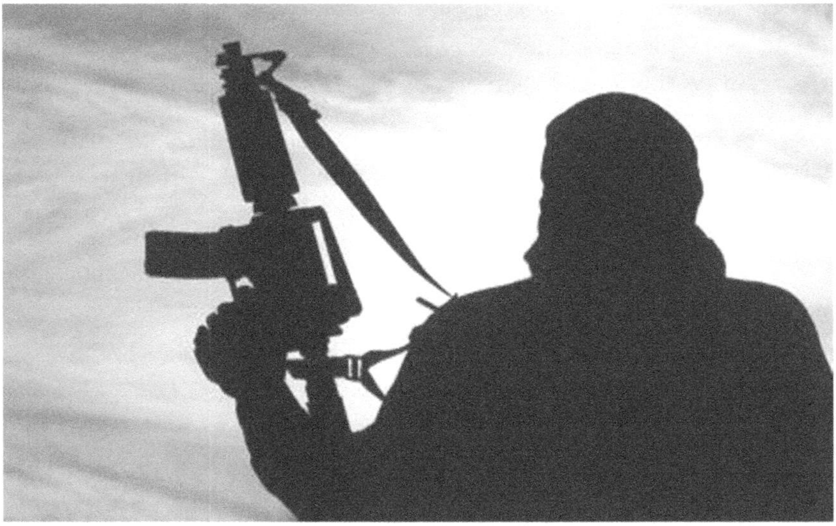

You might associate hostile encounters with survival scenarios, but they can occur in normal times as well. It's hard to read the news without seeing reports of the latest mass shooting by terrorists, the deranged, or the disgruntled. Few believe that they could possibly wind up in the crosshairs of a gunman's sight, but it can happen anytime and anywhere. What would be your response to the "active shooter"?

The natural response for most people is not to do anything, due to what we call "normalcy bias": That's the tendency for people to believe everything follows a pattern and that the day will proceed normally. They're usually right, but when a terrorist event breaks that pattern, the unprepared brain takes time to process the new situation. People will think that the sound of gunfire is a firecracker or a blown tire; anything less threatening than an assassin out to kill them.

In normal times, most citizens believe that law enforcement and homeland security are on the case. While these agencies do the best they can to counter situations like this, most mass shooting events end so quickly that there is little or no chance that help will be there when needed.

Without a plan of action, the average person follows the herd. If fifty people around you drop to the floor, your natural tendency is to do the same. Cowering in fear under a table in plain view of the shooter isn't a recipe for a good outcome. By having a plan, you'll have a better chance of getting out of there in one piece.

Let's suppose you're at the local mall; what would your plan be if you heard gunfire nearby? What would you do first? Run? If so, where? If you couldn't run, what would you do?

These are things you should be thinking about, calmly and rationally, whenever you're in an area where there are a lot of people. It may seem extreme to have to think of these things, but that's the "New Normal".

With an active shooter, what you do in the first few seconds may determine your final outcome. Give yourself a head start by always knowing what's happening around you. We call this "situational awareness". Know where the exits are. Know who appears nervous or suspicious in your immediate area. Know the direction the gunshots are coming from.

Sounds simple, doesn't it? But in this era of people immersed in their smartphones, few are situationally aware. These are the easy targets an assassin is looking for. In survival, your index of suspicion will be higher and the likelihood is that you will be ready to defend yourself. In normal times, most leave their guard down.

Run, Hide, Fight

If you find yourself in the middle of a terrorist event, you should remember these three words: **Run, Hide, Fight**. Just as "**Stop, Drop, Roll**" can save the life of someone on fire, "Run, Hide, Fight" might save the life of someone *under* fire. This represents the order of the actions that you should be taking in the presence of an active shooter.

Most people will hide as their first course of action. You, however, should run away from the direction of gunfire as soon as you hear it. Leave through those exits you've been mentally marking. This will make it less likely that you and the shooter will cross paths. Forget about collecting your stuff, it will only slow you down.

If you're in the line of sight of the shooter, run away at angles that might make yourself a more difficult target. It's not an action you'd naturally take, but most shooters aren't marksmen and will miss a moving target.

A good citizen would yell for others to follow and prevent others from entering the kill zone. Don't spend precious time convincing a reluctant person to leave with you, though. Also, don't try to move or otherwise help the wounded, despite your natural tendency to want to do so. The first priority to get out of there; becoming the next casualty does no one any good. Even the police will leave the injured until after the shooter has been neutralized.

If you see law enforcement arriving on the scene, don't run up and hug them. Get your hands in the air, fingers spread, where officers can see them. They need to know that you're not the threat. Follow any instructions given and leave in the directions the officers came from.

If there's only one exit and the shooter is standing in front of it, running might not be an option. Your next choice is hiding.

You want to quickly get out of the shooter's line of sight. We call this "concealment", but it isn't necessarily "cover". If you're concealed, you can't be seen but a bullet might penetrate to hit you. If you have found cover, it means that you are both hidden and protected from projectiles hurled your way. A leafy bush, for example, is good concealment, but a thick tree trunk might be better cover.

In a building, hiding under a table in the same room as the shooter is a death sentence. Get into another room, preferably one with a door you can lock. If there is no lock, put together a barrier with desks and chairs. Turn off the lights, silence your cell phone, and stay quiet behind an additional barrier like a table or in a closet. If you can *quietly* alert authorities, do so. Don't respond to voice commands unless you're sure the danger is over; sometimes the gunman will try to lure you out of a safe place by yelling "all clear".

By doing everything we just said, you've just made yourself a harder target for someone who wants to do damage as fast as possible. You'll probably be passed by for easier targets.

What if you can't run, and there is no reasonable hiding place? You just might have to fight your way out. This strategy isn't always doomed to failure. You still might be able to subdue an attacker even if unarmed. It's a last resort, but it *can* end without a fatality. If you don't fight, the shooter will have a clear shot to your head and death is likely. If you fight, it might just be harder to be hit with a fatal shot.

Of course, it would be great if you were a martial arts expert, but any type of aggression against the gunman could disrupt their "flow" and possibly put you at an advantage. If you can, approach him from the side or rear; go for his weapon to control where it's pointed.

If you have help, all should attack at the same time from different directions while hurling objects that he has to dodge. This guy is probably not James Bond: he'll be disconcerted and not be able to handle multiple threats at once.

If you've disrupted the shooter or, better, gotten the weapon out of his hands, inflict damage on him until he is dead or has stopped moving. Regardless of how savage it might seem, you must commit to your actions.

Luckily, few people will ever find themselves in the midst of a terrorist shooting, but more are likely in the New Normal. Those with a plan will have a better chance to survive this event and many other disasters in the uncertain future.

PATIENT TRANSPORT

In normal times, your main goal upon encountering an injured or ill person is to transport them to a modern medical facility as soon as possible. These facilities will, unfortunately, be non-existent in many of the scenarios that this book covers.

Standard first aid protocol dictates that you should leave a victim in the position they are found until emergency personnel arrive. When help is not on the way, however, this eventually becomes impractical or impossible. As such, you will have to make a decision as to whether your patient can or cannot be treated for their problem at their present location. If they cannot, you must consider how to move your patient to where the bulk of your medical supplies are.

Before deciding whether to transport, stabilize the patient as much as possible. This means assuring open airways, controlling bleeding, splinting orthopedic injuries, and more. If you are unable to do this with what's on you, consider having a group member get the supplies needed to make transport safer. If possible, gather a team to assist you before you move the victim. If you know the amount of assistance you'll have, you can choose a method of evacuation that will cause the least trauma to both patient and medic.

When moving a patient, you should be concerned about the possibility of a spinal injury, especially if there is:

- Head or neck trauma.
- Altered mental status
- Pain in the head or neck.
- Weakness, numbness, or paralysis in the extremities.
- Loss of bladder control
- Contorted position of head or neck or difficulty moving these areas.

A person with a possible spinal injury should be "logrolled" onto a stretcher as a unit without bending their neck or back if at all possible. A cervical collar and supportive blocks with straps can be used to secure the spine of all patients suspicious for injury. An unstable neck, especially in an unconscious victim, could easily be traumatized even if not involved in the original accident. Keep the head in alignment with the spine during transport.

If you have several helpers, transporting the patient is easier but requires coordination. You, as medic, will serve as leader of the transport team. This entails making sure the patient is transferred to the stretcher safely, but also that all team members lift and move at the same time. Simple "Prepare to Lift", "Lift", and "March" commands should suffice to get everyone on the same page.

To move a patient onto a stretcher, the medic positions the casualty next to it on his back with his arms at his side. Then, one helper slips his arms under the casualty's back and waist and another helper does the same under the hip and knees. Your job is to keep the head in alignment with the spine throughout. Upon your command, the teams lifts and places the victim on the stretcher. An alternative would be to have two helpers carefully turn the patient on their side facing them rather than lift. You would then slip the stretcher underneath. For this, the casualty's arms are placed across their chest.

There are a number of methods available to move the injured patient back to camp. If you don't have the luxury of a vehicle, the next easiest method involves using a stretcher. Many excellent litter systems are available commercially, but stretchers can be improvised with a little ingenuity. Even without any materials to put together a litter, there still exist ways that will allow one, two, or a team of medics to achieve their transport goal.

Transport Using Materials At Hand

In a survival setting, an injury will likely occur without a commercially-made stretcher readily available. However, abandoned residential buildings in urban or rural settings will contain a number of found materials that can serve the purpose. An inside door, blankets, or even an ironing board will be easy finds; after all, who takes their ironing board when them when escaping a disaster? All of these can function as a litter or backboard as long as enough helpers are present to hold the victim in place. Folded-over Paracord, blankets, or rope can be used to serve as handholds and to prevent hanging extremities. Indeed, these items can, in and of themselves, be used as stretchers. Lengths of Paracord, for example, can be crisscrossed using sticks, poles, or knots to form a means of transport.

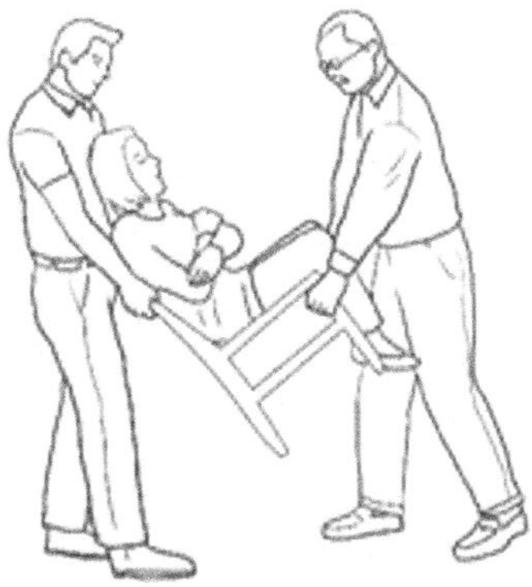

Chair Stretcher

Another example of an easily found item in an abandoned building is a chair. If you have a conscious casualty, a sturdy chair can be used by itself as a reasonable litter. In this method, the patient sits or is placed on the chair. One transporter stands in back of the chair, grasping it from the sides and tilting it back. The second transporter grasps the chair legs in front and both lift using their legs. For short distances, the second transporter can face the victim, but it would be easier for longer distances to face forward.

4 **Person or more blanket stretcher**: Even if you have no backboard, having a blanket and/or sturdy poncho in your backpack can help move a casualty. Simply place the victim on the stretched-out blanket and then roll the sides inward to form handholds to lift and carry.

2 **person blanket stretcher**: With fewer assistants, you'll need some additional support. If you have two long poles or sticks about 6 or 7 feet long and 2 inches or more thick, you could make a litter by placing the sticks so that the blanket is divided into thirds. Fold one of the outer thirds over the stick and then the other outer third over the other stick. The casualty's weight will help keep the blanket in place.

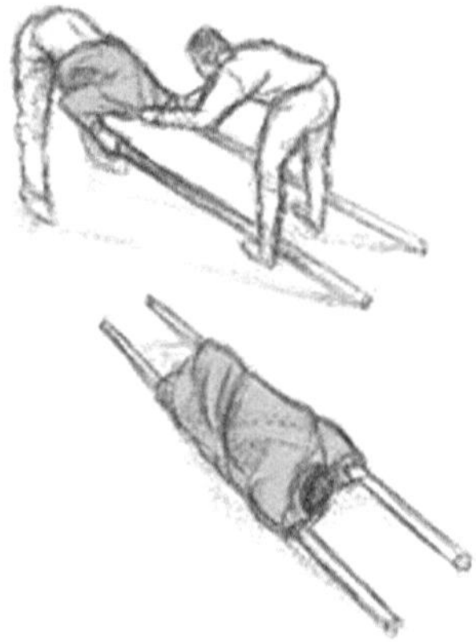

SHIRT STRETCHER

The "**jacket stretcher**" is variation of this method. You'll need two buttoned jackets or shirts, preferably still on the rescuers. While the first transporter is grasping the litter poles, a second pulls the first's garment off, inside out. The jacket automatically moves onto the poles, forming a "bed" for the stretcher. A second shirt or jacket goes onto the other end of the pole when the transporters reverse roles. It should be noted that this method should only be used if the weather is such that rescuers can tolerate the loss of the clothing item during transport.

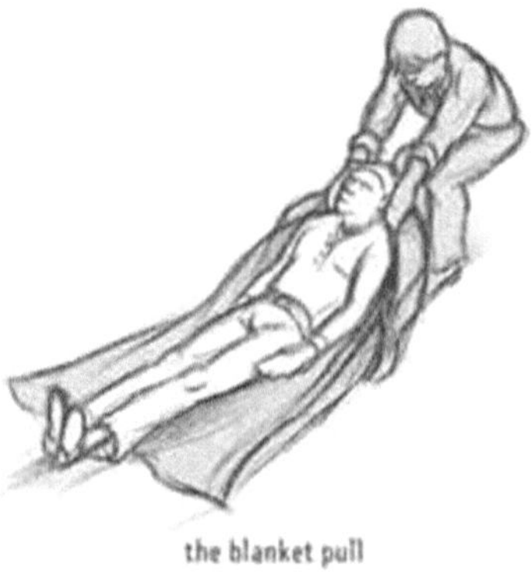

the blanket pull

1 person blanket pull: Sometimes, you might find yourself alone with the victim and can't wait for help to move them. In this case, the blanket can be placed under the patient. Grasp the blanket at one end with both hands and position your forearms to cradle the head. Use your legs to pull instead of your back to avoid injury. Alternatively, you can drag the victim out by the shoulder of his shirt or jacket. Grasp the back of the clothing under the shoulders, and use your legs to pull. Your forearms should cradle the head if done correctly.

Transport Using No Materials

There are circumstances where you might have absolutely nothing at your disposal to help evacuate a patient other than your own muscles. Here are methods to transport a patient without any equipment:

3 person team or more: With a number of assistants, you can form a "**hammock**" that will make for easier lifting and transport. In this method, rescuers kneel on both sides of the victim. You'll reach under the victim to grasp the wrist of the person across from you. Those at each end will use one hand to support the head and feet of the person being moved. Upon command, rescuers will get on one knee, and then stand.

Sometimes, you might have to get a patient onto a higher level than a stretcher on the ground, such as a gurney or an operating table. For this purpose, the "**3 person carry**" is useful to lift a victim for short distances. The transporters, on one knee, roll the patient to his side, facing them. He is then lifted onto their knee, and the team stands on command. The casualty is held on the transporters' chests and they all start the evacuation using the same foot.

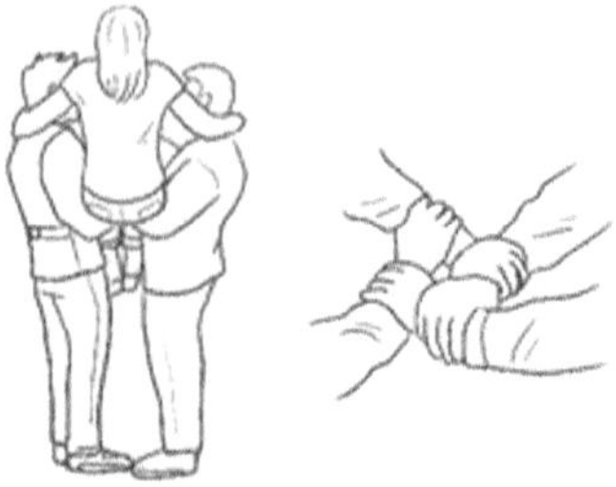

Four-handed Seat Carry

2 persons: When it's you and one assistant, you have a number of options. You can make a "**four-handed seat**" with interlocked wrists if your casualty is conscious and can hold onto your shoulders. With all four wrists interlocked in a square, a wider, more stable seat is formed. If one of the rescuers needs a free hand, 3 wrists can form a triangular seat.

The "**two-handed seat**" is meant to provide a seat with a back for victims that might be less alert. Each rescuer interlocks one wrist to form the seat and uses the other arm to grasp his partner's far shoulder. This forms the back support. All versions start with the transporters squatting on either side of the victim, using their legs to lift instead of their backs.

Another two person lift is the "**crutch**" method. For the conscious victim, this carry allows the victim to walk using the rescuers as a pair of crutches. Each rescuer grabs a wrist and puts the crook of the arm on the back of their neck and over the shoulder, with the other arm around the victim's waist. The victim can then stand with assistance. If unconscious, the waistband or belt can be pulled to help lift the casualty with their legs dragging behind as you move.

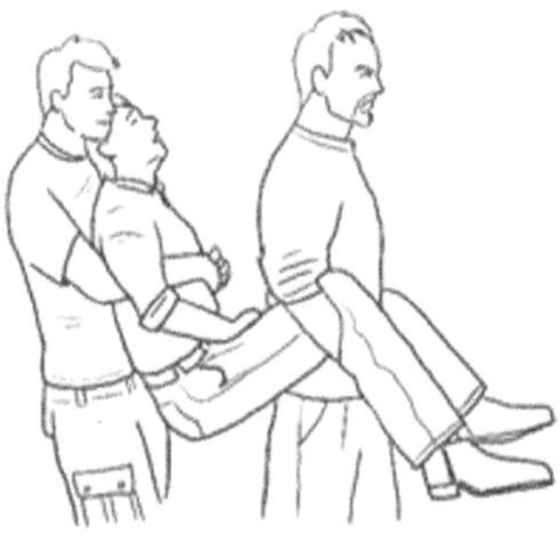

Fore-and-Aft Carry

The "**fore-and-aft**" technique can serve effectively as a long-distance transport method for conscious or unconscious victims. The first rescuer, from behind, puts his arms under the shoulders of a victim lying on his back and locks his hands around the chest. The second rescuer, facing front towards the feet of the victim, uses both arms to grasp underneath each knee. It's more comfortable if the taller transporter is at the patient's head.

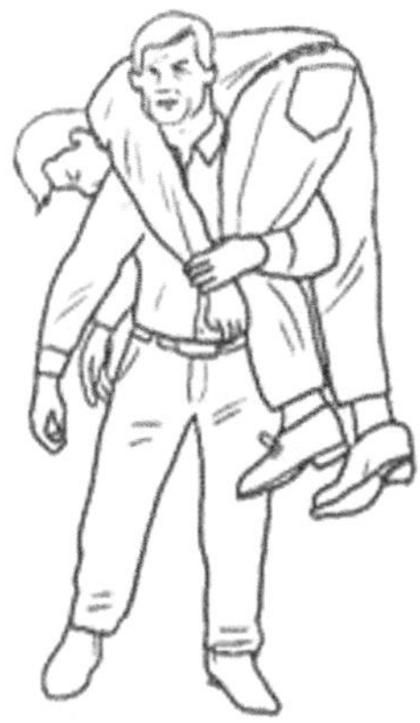

Fireman's Carry

1 **Person:** There are situations where it's just you, there's no equipment, and you have to evacuate a patient. If you are alone with a patient, the "**Fireman's Carry**" is effective and keeps the victim's torso relatively level and stable. To achieve this maneuver: While squatting or kneeling, grasp the person's right wrist with your left hand and drape it over your shoulders. Keeping your back straight, place your right hand between their legs and around the right thigh. Using your leg muscles to lift, rise up; you should end up with their torso over your back and the right thigh resting over your right shoulder. Their left arm and leg will hang behind your back if you have done it correctly. Adjust so as to cause the least strain.

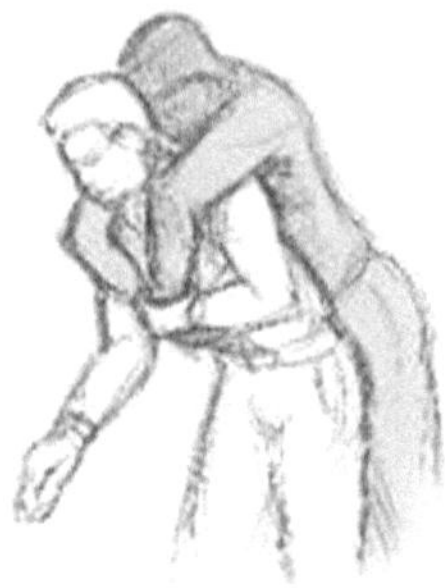

PACK STRAP CARRY

Another option when you are the lone rescuer is the "**Pack-Strap Carry**". With your patient behind you, grasp both arms and cross them across your chest. If squatting, keep your back straight and use your legs and back muscles to lift the victim. Bend slightly so that the person's weight is on your hips and lift them off the ground.

It's important to remember this simple acronym when pulling or carrying a person: **B.A.C.K.**

- Back Straight – muscles and discs can handle more weight safely when the back is straight.
- Avoid Twisting – joints can be damaged when twisting.
- Close to body – avoid reaching to pick up a load; it causes more strain on muscles and joints.
- Keep Stable – the more rotation and jerking, the more pressure on the discs and muscles.

Be sure to check the Video Resources section at the back of this book to see some of these methods being used in real time.

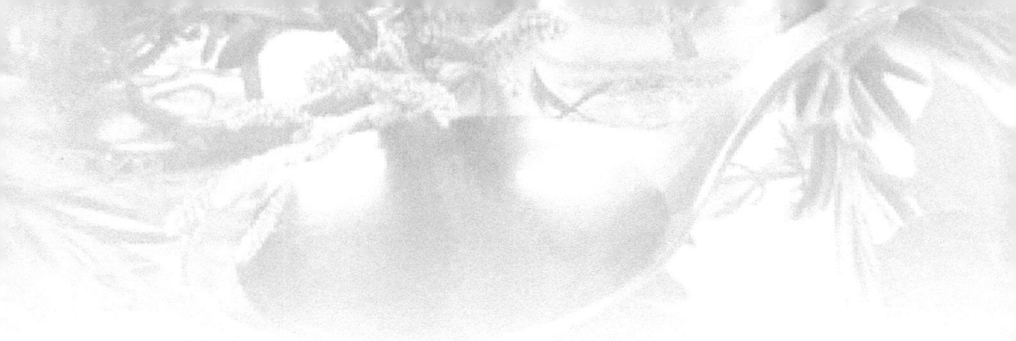

SECTION 3

✚ ✚ ✚

HYGIENE AND SANITATION

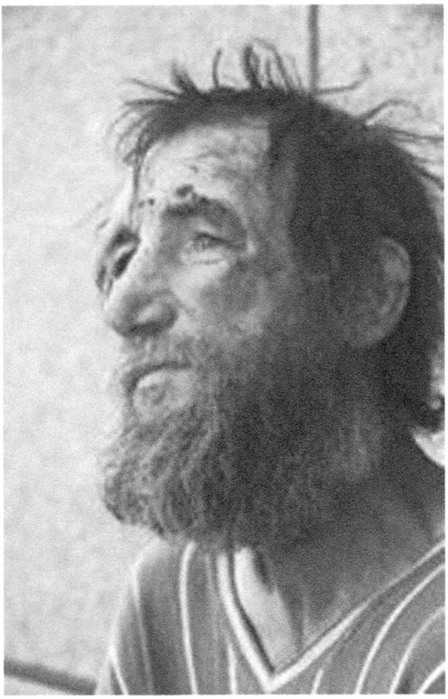

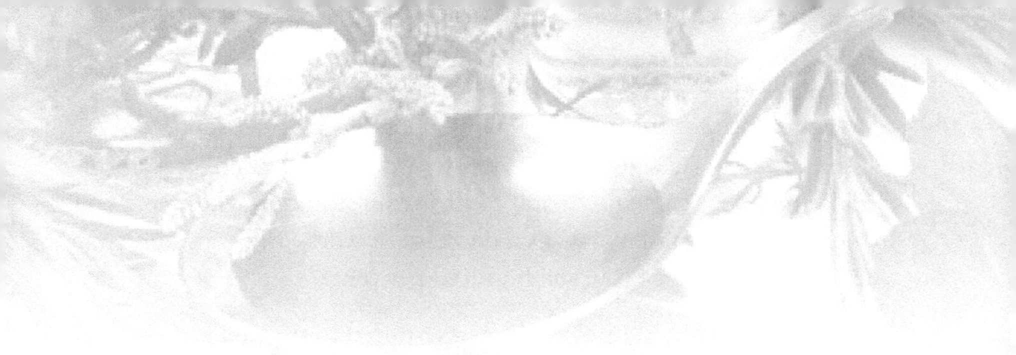

HYGIENE-RELATED MEDICAL ISSUES

In nature, many animals make specific efforts to keep themselves clean by preening and grooming. This instinctual urge eliminates pests and keeps them healthy. The human urge to be clean, although not related to instinct, has done its job as well. Time and effort spent in remaining clean translates into resistance to disease. When humans are under stress, attention to hygiene suffers because all available energy has to be directed to activities of daily survival.

As survival medic, your responsibility is to prevent unsanitary conditions from affecting the health of your family. Indeed, diligence in this matter is one of the major factors that will determine your success as a caregiver.

A person with hygiene issues usually presents with a foul smell. Body odors occur when sweat mixes with bacteria, and certain bacteria can lead to disease. It's up to the medic to ensure that defective hygiene doesn't put their family at risk. Strict enforcement of good sanitation and cleanliness will do more to keep your family healthy than anything a doctor or nurse could do.

Assuring an adequate stockpile of various cleansing items, such as soap or detergent, is also part of your responsibilities. When these are no longer available, the goal of staying clean is difficult to achieve even with the best of intentions.

Important areas where cleanliness will increase your chances of survival include foot care and dental health. Any situation where sore feet or toothaches are present means a decrease in work efficiency at a time where everyone must be at one hundred per cent.

With the increase of physical labor required to succeed in a survival setting, it's a simple fact that we'll get sweaty and dirty. The dirtier and wetter we get, the more prone we will be to problems such as infections or infestations. With careful attention, the medic can improve the chance of avoiding these problems.

LICE, TICKS, AND WORMS

Lice

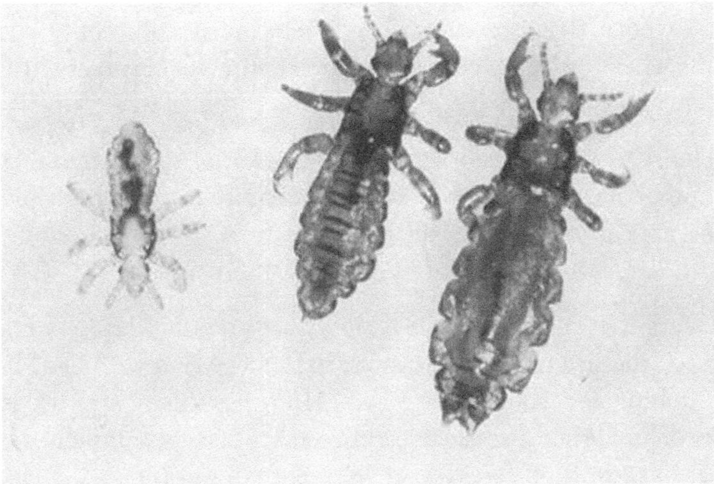

Typical Head Lice

A common health problem that may pertain to poor hygiene is the presence of lice, also known as "**Pediculosis**". Lice (singular: louse) are wingless parasitic insects that feed on blood and are found on many species. On humans, there are three types:

- The **Head Louse** *Pediculus humanus capitis*
- The **Body Louse** *Pediculus humanus corporis*
- The **Pubic Louse** or "Crab" *Pthirus pubis*

Lice are, generally speaking, species-specific: You cannot, as an example, get lice from your dog, like you could get fleas. You get them only from other humans. It's interesting to note that human lice and chimpanzee lice diverged from each other, evolutionarily, about 6 million years ago; this is almost exactly when their hosts went their separate ways.

At present, however, there is no evidence that head or pubic lice transmit diseases to humans. Body lice, however, can. All lice cause irritation that can have major implications for the health of a survival group. For example, irritation and itching caused by lice can break the skin and allow other infections to enter the body.

Major risk factors for lice infestations include crowded, unsanitary conditions or situations where close personal contact is unavoidable. In normal times, these conditions most commonly occur in schools where ordinarily clean children come into contact with those who have lice.

The sharing of personal items can also lead to louse infestations. Clothing, combs, bedding, and towels that are used by multiple individuals are common ways that lice spread from person to person. These risks are even more pronounced in survival settings.

Head lice (*Pediculus humanus capitis*) are greyish-white as adults and can reach the size of a small sesame seed. Infestation with head lice can cause itching and, sometimes, a rash. However, this type of lice is not a carrier of any other disease. Head lice are relatively common, so much so that 6-12 million cases a year are reported, mostly among children, in the United States.

With their less developed immune systems, kids often don't even realize they are infested with lice. Adults, however, are usually kept scratching and irritated unless treated. An interesting fact is that African-Americans are somewhat resistant to head lice, possibly due to the shape and width of the hair shaft.

The diagnosis is made by identifying the presence of the louse or its "**nits**" (eggs) on the head. Nits look like small bits of dandruff that are stuck to hairs. They are more easily seen when examined using a "black light". This causes them to fluoresce as light blue "dots" attached to the hair shafts near the scalp.

As black lights will be rare commodities in a collapse, a fine-tooth comb run through the hair is more practical to reveal the adult lice and nits. These special combs are used to remove as many lice as possible before treatment and to check for them afterwards. Look at "hot spots" where lice seem to concentrate, like the nape of the neck, around the ears, and the crown of the head. The diligence required to do this effectively led to the coining of the term "nitpicking".

You will find the nits firmly attached to the hair shaft about ¼ inch from the scalp. Nits will generally appear as yellowish white and oval-shaped. The application of olive oil to the comb may make them easier to remove. Many prefer the metal nit combs sold at pet stores for animals to plastic ones sold at human pharmacies.

In normal times, wash and dry all clothes in hot temperatures or, alternatively, place in the freezer to kill the lice. If you are off grid, place clothing and personal items in a plastic bag for two weeks. Adult head lice can only live a few days off the host.

Body lice (*Pediculus humanus corporis)* are latecomers compared to head lice, probably first appearing when humans began to wear clothes about 170,000 years ago. As the concept of doing laundry occurred somewhat later than that, you can imagine that constant contact with dirty clothes caused frequent infestations.

Body lice, unlike head lice, have been linked to infectious diseases such as typhus, trench fever and epidemic relapsing fever. Continuous exposure to body lice may lead to areas on the skin that are hardened and deeply pigmented, a condition previously known as "vagabond's disease".

Infestations may be an issue common only with the homeless or in underdeveloped countries today; body lice will, however, likely become an epidemic in settings where regular bathing and washing of clothes isn't possible.

Body lice are slightly larger than head lice; they also differ in that they live on dirty clothes (especially the seams), not on the body. They go to the human body only to feed. Also, they are sturdier than their cousins and can live without human contact for 30 days or so. Examination of clothes and bedding seams usually pinpoints the problem.

Destruction of the infested clothing, if possible, is the appropriate strategy here. Sometimes, using medication is unnecessary as the lice have left with the clothes (don't bet on it, however). .

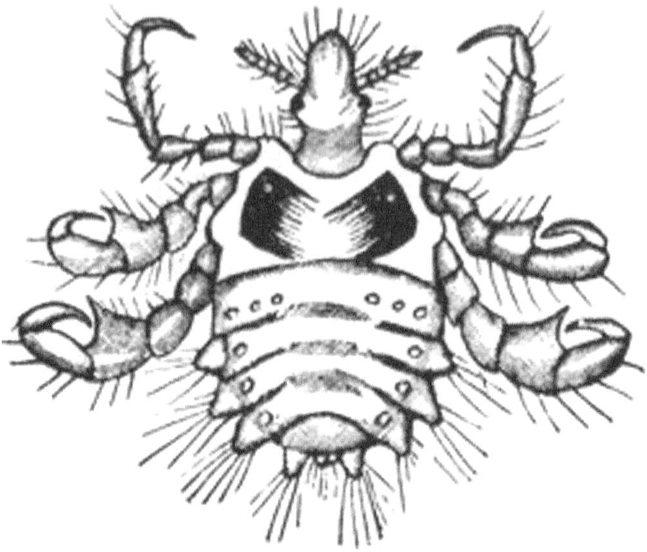

Crab Louse

Pubic infestations may be either caused by lice or mites. **Pubic lice** (Pthirus pubis), also known as **"crabs"**, usually start in the pubic region but may eventually extend anywhere there is hair. They are most commonly passed by sexual contact. Severe itching is the main symptom and can involve the axillary (armpit) hair or even the eyelashes.

Although they are sometimes seen in a patient that has other sexually transmitted diseases, pubic lice do not actually transmit them and are not the cause. It should be noted that pubic lice infestations are one of the few sexually transmitted diseases that is not prevented by the use of a condom.

Scabies is often confused with "crabs", but is caused by another creature entirely, tiny eight-legged mites of the species *Sarcoptes scabiei*. Like pubic lice, scabies can be passed through sexual contact or other direct skin-to-skin contact with another human but not from animals.

Unlike lice, however, the mites do not live and reproduce on hair shafts but burrow through the skin forming small raised red bumps that may become crusted. These bumps may hold hundreds of mite eggs. Itching is usually severe and most intense at night. It should be noted that Scabies can affect skin folds, even those with little hair such as the folds of the wrists, elbows, or between fingers and toes.

Infestations with lice and mites can be treated with medications called "Pediculicides". They usually come in lotions and shampoos:

- Pyrethrin (brand name Rid shampoo, a natural product also found in chrysanthemum flowers)
- Permethrin 1% (brand name Nix lotion, a synthetic pyrethrin)
- Lindane (prescription brand Kwell)
- Spinosad (brand name Natroba, a natural insecticide derived from soil bacteria – only for head lice in children 4 years or older
- Ivermectin 0.5% (brand name Sklice, also from soil bacteria and only for head lice in children 6 months or older). Ivermectin also comes in as an oral medication by prescription only.

Nix lotion (permethrin) will kill both the lice and their eggs. Rid shampoo will kill the lice, but not their eggs; be certain to repeat the shampoo treatment 7 days later. This may not be a bad strategy with the other treatments as well, so thoroughly examine the area in question for persistent nits and adults.

You might ask your physician for a prescription for Kwell (lindane) shampoo to stockpile. It is a much stronger treatment for resistant cases. It may cause neurological side-effects in children, so avoid this medicine in pediatric cases and also in pregnant women. Here are general instructions for the above products:

- Start with dry hair. If you use hair conditioners, stop for a few days before using the medicine. This will allow the medicine to have the most effect on the hair shaft.
- Apply the medicine to the hair and scalp.
- Rinse off after 10 minutes or so.
- Check for lice and nits using a comb in 8 to 12 hours.
- Repeat the process in 7 days

Scabies may be resistant, but can be eliminated with oral Ivermectin (brand name Stromectol) and also with a higher strength of Permethrin (5%, brand name Elimite), by prescription only.

Wash all linens that you don't throw away in hot water (at least 120 degrees). Unwashable items, such as stuffed animals, that you cannot bring yourself to throw out should be placed in plastic bags for 2 weeks (for head lice) to 5 weeks (for body lice). The bags are then opened to air outside and shaken out.

Combs and brushes should be placed in alcohol or very hot water. Your patients should change clothes daily, although this may be problematic in austere settings. It would be wise for any item that might have been exposed to be treated, even if it belongs to unaffected family members. Have enough pediculicide products to treat the entire group.

Over time, commercial medications may run out, but natural remedies for lice have existed for thousands of years. Even commercial medications like Rid Shampoo use pyrethrin, a substance extracted from the chrysanthemum flower. Another favorite anti-lice product is Clearlice, a natural product containing peppermint, among other things.

A combination used for lice utilizes tea tree and neem oils. One topical therapy mixes a blend of vinegar, tea tree oil, and neem oil, which is applied daily for 21 days. A mixture of Witch Hazel and tea tree oil applied daily after showering for 21 days has also been reported as effective against hair lice.

A triple blend of tea tree, lavender, and Neem oil applied to the public region for 21 days may be effective in eliminating Scabies. Every natural method used to eliminate infestations require diligent removal of nits and adult lice beforehand by combing.

Although there are recommendations to "suffocate" head lice with mayonnaise, lard, butter, or coconut/olive oil, there isn't enough evidence to be certain that this method will work. Besides, you might just need those products for survival purposes. If you decide to use them, you would generously apply to the head, place a shower cap overnight, and rinse out in the morning.

Ticks

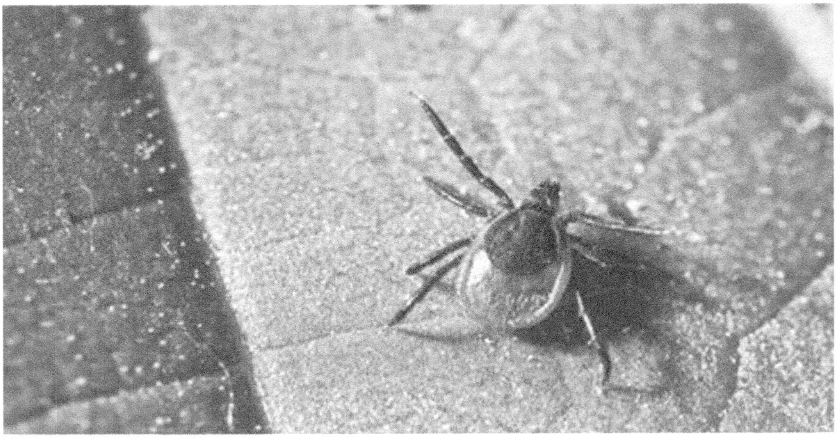

Common Deer Tick

Although ticks are commonly thought of as insects, they are actually eight-legged arachnids like scorpions and spiders. One species or another of this parasite is found just about everywhere in the U.S. and Southern Canada, and a number of species seem to be extending their range over time.

Although not as clearly associated with poor hygiene as lice, ticks are often first detected while bathing. This means that failure to bathe may allow them to remain on the body and increase the chances of disease transmission. As many tick-borne illnesses are most treatable in the early stages, you must, as family medic, know how to quickly identify and treat these conditions.

Ticks bite humans and animals to obtain a blood meal. Although the bite itself is not a major medical issue, ticks serves as vectors for many organisms that cause illness, including bacteria, viruses, parasites, and more. As examples, the American dog tick carries the microbe for Rocky Mountain spotted fever and the blacklegged tick, also known as the deer tick, carries the parasite that's responsible for Lyme disease. Other illnesses carried by ticks include Babesiosis, Anaplasmosis, Erlichiosis, and Tularemia. Many of these present similarly to influenza with regards to symptoms and, as such, are often misdiagnosed by medical professionals.

Ticks don't jump like fleas do and they don't fly like, well, flies. The larvae (juveniles) like to live in leaf litter, and they latch onto your lower leg as you pass by. Adults live in shrubs along game trails (hence the name Deer Tick) and appear less likely to transmit disease. Near inhabited areas like your yard, you might find them in shaded woodpiles, leaf piles, or tall grass. Ticks like areas where there is a significant deer or rodent population.

Lyme disease

Lyme disease is caused by the bacterium *Borrelia Burgdorferi* and is thought to be the most common disease transmitted by another species to humans.

Most active during summer, the microbe is carried and transmitted by the larval (juvenile) stages of the deer tick. These are not much bigger than a pinhead, making them difficult to spot. There are a number of larval stages, each of which feeds only once, very slowly, over several days.

Although deer ticks are most common in the Northeastern U.S., they are making their way further South and West every year, including Texas, Wisconsin, and Florida.

Tick bites will first present as a small red bump. By itself, the bite doesn't represent disease of any sort, but about 20% will contain the Lyme disease microbe. Acute Lyme disease is characterized by the onset of a flu-like syndrome often accompanied by a ring-like rash that expands over time. You can expect to see this anywhere from 3 to 30 days after the bite. This rash, along with the original red bump, looks like a "bulls-eye" and has the scientific name "Erythema Migrans". The patient may or may not experience itchiness or pain.

Other than the bulls-eye rash of Lyme disease, most tick-borne illnesses look very similar. You can expect to see fever, chills, head and body aches, fatigue, and sometimes nausea and vomiting.

The condition can be cured if identified quickly with a course of antibiotics. Amoxicillin (500mg three times a day for two weeks) and Doxycycline (100mg twice a day for two weeks) are the drugs of choice. Symptoms may linger for a time even after successful treatment.

If untreated, the condition may progress to chronic Lyme disease in a matter of weeks to months. You may see:

- Joint pain, especially the knees
- Chronic fatigue
- Rashes
- Nerve damage
- Irregular heartbeats
- Eye inflammation
- Liver inflammation (also called "hepatitis")
- Inflammation of the spinal cord/brain lining (also called "meningitis")

No proven cure or treatment for those with long-term symptoms of Lyme disease exists at present.

Preventing tick bites

Many people don't think to protect themselves outdoors from exposure to ticks. If you're going to spend the day in the fresh air, you should be taking some precautions:

- Don't leave skin exposed below the knee.
- Wear thick socks (tuck your pants into them).
- Wear high-top boots
- Walk in the center of trails
- Use insect repellants like DEET on skin and/or clothing
- Apply Permethrin 0.5% insecticide on clothing

It should be noted that 0.5% Permethrin deactivates quickly on skin and, as such, is of limited use there. On clothing, however, it can last several weeks if enough is used to moisten the fabric, then allowed to dry. Permethrin is thought to even withstand laundering if applied correctly.

As a repellant, DEET is a reasonable option for skin. A natural alternative is Citronella, which can be cultivated in some areas. With Citronella, simply rub the leaves on your skin. Other natural products thought to be effective include Eucalyptus and Soybean oil.

Ticks sometimes don't latch onto your skin for a few hours, so showering or bathing after a wilderness outing might simply wash them off. Examine children and pets after a day outdoors, especially near skin folds.

Tick removal

It is important to know that your risk of Lyme disease or other tick-borne illness increases the longer it feeds on you. Transmission of the disease is rare in the first 24 hours. The highest chance for infection occurs after 48 hours. Therefore, it makes sense to remove the tick as soon as possible. There are a number of ways to accomplish this goal:

- Using a fine set of tweezers, grab the tick as close to the skin as possible. Pull the tick straight up to remove it intact. If removed at an angle or twisted, the mouthparts may remain in the skin. This causes an inflammation at the site but will prevent Lyme or other diseases.
- Besides tweezers, other variously-named instruments are commercially available that isolate the tick and easily remove it.
- Unwaxed dental floss can be used to loop under the tick, tighten, and lift the tick off the body.

Afterwards, wash the area with soap and water, and consider applying some antibiotic ointment. Don't forget to dispose of the tick in a small amount of rubbing alcohol.

We're sure you've heard about other methods of tick removal, such as smothering it with petroleum jelly or lighting it on fire. No method, however, is more effective that simply pulling it out.

Parasitic Worms

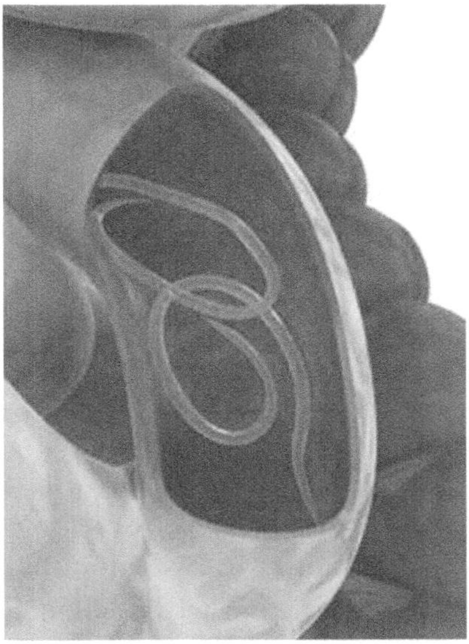

It's important to realize that there are infections not commonly seen today that may become major issues if a disaster throws you off the grid. Knowing which disease-causing organisms exist in your area, even if they are not major problems today, will be important to keep your loved ones healthy.

The word "parasite" comes from the Greek word *Parastos*, meaning "someone that eats at someone else's table". When we think of parasites, none give us the creeps more than having worms.

Parasites like ticks, fleas, mites, and lice live on our skin or just beneath; these are called ectoparasites. Worms, also known as **helminths**, are endoparasites. They live deep in our intestines or other core organs, often gaining sustenance by sharing our partly-digested food. They are also egg-laying machines, with some depositing tens of thousands a day into their host.

Worms can be nematodes, trematodes, flatworms, flukes, or others. The diseases they cause are a major health issue in underdeveloped countries due to difficulties with sanitation. Even in developed nations, a disaster that impairs access to safe food and water could cause cases of parasitic worms to skyrocket anywhere.

Worm infestation is caused by ingesting soil that contains their eggs. While this may seem unlikely to you, areas where people defecate openly and fail to wash their hands leads to contaminated soil. Some of this soil ends up on people's hands, and then to their mouth.

Parasitic worms range in size from microscopic to very long, depending on the species. The most common infection we'll see in the U.S. is the tiny Pinworm, which affects 40 million Americans. However, almost a quarter of the world's population has some type of worm infestation. Children are especially vulnerable and experience stunted growth and developmental problems as a consequence.

Worm eggs or larvae enter the body through the mouth, nose, anus, or breaks in the skin. Amazingly, many helminths actually *require* your stomach acid to dissolve their egg shells to allow them to hatch. Once hatched, the acid-immune larvae travel from the stomach and attach themselves to the walls of the intestinal tract. Some species infest the liver and lungs as well.

Colonization by worms may be asymptomatic or, in the case of pinworms, just involve some itching in the anal area. With some species, however, a large concentration of organisms can cause serious problems.

Each type of worms cause different symptoms, but you should suspect their presence in unexplained cases of:

1. Constipation, diarrhea, abdominal swelling, cramping, or gas.
2. Nausea and vomiting
3. Weight loss.
4. Constant urge to have a bowel movement.
5. Unexplained skin rashes or sores.
6. Anal itching
7. Difficulty sleeping.
8. Constant fatigue.
9. Chronic muscle and joint aches.
10. Malnutrition

In rare cases, the population of internal parasites is so high that it causes an obstruction of the bowels. Worm species that invade the liver or lungs can cause respiratory distress or a weakened metabolism. All of these complications may result in the death of the patient.

Your body knows when it has been invaded and sets up an immune response against the worm. It is unlikely to kill the invader, however, and all the energy put into defense may weaken the ability to fight other, "secondary" infections that may occur. The more issues the body has to deal with, the less effective it is in fighting them.

Some worms actually compete with your body for the food that you take in. A species known as Ascaris, for example, will attach to the wall of your intestine and eat partially digested food that comes its way. This competition prevents you from absorbing nutrients effectively, and anemia and malnutrition results.

Types of worms

There are numerous types of helminthic infections based on the species involved. Infections are often termed by the species and the suffix "-asis" (for example, ascariasis), as opposed to other infections which often end with the body part affected and the suffix "-itis" (for example, tonsillitis).

Although there many worms that infect humans, some of the more common types are:

Pinworms

Pinworms are a type of nematode called a roundworm. Reaching only 1/3 inch in length, they lay eggs around the host's anus, usually at night. This leads to an itching sensation which can become severe. Pinworms are the most common parasitic worm infection in the United States.

A cycle then develops where contaminated fingers from scratching come in contact with the mouth. This transports the eggs inside the body where they hatch.

You can easily test for pinworms simply by placing adhesive tape on the anal region of the patient. Inspect the tape for worms (eggs may also be seen with a low-power microscope) after a few hours.

Hookworms

Hookworms are another roundworm and one of the most common helminth infections worldwide. The parasite feeds on blood from vessels in the intestinal walls. Hookworm infestation is sometimes asymptomatic, but can cause anemia as well as abdominal symptoms.

Occasionally, a larval (juvenile) hookworm that uses a non-human host may penetrate the skin of a human. Although it can't go into the organs, it can cause a skin disease called "Larva Migrans", once known as "creeping eruption".

With Larva Migrans, you can see serpentine vein-like lesions with itching in the skin. As the larva move, areas where they previously were may become crusty and very itchy.

Ascaris

The largest intestinal roundworm, reaching 14 inches, is known as Ascaris. It is thought that there are 2 billion people that carry this worm, mostly in poorly developed countries.

Ascaris eggs, when ingested, become a larvae that enters the bloodstream through the small intestine. It reaches the lung, where it leaves the circulation and is eventually coughed up, swallowed, and goes back to the intestine, where it matures. Once mature, the female worm can produce up to 200,000 eggs a day.

Ascaris effects may include bloody phlegm, fever, cough, and abdominal symptoms. If the concentration of worms is high enough, they may begin to leave the body through the anus, nose, or mouth.

Tapeworms

Tapeworm is a type of infection caused by a flatworm that lives mostly in Asia and Africa. The worm is, indeed, flat. Tapeworm eggs can form walled-off "cysts" in body tissues and organs. If larvae are ingested, however, they will mature into adult tapeworms in the intestines. The adults are segmented and reach prodigious lengths up to 55 feet long.

Symptoms are typical for other helminth infections but symptoms related to the infested organ may also be seen.

Treatment

Medications that can kill parasitic worms are called "**vermiculicides**". All are prescription drugs, although persons with travel plans to underdeveloped countries shouldn't have trouble getting these from their physician.

- Albendazole (brand name Albenza for roundworms) 400 mg once or twice.
- Mebendazole (only available in generic form; most specific for pinworm infestation) 100 mg twice a day for 3 days or 500 mg once.
- Pyrantel pamoate (common ingredient in heartworm meds for dogs) 11 mg/kg once, some species once daily up to 3 days.
- Praziquantel (brand name Biltricide for tapeworms, various dosages depending on worm species)

Dosing may vary with some of these medications dependent on the type of worm. A second course of therapy is administered if the patient is not cured in 2-4 weeks.

Natural anti-helminthic plants also exist. Wormwood, Clove, and Plumeria have been reported as effective. Interestingly, some believe that tobacco may help eliminate worms.

Careful attention to hygiene and, among medical providers, strict glove use will decrease the likelihood of contagion. Hand washing, especially before preparing food, is considered especially important in preventing community-wide outbreaks.

DENTAL ISSUES

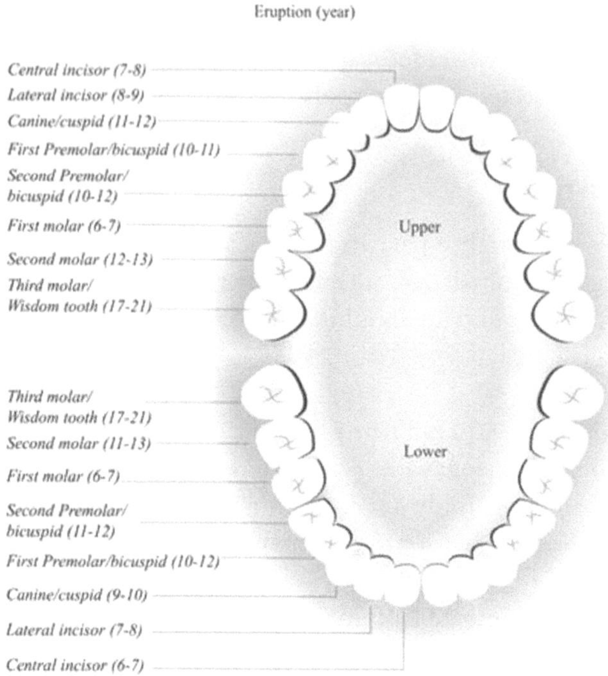

Many of our readers are surprised that a book on survival medicine devotes a portion of its pages to dental issues. Indeed, few who are otherwise medically prepared seem to devote much time to dental health. Poor dental health, however, can cause issues that affect the work efficiency of members of your group in survival settings. When your people are not at 100% effectiveness, your chances for survival decrease.

History tells us that problems with teeth take up a significant portion of the medic's patient load. In the Vietnam War, medical personnel noted that close to half of those who reported for daily sick call came with dental complaints. In a long-term survival situation, you certainly will find yourself as dentist as much as nurse or doctor.

Anyone who has had to perform a task while simultaneously dealing with a bad toothache can attest to the effect on the amount and quality of work done. If your teeth hurt badly, it's unlikely that your mind can concentrate on anything other than the pain. Therefore, it only makes sense that you must learn basic dental hygiene, care, and procedures to keep your people at full work efficiency. It could easily be the difference between success and failure in a collapse.

A survival medic's philosophy should be that an ounce of prevention is worth a pound of cure. This thinking is especially apt when it comes to your teeth. By enforcing a regimen of good dental hygiene, you will save your loved ones a lot of pain (and yourself a few headaches).

This section will discuss procedures that are best performed by someone with experience. Unfortunately, you're probably not going to have a dentist in your party. The information here will give you a basis of knowledge that may help you deal with some basic issues.

Dental Anatomy And Hygiene

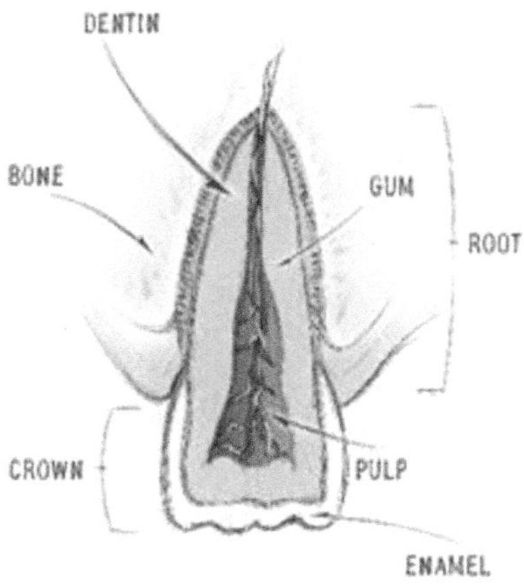

TOOTH ANATOMY

The anatomy of the tooth is relatively simple for such an important part of our body. The part of the tooth that you see above the gum line is called the "crown". Below it, you have the "root". The bony socket that the tooth resides in is called the "alveolus". Teeth are anchored to the alveolar bone with ligaments, just like you have ligaments holding together your knee or shoulder.

The tooth is composed of different materials:

- Enamel: The hard white external covering of the tooth crown.
- Dentin: Bony yellowish material underneath the enamel and surrounding the pulp.
- Pulp: Tissue containing blood vessels and nerve endings in the central portion of the tooth. When the nerve dies, the tooth dies.

Most dental disease is caused by bacteria. Your mouth is chock full of them, so anything that decreases the amount of bacteria there will reduce the chance of developing dental disease. By ensuring good oral hygiene, a person will decrease their risk of an appointment at the survival dental office.

A daily brushing routine is essential, but at one point or another you will run out of toothbrushes. As an alternative, you can use your finger with a little toothpaste in a circular motion; this method will work long-term, or at least as long as you have fingers. A piece of cloth can also be utilized for this purpose.

Another option is to chew on the end of a live twig until it gets fibrous and use that to clean your teeth. Any bendable twig will serve the purpose (dead wood will just fall apart in your mouth). Native Americans prized black birch (also known as "sweet birch") due to its mild minty taste. Your twig toothbrush can serve dual purposes in that you could use the other end as a toothpick.

Eventually, commercially-made toothpaste will no longer be available and you will have to improvise. Baking soda is an excellent alternative: It is inexpensive and less abrasive to dental enamel than manufactured silica-based toothpaste. It's a reasonable choice in normal times as well, especially for those concerned about the effects of fluoride.

Fluoride is sometimes useful as a direct treatment to strengthen teeth in those less than 12 years old, but adults really get very little benefit from it. There is even a school of thought that there are major medical risks associated with long term exposure to it. Years after its introduction in drinking water, it's still a controversial topic to some.

Every time you eat a meal and, especially before going to bed, you should be brushing your teeth or at least rinsing your mouth with warm saline solution or a good antibacterial rinse. This will decrease inflammation in the gums, foul breath, and the risk of infection.

Although most don't include mouth rinses as part of their survival storage, they're a great way to prevent tooth issues. An effective and inexpensive option would be to use a solution made of equal parts water and 3% hydrogen peroxide. Swish it around in your mouth for one or two minutes to obtain the full effect. Beware of higher concentrations of hydrogen peroxide, as these could burn the inside of your mouth.

Salt water can be made into a reasonable mouthwash. Take eight ounces of warm water with one teaspoon of salt and two teaspoons of baking soda. Use two-three times daily.

Many people swear by coconut oil as an option to decrease bacteria in and lower the risk for gingivitis (gum inflammation) and tooth decay.

"Oil pulling" is accomplished by swishing a tablespoon of coconut oil around in your mouth. As oil is a fat and bacterial walls have fatty substances in their membranes, they stick to each other. As the oil hits your teeth and gums, germs are picked up like iron fillings by a magnet. The action of swishing ("pulling") extracts bacteria from crevices in the gums and teeth.

Another method of preventing tooth decay is the use of dental floss. It may be inconvenient for some, but a lot of bacteria accumulate between your teeth. Flossing not only dislodges microbes but is also useful for removing foreign objects, such as food particles. Tie a simple knot in the floss if a particle is particularly difficult to remove.

How Teeth Decay

Just as you, the medic, should know the causes of medical illness, it's important to understand how bacteria cause dental disease. Bacteria live in your mouth and colonize your teeth. They accumulate in the crevices on your molars and at the level where the teeth and gums meet. These colonies form an irregular thick film on the base of your enamel known as "tartar" or "plaque". The more tartar you have, the less healthy your gums and teeth are.

When you eat, these bacterial colonies also have a meal; they digest the sugars you take in and produce a toxic acid. Acid has the effect of slowly dissolving the enamel of your teeth (the outside of the tooth that's shiny). This process is called "decay" and especially happens around areas where you've had dental work before, like the edges of fillings and under crowns. More than two billion people suffer from active tooth decay.

Once the enamel has broken down, you have what is called a "cavity". Development of a cavity could take just a few months to cause problems or could take two or three years. Once the decay becomes deep enough to invade the soft inner part of the tooth (the pulp), the process speeds up and, due to the living nerves in each tooth, starts to cause pain. If the cavity isn't dealt with, it can lead to infection once the bacteria dig deep enough into the nerve or the surrounding gum tissue.

The gums, or "**gingiva**", are the pink soft tissue covering the tooth-bearing part of the jaw. Tooth loss occurs over time if the gums aren't healthy. Inflammation of the gums is referred to as "gingivitis". Gingivitis is very common once you reach adulthood; you can expect to see it frequently in a survival setting if dental hygiene isn't enforced.

Inflamed gums have a distinctive appearance: They'll look red and swollen and will bleed easily during tooth brushing. As the condition worsens, it easily leads to infection. If an infection affects the gums, bacteria may spread to the roots of teeth or even the bony socket.

Once the root of the tooth is involved, you could develop a particularly severe infection called an "**abscess**". This is an accumulation of pus and inflammatory fluid that causes swelling and can be quite painful. Once an abscess has formed, you will need antibiotic therapy to tame the infection and/or a procedure to drain the pus that has accumulated. The tooth will likely be unsalvageable at this point and require extraction.

Diet plays an important part in the process of cavity formation. A diet that is high in sugar causes bacteria to produce the most acid. The longer the microbes in your mouth are in eating mode, the longer that acid is digging into your teeth.

The two most important factors that cause cavities are the number of times per day and the duration of time that the teeth are exposed to this acid. Let's say you have a can of soda in your hand. If you drink the entire thing in 10 minutes, you've had one short episode in which your mouth bacteria are producing high quantities of acid. The acid level drops after about 30 minutes or so.

If you nurse that soda, however, and sip from it continuously for hours, you've increased both the number of exposures to sugar and the amount of time it's swishing around in your mouth. The acid level never really gets a chance to drop, and decay ensues.

The Survival Dental Kit and Exam

The prepared medic will have included dental supplies in their storage, but what exactly would make sense in austere settings? You would want the kit to be portable, so dentist chairs and other heavy equipment wouldn't be practical.

We've mentioned that gloves for medical and dental purposes are one item that you should have in quantity. Don't ever stick your bare hands in someone's mouth. Buy hypoallergenic nitrile gloves instead of latex. For additional protection, masks should also be stored and worn by the medic.

Other items that are useful to the survival "dentist" are:

- Dental floss, dental picks, toothbrushes, toothpaste or baking soda.
- Dental or orthodontic wax as used for braces; even candle wax will do in a pinch. Use it to splint a loose tooth to its neighbors.
- A Rubber bite block to keep the mouth open. This provides good visualization and protection from getting bitten. A large eraser would serve the purpose.
- Cotton pellets, Cotton rolls, Q tips, gauze sponges (cut into small squares)
- Commercial temporary filling material, such as Tempanol, Cavit, or Den-temp.

- Oil of cloves (eugenol), a natural anesthetic. Often found in commercial preparations:
  -Red Cross Toothache Medicine (85% eugenol)
  -Dent's Toothache Drops (benzocaine in combo with eugenol)
  It's important to know that eugenol might burn the tongue, so be careful when touching anything but teeth with it.
- Oral analgesics like Hurricaine or Orajel (Benzocaine)
- Zinc oxide powder; when mixed with 2 drops of clove oil, it will harden into temporary filling cement.
- Spatula for mixing (a tongue depressor will do)
- Oil of oregano, a natural antibacterial.
- A bulb syringe to blow air and dry teeth for better visualization, and as a diagnostic tool to elicit discomfort in damaged teeth.
- An irrigation syringe to clean areas upon which work is being done
- Scalpels (#15 or #10) to incise and drain abscesses
- Dental probes, also called "explorers".
- Dental tweezers
- Dental mirrors
- Dental scrapers/scalers to remove plaque and probe questionable areas.
- Spoon excavators. These instruments have a flat circular tip that is used to "excavate" decayed material from a tooth. A powered dental drill would be a much better choice, but not likely to be an option off the grid.
- Elevators. These are thin but solid chisel-like instruments that help with extractions by separating ligaments that hold teeth in their sockets. #301 or #12B are good choices. In a pinch, some parts of a Swiss army knife might work.
- Extraction forceps. These are like pliers with curved ends. They come in versions specific to upper and lower teeth and, sometimes, left and right.

  Although there are more types of dental extractors than there are teeth, you should at least have several. Although every

dentist has their preferences, you should consider including the following in your dental kit:
-#151 or #79N for lower front teeth
-#150A or #150 for upper front teeth.
-#23, best for lower right or left molars
-#53R, best for upper right molars
-#53L, best for upper left molars

- Blood-clotting Agents: There are a number of products, such as Act-Cel, that help control bleeding in the mouth after extractions or other procedures. Act-Cel comes in a fabric square that can be cut to size and placed directly on the bleeding socket or gum.
- Sutures: A kit consisting of a needle holder, forceps, scissors, and suture material is helpful for the control of bleeding after extraction or to preserve the normal contour of gum tissue. We recommend 4/0 Chromic catgut as it is absorbable and delicate enough for the oral cavity but large enough for the non-surgeon to handle. Don't forget a small scissors to cut the string. More information on suture materials can be found later in this book.
- Pain medication and antibiotics. Medications in the Penicillin family are preferred if not allergic. For those allergic to Penicillin, Erythromycin can be used. For tooth abscesses, Clindamycin is a good choice. Antibiotics are discussed in detail in the section dedicated to them in this book.

Because your hands and your patient's mouth are colonized with bacteria, every exam should begin with hand washing and the donning of gloves. All instruments should have been thoroughly cleaned or sterilized between exams. If an instrument has touched blood, consider using heat in the form of boiling water (or steam from a pressure cooker) as previously described in this book. Alcohol or bleach solution may be sufficient in cases where there was no blood involved.

Have your patient open their mouth so that you can investigate the area. A dental mirror and dental probe, also called an "explorer", are good tools to start with. Does the patient have any problems opening and closing their mouth? Are there sores at the corner of their mouths (sometimes seen in vitamin B2 and other nutritional deficiencies)?

Evaluate the cheek linings, roof of the mouth, the tongue, tonsils, and the back of the throat. Are the gums pink, or are they red and swollen? Do they bleed easily when lightly touched by the probe?

Are there "canker" or "cold" sores? Contrary to popular opinion, these are not the same thing. Cold sore, or fever blisters, start off as small blisters and are caused by Herpes type I virus. They mostly affect the hard gums and the roof of your mouth. Canker sores are less certain in origin.. They are shallow ulcers that affect soft parts like the inside of your lips and cheeks, the floor of the mouth, and the underside of the tongue.

Other soft tissues to check out include the tonsils. Are they enlarged? Are they or the back of the throat reddened and dotted with pus? These can be signs of tonsillitis or Strep throat.

Once you have checked the soft tissues inside the mouth, it's time to examine the teeth. Using your dental explorer, carefully look around for any obvious cavities. A cavity will appear as a dark pit where bacteria has demineralized the enamel. Search for fractures, missing fillings, or other irregularities. Even if there is nothing visible, however, there may still be serious decay between teeth or below the gums. Patients with this issue may have pain, otherwise known as "toothache".

Toothache

One of the most common problems you'll deal with as a medic in tough times will be toothache. Treatment of a toothache starts with finding the bad tooth. In many cases, it will be evident by the presence of a cavity of dark decay that has demineralized the enamel and exposed the dentin.

If your examination doesn't reveal an abnormal area, identification of the problem is still possible. Touch the teeth in the area of the toothache with something cold. The bad tooth will be painful. Now, touch it with something hot. If there is no sensitivity to heat, the tooth may be salvageable.

A tooth that is probably beyond hope will cause significant pain when you touch it with something hot (only touch the tooth in question). It will continue to hurt for 10 seconds or so after you remove the heat source. This is because the nerve has been irreversibly damaged. Once the nerve is damaged at the level of the root, you might not feel either hot or cold. It will, however, be painful to even the slightest touch.

The basis of modern dentistry is to save every tooth if at all possible. The technology has advanced so far that many damaged teeth can be salvaged with root canal procedures. In the old days, however, the main treatment for a diseased tooth was extraction. By "the old days", we're not talking about Roman times; we mean just 60 or 70 years ago. In survival settings, we might be thrown back to the era where extraction was the mainstay of dental care.

If you delay extracting a severely decayed tooth, it will likely get worse. Decay could spread to other teeth or cause an infection that could spread to your bloodstream and become life-threatening. The good (and bad) news is that 90% of all dental emergencies can be treated by extracting the tooth.

Temporary Fillings

Some tooth decay can be treated by placing a filling. As long as there is no evidence of an abscess, pain is not constant and severe, and the tooth is not tender to heat or a light tap, it might be a candidate for less drastic measures than extraction.

The purpose of placing a filling is to stop the decay from progressing deeper into the tooth and to stop air, food, and water from entering the area that has lost its protective enamel. To place a filling:

Examine the extent of the decay: Use your probe and dental mirror to explore the tooth in question. Look for weak, demineralized areas on the sides and the depth of the decay. This may be somewhat painful, and local anesthetics like lidocaine, if available, would be useful.

Keep the area dry: Temporary filling cement will last longer if placed in a dry area. Cotton rolls or small gauze squares are helpful if placed on the cheek, or "buccal", side of the damaged tooth. If you are treating a tooth on the lower jaw, place an additional roll on the tongue, or "lingual", side as well. Replace when saturated with saliva. Small cotton pellets can be used with tweezers to dab the tooth dry. Blasts of air from a bulb syringe will also help remove moisture.

Remove the decay: In austere settings, it is difficult to completely remove all decay. It's important, however, to make sure that you eliminate the decay on the edges of the cavity. If you can do this, you can prevent food and bacteria from entering the tooth. A dental scraper is helpful for this purpose and to eliminate thin edges that would not hold the filling material well. Use the spoon excavator to remove the softer decay from the inside of the cavity.

Making a temporary filling: Take 2 drops of Oil of Cloves (eugenol); mix it with zinc oxide powder until you make a paste. If the cavity is deep and close to the pulp, calcium hydroxide (Dycal) is used as a "cap" to protect the nerve before placing the cement. Of course, commercial temporary filling cement such as DenTemp is another option.

Quickly apply the paste to the cavity: Roll the paste you made into a ball and apply it to the entire cavity. The mixture will harden while relieving the discomfort. If the cavity is large, this may take more than one application. Be aware that decay will return in any areas without enamel that is not covered by the filling material. Remove any excess with a scraper so that the person can close their teeth normally when they bite.

It should be noted that, if a cavity is located between two teeth, that some kind of barrier should be placed between them. In modern dentistry, a very thin metal band is used around the tooth that provides support during the procedure and protects the gum.

Eliminate excess filling material: Too much filling material causes the bite to cause undue pressure on the repair. To identify excess cement, use carbon paper or paper on which you have rubbed a pencil. Have your patient bite down and the carbon or graphite will stain the excess filling material on the tooth dark. Scrape it off until smooth and the bite is comfortably even. Use your probe to remove any loose material.

It should be noted that we are talking about temporary measures for survival scenarios. Until modern dentistry becomes available again, you will likely have to replace temporary fillings multiple times.

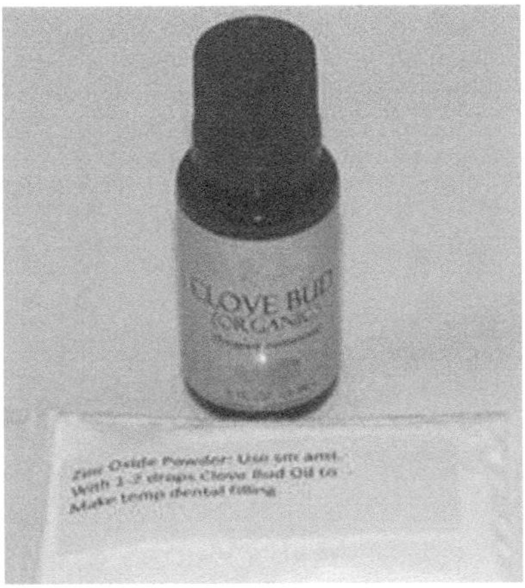

Clove Bud Oil And Zinc Oxide

There are other methods using longer-lasting materials, such as the glass ionomer GC Fuji IX. This product has been used by the military in the field and on humanitarian missions. While the end result is superior, none of these methods are as simple and inexpensive as the one just described.

Dental Trauma

Today's dentists have high technology on their side, but this technology won't be available if things go south. Therefore, we look to historical methods of treating dental problems. Some of these methods may not currently be in use, but they may, at least temporarily, suffice to deal with emergencies in times of trouble. Of these emergencies, some will be related to trauma.

Dental trauma may appear in various forms. After an injury to the oral cavity, a person may have:

- **A Dental Fracture**: a portion of a tooth chipped or broken off
- **A Dental Subluxation**: a loose tooth
- **A Dental Avulsion:** a tooth knocked out completely

Dental fractures

When a portion of a tooth is broken off, it is categorized based on the number of layers of the tooth that are exposed. Classically, dentists have referred to these as Ellis class 1, 2, and 3 fractures.

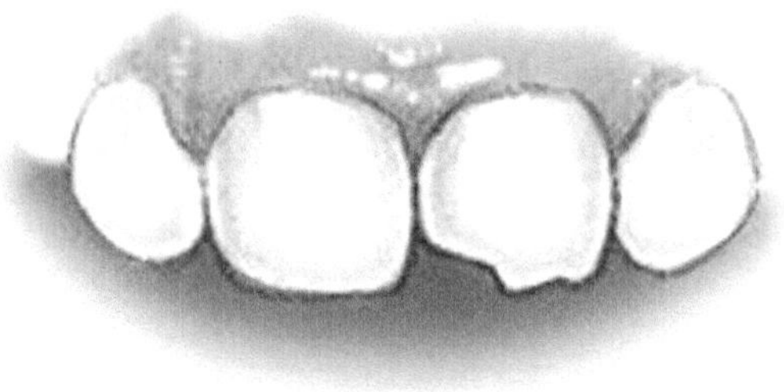

ELLIS no.1

- **Ellis 1 fractures**: In a Ellis 1 fracture, only the enamel has been broken and no dentin or pulp is exposed. This is only a problem if there is a sharp edge to the tooth. You can consider filing the edge smooth or using a mixture of Oil of Cloves, also known as eugenol, and zinc oxide powder as temporary cement or other materials previously mentioned.

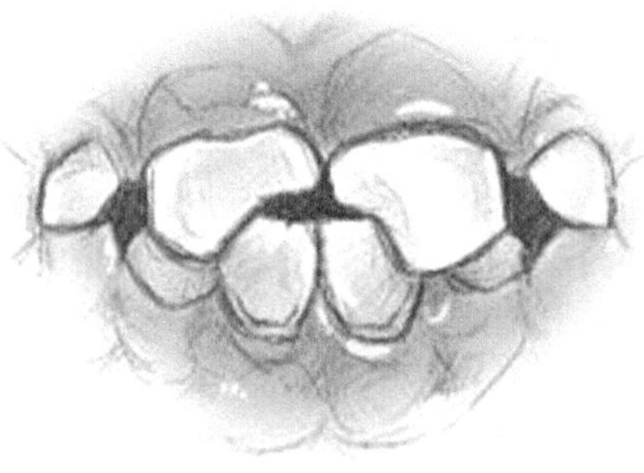

ELLIS no.2

- **Ellis 2 fractures**: Ellis 2 fractures show yellow or beige dentin under the enamel. This area may be sensitive and should be covered if possible. The composition of dentin is more porous than enamel and allows bacteria to enter and infect the tooth. This is especially the case with pediatric dental trauma.

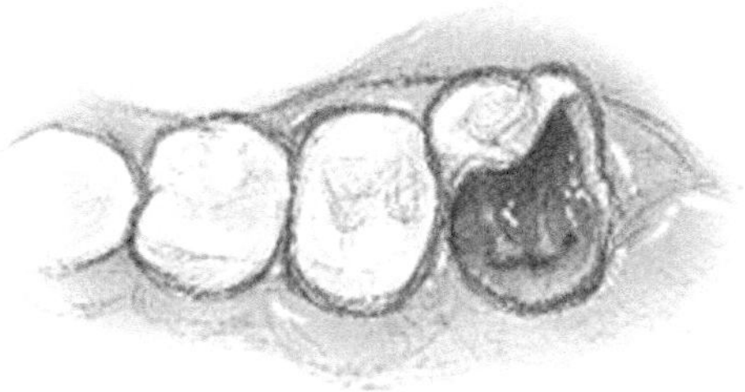

ELLIS no.3

- **Ellis 3 fractures**. Here the pulp and dentin are both exposed. Ellis 3 fractures can be quite uncomfortable and, if the pulp is exposed, may bleed. The risk of permanent damage is most likely here, so protective coverings will be very important.

When you identify a fracture of a tooth, you should evaluate the patient for associated damage to the face, inside of the cheek, tongue, and jaw. On occasion, a tooth fragment may be lodged in the soft tissues and require removal.

There is likely to be blood due to the trauma, so thoroughly clean out the inside of the mouth with water from an irrigation syringe for easier evaluation. Then, using your gloved hand or a cotton applicator, lightly touch the injured tooth to see if it is loose. Don't forget your bite block, as pain may cause the patient to bite down.

For sensitive Ellis II fractures of dentin, cover the exposed surface with a calcium hydroxide composition (commercially sold as "Dycal"), a fluoride dental varnish, clear nail polish, or medical glue such as Dermabond to decrease sensitivity. Provide pain medications and instruct the patient to avoid hot and cold food or drink.

Ellis III fractures into pulp are more problematic, partially due to the high risk of infection. Calcium hydroxide on the pulp surface coupled with additional temporary cement can be used as coverings. In this circumstance, antibiotics may be appropriate. Penicillin and Doxycycline are acceptable options. Pain relief will be needed in many cases as well. Despite all this, the prognosis isn't favorable without modern dental intervention.

A particularly difficult dental fracture involves the root. Sometimes, it is not until the gum is peeled back that a fracture in the root is identified. If this is the case, the tooth is likely unsalvageable (especially in vertical fractures) and, off-grid, should be extracted.

Teeth knocked loose or out

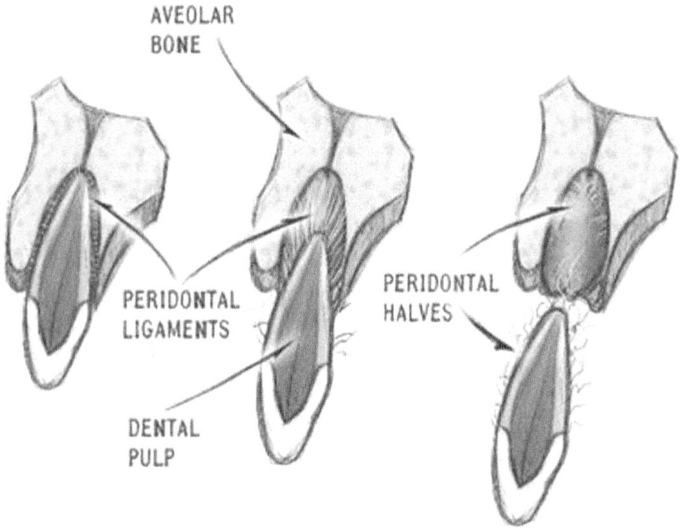

TOOTH AVULSION

A tooth that is knocked loose but not out of its socket is called a "**subluxation**". Use your gloved fingers or a cotton applicator lightly to identify it. Often, these injuries will appear to bleed slightly from the border between the tooth and gum.

Minimal trauma may require no major intervention, although the tooth may benefit from support. The loose tooth should be pressed back into the alveolus (socket) and "splinted" to neighboring teeth for stability. Dentists use wire or special materials for this purpose, but you might have to use soft wax if professional help is not at hand. If you can, use enough wax to anchor the loose tooth to neighboring teeth both in front and in back. Prevent further trauma by placing your patient on a liquid diet for a time. Puddings, gelatins, or soft cereals are also ok.

Occasionally, the trauma may be severe enough to completely knock the tooth out of its socket. This is called an "**avulsion**". The most favorable situation when a tooth is knocked out is when it comes out in one piece, including the root and ligaments. In this circumstance, time is a very important factor in possible treatment success. If the tooth is not replaced or preserved in a solution, the success of re-implantation drops 1% every minute the tooth is not in its socket.

A good preservative for teeth that have been knocked out is "Hank's Solution". This is a balanced salt solution that has been used to culture living cells, and it helps protect raw ligament fibers for a time. Hank's Solution is available commercially as "Save-a-Tooth". Although you can make your own Hank's Solution, it is a fairly complex process.

If you are not at your retreat at the time of injury:

- Find the tooth
- Pick it up by the crown, avoid touching the root as it will damage already-compromised ligament fibers.
- Flush the tooth clean of dirt and debris with water or saline solution. Don't scrub it, as it will further damage the ligaments.
- If you don't have preservation solution, place the tooth in milk, saline solution, or saliva (put it between your cheek and gums or under your tongue). This will keep the ligament cells viable longer than plain water.

If the tooth has been out for less than fifteen minutes, you may attempt to re-implant it. Flush the tooth and the empty socket with Hank's solution (Save-a-Tooth). Replace the tooth, hold in place for five minutes, and make sure the tooth is level with its neighbors. Cover with cotton or gauze, and have the patient bite down firmly to keep it in place. After a while, splint the tooth with soft wax to the teeth on either side for support. Place your patient on a liquid diet and consider antibiotics such as Penicillin (veterinary equivalent: Fish-Pen) or doxycycline (Bird-Biotic) to prevent infection. Antibiotics and their veterinary equivalents will be discussed later in this book.

If the tooth has been out longer than 15 minutes, you may have to soak the tooth for a half hour or so in Hank's Solution before you replace it. The longer you wait to replace the tooth, the more painful it will likely be to replace, so make sure you have pain meds available in your supplies.

After a couple of hours of being out, the ligament fibers dry out and die, and the tooth is for most intents and purposes dead. Replacing it at this point is likely to be unsuccessful, as the pulp will decay like all dead soft tissue does. This causes a chronic inflammation causing the dead tooth (which may turn dark in color) to scar down into its bony socket, almost like a dental implant. This is called "Ankylosis". Don't replace "baby teeth", because the scarring process may prevent the permanent teeth from emerging.

It's important to know that, in mature permanent teeth, the pulp rarely, if ever, survives the injury even if the ligaments do. As such, without the availability of root canal procedures to remove dead tissue, even your best efforts may be unsuccessful. If a serious infection arises in the dead pulp, your patient may be in a worse situation than just missing a tooth.

Dental Extraction

Life with dentists may be unpleasant sometimes, but life without dentists will often leave us with few options. In such circumstances, we may have to return to tooth extraction as the treatment of choice for dental disease or emergencies.

You, as medic, will eventually find yourself in a situation where you have to remove a diseased tooth. 90% of all dental emergencies can be treated by extracting the tooth.

Tooth extraction is not an enjoyable experience as it is, and will be less so in a long-term survival situation with no power and limited supplies. Unlike baby teeth, a permanent tooth is unlikely to be removed simply by wiggling it out with your (gloved) hand or tying a string to it and the nearest doorknob and slamming. Knowledge of the procedure, however, will be important for anyone expecting to be the medical caregiver in the aftermath of a major disaster.

Before we go any further: It is illegal and punishable by law to practice dentistry without a license. The lack of formal training or experience in dentistry may cause complications that are much worse than a bum tooth. If you are lucky enough to have access to modern dental care, seek it out.

Proper positioning will help you perform the procedure more easily. For an upper extraction (also called a "maxillary extraction"), the patient should be tipped at a 60 degree angle to the floor. The patient's mouth should be at the level of the medic's elbow. For a lower extraction, (also called a "mandibular extraction"), the patient should be sitting upright with the level of the mouth lower than the elbow.

Right-handed medics should stand to the right of the patient; left-handers stand to the left. For uppers and most front lower extractions, it is best to position yourself in front. For lower molars, some prefer to position themselves behind the patient.

To begin with, you will want to wash your hands and put on gloves, a face mask, and some eye protection. You will want to keep the area around the tooth as dry as possible, so that you can see what you're doing. There will be some bleeding, so you might want to place cotton balls or rolled gauze squares around the tooth to be removed. These may have to be changed from time to time.

Teeth are held in place in their sockets by ligaments, which are fibrous bands of connective tissue. These ligaments must be severed to loosen the tooth. This goal is best accomplished with a dental elevator, an instrument which looks to some like a screwdriver with a very small head or a tiny chisel.

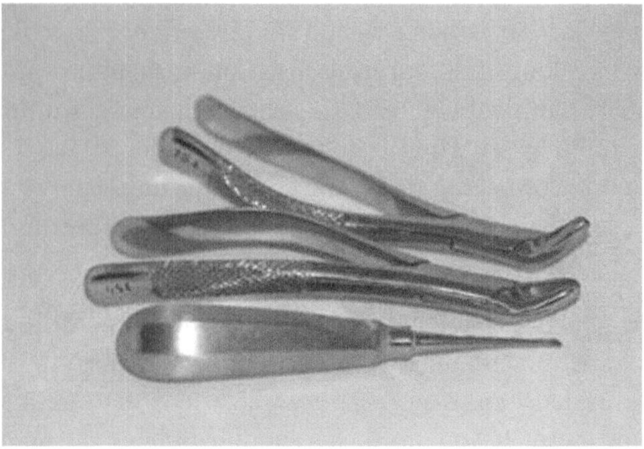

Dental Extractors and Elevator (bottom)

Once positioned, you will:

Separate the gum from the tooth: Use your spoon excavator between the tooth in question and the gum on all sides to separate the two. If this is not done, the gum may tear during the extraction and cause bleeding and slow healing.

Loosen the tooth: Use a dental elevator to go between the tooth and the bony socket. Use your index finger for support against the tooth in front of the one being extracted, and apply pressure with the head of the elevator to get down to the root area. Your goal is to sever the ligaments holding the tooth in place. Expect some bleeding.

Extract the tooth: Take your extraction forceps and grasp the tooth as far down the root as possible. This will give you the best chance of removing the tooth in its entirety the first time.

For front teeth (which have one root), exert pressure straight downward for uppers and straight upward for lowers.

For teeth with more than one root, such as molars, a gentle rocking motion will help loosen the tooth further as you extract. Once loose, avoid damage to neighboring teeth by extracting towards the cheek rather than towards the tongue. This is best for all but the lower molars that are furthest back (wisdom teeth).

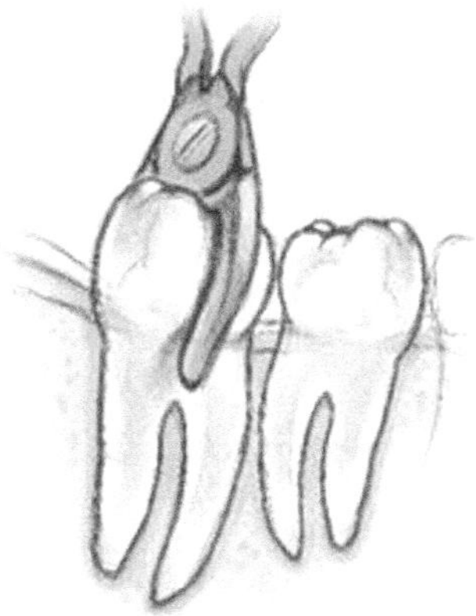

DENTAL EXTRACTOR
GRASPING ROOT

Not uncommonly, a tooth might break during the extraction. In this case, use your elevator to identify and further loosen the root. Then, push it outward using the instrument as a lever.

Control bleeding: Place some gauze on the bleeding socket and have the patient bite down. In most cases, bleeding should be light. If excessive bleeding occurs, a product known as Actcel hemostatic gauze can be used. Cut the gauze into small moistened squares and place directly on the bleeding area. It should form a gel which can be rinsed away with water in 24 hours.

Occasionally, a suture may be required if bleeding is heavy and direct pressure with gauze fails. Use 4-0 chromic catgut absorbable suture material in this case. Methods of wound closure are covered later in this book.

In a recent Cuban study, veterinary super glue (N-butyl-2-cyanoacrylate) was used in over 100 patients with good success in controlling both bleeding and pain. Dermabond, a prescription medical glue, has been used in some cases in U.S. emergency rooms.

Hot liquids and hard foods should be avoided for 24-72 hours. Expect some swelling, bruising, and pain over the next few days. Cold packs will decrease swelling for the first 24-48 hours; afterwards, use warm compresses to help with jaw stiffness. Also, consider antibiotics, as infection is a possible complication. Liquids and a diet of soft foods should be given to decrease trauma to the area.

Use medicines such as (NSAIDS) such as Ibuprofen and Acetaminophen for pain. You can use warm salt water rinses after six to eight hours.

Stay away from aspirin, as it may hinder the blood clot that naturally forms in the socket.

That blood clot is your friend, so make sure not to smoke, spit, or use straws. These actions might dislodge it and cause a painful condition called Alveolar Osteitis or "**dry socket**". With this condition, you will notice that the clot has disappeared and has been replaced by foul breath. Antibiotics and warm salt water gargles are useful here; a solution of water with a small amount of Clove oil may serve to decrease the pain. Don't use too much, however, as it could burn the mouth.

In a long-term survival situation, difficult decisions will have to be made. If modern dentistry is gone due to a mega-catastrophe, the survival medic will have to take on that role as well as the role of medical caregiver. Performing dental procedures without training and experience, however, is a bad idea in any other scenario. Never perform a dental procedure on someone if you have modern dental care available to you.

RESPIRATORY INFECTIONS

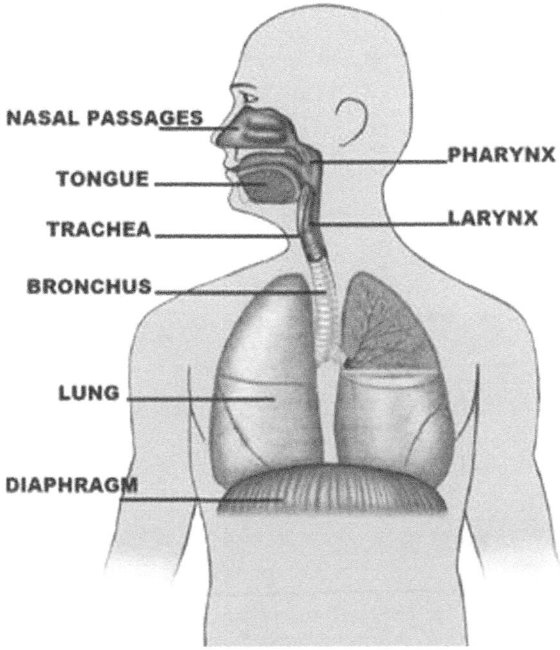

Upper and Lower Respiratory System

Even with modern medical technology, most of us can't avoid the occasional respiratory infection. Without strict adherence to hand washing and **respiratory hygiene**, it would be very easy for your entire survival community to come down with colds, influenza, or even pneumonia. Although not all of these medical illnesses are life-threatening, they can affect work efficiency at a time when everyone must be at one hundred per cent.

Human illness involves the respiratory tract more commonly than any other organ system. Germ-laden droplets are expelled during coughs and sneezes and enter the nose, mouth, or eyes of others. As a result, these infections are often highly contagious. Most respiratory infections are associated with viruses, although there are a number that are bacterial in origin.

We classify respiratory infections as upper or lower. Upper respiratory infections involve the throat, nasal passages, sinuses, and larynx (voice box). Lower respiratory infections involve the trachea (windpipe), bronchi, and lungs.

Upper respiratory infections are the most common and include:

- Common colds
- Influenza
- Throat infections (also called "Pharyngitis")
- Sinusitis
- Laryngitis
- Croup (Laryngotracheitis)

Lower respiratory infections include:

- Tracheitis (sometimes categorized as upper)
- Bronchitis
- Pneumonia

Many of these infections present with similar symptoms and you, as medic, must determine the diagnosis without an arsenal of lab tests, X-rays, and other high technology at your disposal.

Upper Respiratory Infections

The Common Cold

The most frequently seen respiratory infection is the common cold. It is responsible for more work and school days lost in the United States than any other illness. Colds can be caused by over 200 different viruses, most of them in the Rhinovirus family.

Symptoms usually appear one to three days after exposure. You can expect to see:

- Nasal congestion
- Sore throat
- Coughing and sneezing

- Low-grade fever
- Muscle aches
- Fatigue

There are many viruses that cause symptoms that can be confused with the common cold. The most likely is influenza, but another one that has caused community-wide pediatric outbreaks in the U.S. is Enterovirus D68. It's a member of the *Picornaviridae* family, the same family that contains the polio virus.

Enterovirus D68 infection starts off looking just like the common cold, and that's as far as it goes in most cases. Sometimes, however, it can quickly progress to a syndrome which includes nausea and vomiting and severe breathing difficulties. Advanced support is needed in some cases and long-term nerve damage may occur.

Influenza

You probably won't die as a result of getting a cold, but influenza is one of the great killers of modern times. It has been responsible for world-wide outbreaks called "pandemics". The "Spanish Flu" of 1918 is thought to have caused 50-100 million deaths around the globe.

Some recent influenza pandemics:

- The Russian Flu in 1889-90 (1 million deaths)
- The Spanish Flu in 1918 (50-100 million deaths)
- The Asian Flu in 1957-8 (1-1.5 million deaths)
- The Hong Kong Flu in 1968-9 (750,000 deaths)
- The Swine Flu in 2009-2010 (18,000 deaths)

Influenzas are usually caused by Influenza type A (the most common) and Type B viruses. They are classified according to the proteins that exist on their surface. These are called *Hemagglutinins (HA)* and *Neuraminidases (NA)*. There are more and more different HA and NA subtypes discovered every year. The Swine flu, for example, is H1 N1. The Hong Kong flu was H2 N2.

Although certain viruses rarely seen in humans, like bird flus, have a high death rate, today's influenza cases aren't usually fatal. Victims who succumb are often elderly or very young. Any influenza virus, however, can mutate. Bird flu is almost never transmitted to humans unless they work in close contact with, say, poultry. If the bird flu virus mutates one day to pass more easily to humans, it will become a candidate for the next great pandemic.

With a viral mutation, the effect on the human population depends on how different it becomes compared to the previous year's virus. When a new virus is significantly changed, there are often more deaths because the community hasn't yet developed immunity or resistance to it. A good example is the high Native American mortality when first exposed to Smallpox virus introduced by the first European settlers.

Symptoms of influenza begin anywhere from one to four days after exposure. They are similar to the common cold and include:

- High fever
- Cough
- Headache
- Severe fatigue
- Severe muscle aches

Colds vs. Influenza

With similar symptoms, a cold may be difficult to differentiate from the flu. Here are some subtle hints:

Symptom	Cold	Influenza
Fever	Rare, Low	Common, High
Headache	Rare	Common
Nasal Congestion	Common	Occasional
Sore Throat	Common	Occasional
Cough	Mild	Severe
Aches and Pains	Common	Severe
Fatigue	Mild	Severe

Colds will resolve themselves over a week or so, but influenzas will last longer. The flu could weaken you enough that secondary bacterial respiratory infections will set in. Indeed, these secondary infections are the most probable causes of death related to flu cases. If this happens, you'll notice that you are getting worse, not better, over time despite the usual treatments.

Pharyngitis

Throat inflammation due to pharyngitis, or "sore throat", is part and parcel of many respiratory syndromes. Most pharyngitis is viral in nature, but "Strep throat" is caused by the bacteria *Streptococcus pyogenes*, also known as group A streptococcus. It can affect the throat, tonsils, sinuses, and ear canal.

To tell the difference, put on a mask and gloves and look at the back of the oral cavity. Strep throat will reveal swollen tonsils with white spots or red spots on the back of the throat. Combine this with a high fever and headache in a child (in the absence of a cough or runny nose) and it should give you the diagnosis. Amoxicillin 500mg orally 3 times a day for 7-`10 days or Cephalexin 500mg orally 4 times a day for 7-10 days are used to treat Strep throat. Clindamycin 300mg orally 4 times a day can be used in those who are allergic to the Penicillin family of drugs.

Near the same area exists a structure known as the epiglottis. It's essentially a flap that helps keep food from going into the windpipe. Certain viruses, bacteria, and even allergies can cause inflammation and swelling that decreases the ability of air to pass into the lungs. A child with "epiglottitis" tends to sit forward in an effort to get air. Drooling may also be seen due to the blockage.

If severe enough, the swelling can be life-threatening. Look for fever coupled with hoarseness and difficulty breathing. A high-pitched whistle when breathing may represent "**stridor**", a sign of partial airway blockage. These patients may need advanced care to keep the airway open such as endotracheal tubes, IV antibiotics, and even tracheotomy (discussed later in this book).

Sinusitis

Your sinuses are several paired air-filled spaces in the skull that surround the nose. Sinus infections (also called "**sinusitis**") occur when germ-laden fluid fills these compartments. Sinusitis can be caused by viral or bacterial infection or may be related to non-infectious causes like allergies.

Common signs include thick mucus congestion (sometimes green or yellow in color), facial pain, low-grade fever, bad breath, and cough. Some notice a loss of the sense of smell. Pain may be localized over the particular sinus infected:

- Maxillary sinusitis: Pain or pressure in the area of the cheek. Sometimes caused by dental infections.
- Frontal Sinusitis: Pain or pressure in the forehead area.
- Ethmoidal Sinusitis: Pain or pressure between or behind the eyes or around the bridge of the nose.
- Sphenoidal Sinusitis: Pain or pressure behind the eyes, the top or back of the head, or behind the ears.

Discomfort may worsen when lying down or bending over. Symptoms of sinusitis may last from 4 weeks in acute cases to more than 8 weeks in chronic cases. They may recur several times a year.

Viral sinusitis is shorter in duration than bacterial sinusitis. Besides treating the symptoms with decongestants, chronic bacterial sinusitis is treated with antibiotics like Amoxicillin 500mg orally 3 times a day for 10-14 days.

Laryngitis

Laryngitis is an inflammation of the larynx or voice box. Symptoms include hoarseness or loss of the ability to speak due to irritation and swelling of the vocal cords. Laryngitis may be caused by viral or bacterial organisms and is characterized by redness in the area (only visible with special instruments).

Tracheitis

Although tracheitis involves part of the lower respiratory system, it is often categorized as an upper respiratory infection. Symptoms include a dry "barking" cough, stridor, and fever. When not caused by a virus, *Staphylococcus Aureus* is probably the causative agent.

Laryngotracheitis (Croup)

A common pediatric infection of this area is Laryngotracheitis or "croup". Croup is usually viral but can be mimicked by bacterial tracheitis.

Fairly common in young children, croup presents as a distinctive cough that sounds like a dog or seal barking. Other symptoms include stridor, hoarseness, nasal congestion, fever, and difficulty breathing. These symptoms often worsen at night.

Difficulty breathing is also called "**dyspnea**" and often causes a fearful child to become agitated. This creates a worsening cycle that can lead to a significant narrowing of the airways. The presentation of the illness makes diagnosis fairly straightforward, but the oral cavity should be examined to rule out a foreign object or epiglottitis causing a partial obstruction.

Other than keeping the child calm and treating symptoms, relief may be given with an oral steroid or epinephrine via nebulizer. Oxygen is administered in the worst cases. When these options aren't available, steam inhalation may improve breathing. Croup normally resolves itself in one or two days.

Lower Respiratory Infections

Bronchitis

The bronchi (singular: bronchus) are the airway tubes that branch out below the trachea to serve the lungs. Acute bronchitis occurs at least once a year in more than 5% of the population and often follows a cold or flu. Once known as a "chest cold", bronchitis is caused by viruses in 90% of cases.

When the bronchi that carry air into your lungs become inflamed, their lining swells and the breathing passages narrow. The inflamed lining also produce mucus or phlegm, which can sometimes cause difficulty breathing.

In acute bronchitis, you'll see:

- Cough
- Phlegm (ranging from clear-white to yellow-green)
- Wheezing
- Shortness of breath
- Mild fever
- Fatigue

Examination of the lungs with a stethoscope may reveal high pitched "musical" noises (wheezes) or lower, coarse "snoring" sounds (rhonchi). As medic, you should listen to normal lungs frequently; this will help you identify when there are abnormal (or no) sounds.

Unlike colds or most influenzas, the cough in bronchitis tends to linger for weeks after the rest of the symptoms disappear. If the cough fails to go away after that time or recurs frequently over the course of time, you should consider chronic bronchitis as a possibility.

Chronic bronchitis may also be caused by long-term exposure to dust or other pollutants and may cause permanent damage to the lungs. Cigarette smoke is thought to be the culprit in most cases.

Steroids are often used to treat the condition, in addition to medications that open your airways called "bronchodilators". Other meds to treat specific symptoms like fever are used, but antibiotics are reserved for suspected bacterial cases only. Amoxicillin 500mg orally 3 times a day or Doxycycline 100mg orally twice a day are options.

Pneumonia

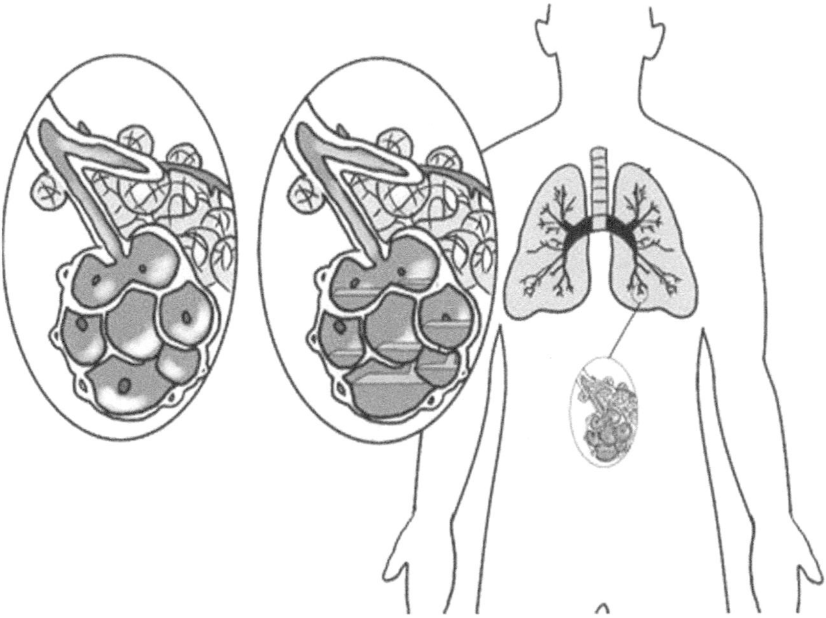

Normal Alveoli and Fluid-Filled Alveoli in Pneumonia

Pneumonia is an infection affecting the part of the lungs that absorbs oxygen from the atmosphere. Inhalation brings air to tiny sacs in the lungs called "**alveoli**". In pneumonia, these air sacs fill with fluid or pus and prevent oxygen from entering the body. Pneumonia may be a viral, bacterial, or fungal infection. Most cases in adults are bacterial but viral pneumonia is more common in children less than five years of age. Pneumonia appears, at first, similar to the flu. Signs and symptoms may include:

- High fever
- Cough
- Phlegm
- Shortness of breath
- Chest discomfort
- Fatigue

When a respiratory infection with the above symptoms fails to improve over time despite treatment, suspect pneumonia as the primary diagnosis or as a secondary infection caused by a weakened immune system.

The infection usually starts by affecting a portion of one lung (a "**lobe**") before spreading to the entire organ. Air passage through fluid-filled alveoli cause bubbling and crackling sounds called "rales" over the infected area during inhalation. If enough fluid clogs the air sacs, it's possible that you won't hear any lung sounds at all.

Antibiotics are commonly used to treat pneumonia, as most cases are bacterial in origin. Some effective drugs would be:

- Amoxicillin
- Doxycycline
- Azithromycin
- Cephalexin
- Erythromycin
- Ampicillin
- Clindamycin

Dosages of each of these drugs can be found in the antibiotics section of this book. It should be noted that cases of antibiotic resistance have been seen for a number of the medications listed.

Occasionally, the organism that causes pneumonia may be a fungus. One example is Coccidioidomycosis, also known as Valley Fever. Common in the Southwestern U.S., symptoms include persistent cough, fever, headaches, fatigue, and shortness of breath. The treatment most often used is the oral prescription antifungal drug Fluconazole 400mg-800mg/day. Other drugs used are Ketoconazole, Itraconazole, and Amphotericin B.

It's important to know that inflammation of the lungs may occur as a result of reasons other than infection, such as inhaling food, drink, or vomit into the lungs. This is called "**aspiration pneumonia**" and can be life-threatening.

Treating viral respiratory infections

Most respiratory infections are viral in nature. As such, antibiotics will be ineffective. There are, however, a few anti-viral medications for infections like influenza. The administration of antiviral medications such as Oseltamivir (Tamiflu) or Zanamivir (Relenza) will shorten the course of the infection if taken in the first 48 hours after symptoms appear. After the first 48 hours, less medicinal effect is noted.

For colds, concentrate your treatment on the particular symptom: for example, nasal decongestants for runny noses or sore throat lozenges for pharyngitis. Ibuprofen or Acetaminophen will alleviate muscle aches and fevers. Steam inhalation may help breathing. Good hydration can thin out thick phlegm. If available, oral steroids, Intravenous fluids, IV medications, and oxygen are useful tools.

Cough suppressants may sometimes (but not always) be helpful. Coughing helps remove thick mucus and should not be suppressed unless it is so severe that breathing is difficult, causes vomiting, or prevents sleep.

Although the use of antibiotics should be discouraged unless absolutely necessary, the serious nature of pneumonia leads many practitioners to use them more often. The patients who are at risk will appear to have worsening shortness of breath or thicker phlegm over the course of time despite the usual therapy. There is a school of thought that recommends more liberal use of antibiotics in sick persons over the age of 60 or those with serious medical conditions. This population has a higher risk of death because of decreased resistance to secondary bacterial infections.

Both upper and lower respiratory infections are different than asthma, which is a condition where the airways become constricted in a type of spasm. Asthma may occur as an allergic response, or may be associated with some respiratory infections, such as childhood "croup". Treatment sometimes involves different medicines than those used with colds or flus. Asthma is discussed later in this book.

Natural Remedies for Respiratory Infections

Many of the strategies and treatments described above will deal with respiratory infections quite well, but what if modern pharmaceuticals are not available or are no longer produced due to a major catastrophe? In that circumstance, you must look to natural substances that might help alleviate various respiratory symptoms and strengthen the body's immune response.

Historically, Vitamin C, Vitamin E, and other antioxidants taken regularly are supposed to decrease the frequency and severity of respiratory infections. Many studies confirm their usefulness, although the amount of down time due to colds or flus per year was only decreased 1 day in one study. Despite this, antioxidant support of the immune system should be encouraged.

Most natural remedies are meant to target individual symptoms, such as nasal congestion or fever. There are, however, a number of alternative remedies that are reported to help stimulate the entire immune system. Consider these essential oils:

- Geranium
- Clove Bud
- Tea Tree
- Lavender

To use these oils, you would use a procedure called "direct inhalation therapy". Place 2-3 drops on the palm of your hand. Warm the oil by rubbing your hands together, and then bring your hands to your nose and mouth. Breathe 3-5 times slowly and deeply. Relax and breathe normally for 2 minutes, then repeat the process. Wipe any excess oil onto your neck and chest.

Many herbs may be helpful when ingested as a tea. Popular ones for general respiratory immune support are Elderberry, Echinacea, Licorice root, Goldenseal, Chamomile, Peppermint, and Ginseng. Additionally, antibacterial action has been found in Garlic and Onion oil, fresh Cinnamon, and powdered Cayenne Pepper. Other options include raw unprocessed honey, lemon, and apple cider vinegar, which are often added to one of the above teas.

Other than general treatments, there are several good remedies to treat specific symptoms associated with colds and flu. To treat fever, for example, consider teas made from the following herbs:

- Echinacea
- Licorice Root
- Yarrow
- Fennel
- Catnip
- Lemon Balm

The underbark of willow, poplar, and aspen trees are known to be a source of Salicin, the essential ingredient in aspirin. Strip off the outer bark, then take several strips of the green underbark and make a tea out of it. It should work as aspirin does to decrease fever.

Other strategies to combat fever include sponge baths with water and vinegar. In the same vein, many have used herbal aerosol "spritzers": Combine several drops of Chamomile, Lavender or Thyme essential oil with water and spray on the chest, back, arms, and legs (avoid spraying the face). The cooling effect alone will be beneficial in those with fevers.

To deal with the congestion that goes along with most respiratory infections, consider using direct inhalation therapy (described above) or chest salves with these essential oils:

- Eucalyptus
- Rosemary
- Anise
- Peppermint
- Tea Tree
- Pine
- Thyme

Another inhalation method of delivering the above herbs or even traditional medications involves the use of steam. Steam inhalation is beneficial for many respiratory ailments and is easy to implement. Just place a few drops of essential oil into steaming water and lower your face to inhale the vapors. Cover the back of your head with a towel to concentrate the steam.

Herbal teas that relieve congestion include: Stinging Nettle, Licorice Root, Peppermint, Anise, Cayenne Pepper, Sage, and Dandelion. Mix with honey and drink 3-4 times per day as needed. Fresh horseradish is used to open airways by taking ¼ teaspoon orally 3 times a day.

Plain sterile saline solution (via nasal spray or in a "**neti pot**") is also used by both conventional and alternative healers. Be aware that failure to assure sterility of the solution may cause serious infections.

For aches and pains due to colds, try using salves which contain essential oils of:

- St. John's Wort
- Eucalyptus
- Camphor
- Lavender
- Peppermint
- Rosemary
- Arnica

Helpful teas to relieve muscle ache include: Passionflower, Chamomile, Valerian Root, Willow under bark, Ginger, Feverfew, and Rosemary. Drink warm with raw honey 3-4 times a day.

For the occasional sore throat, time-honored remedies include honey and garlic "syrups" and ginger, Tilden flower, or sage teas. Drink warm with honey and perhaps lemon several times a day.

Gargling with warm salt water will also bring relief. Licorice root and honey lozenges are also popular to decrease painful swallowing.

A study in Israel evaluated a substance found in black elderberries known as Sambucol. It found that those who were given it had substantially shorter periods of flu symptoms than those given placebos. Sambucol is thought to have strong antioxidant properties and strengthen the immune system.

It's important to remember that individual response to a particular herbal product differs from person to person. Stop using it immediately if you notice any negative effects. Also, the quality of an essential oil may differ dependent on various factors, including rainfall, soil conditions or the time of year harvested.

Prevention of Respiratory Infections

Good respiratory hygiene is necessary to prevent patients with respiratory infections from transmitting germs to others. If you are the caregiver:

- Perform rigorous hand hygiene before and after contact. Wash soiled hands with soap and warm water for 15 seconds or clean your hands with alcohol-based hand sanitizer.
- Wash down all possibly contaminated surfaces, such as kitchen counters or doorknobs, with an appropriate disinfectant (dilute bleach solution will do).
- Isolate sick individuals in a specific quarantine area, especially those with a high fever.
- Wear gloves and a mask at all times when treating someone with a contagious respiratory illness.
- Don't self-medicate, especially with antibiotics, unless modern medical care is not accessible for the foreseeable future.

If you are the patient:

- Cover your mouth and nose with tissues and dispose of those tissues safely.
- Use a mask is you're coughing or sneezing a lot. Although your caregivers may wear masks, it's more important for you to wear one.
- Keep at least four feet away from healthy people. This is the average distance that air droplets will spread during a cough or sneeze.

Many people think that they can avoid respiratory infections by staying inside out of the cold. Actually, being in crowded, closed spaces increases the germ count in the air and, therefore, your chances of being infected.

Others believe that Vitamin C and zinc will prevent colds and flus. They might decrease the duration of the illness, but don't do anything to prevent exposure to the virus.

Guide To Protective Masks

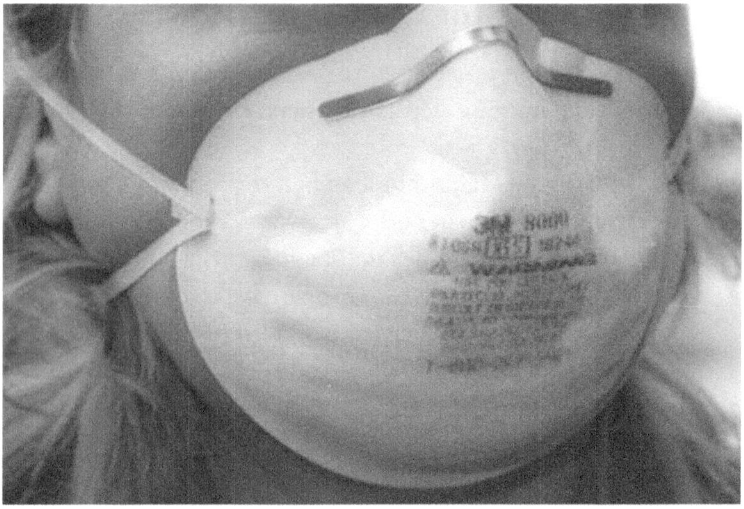

Tightly Fitted N95 Mask

Throughout history, infectious diseases have been part and parcel of the human experience. Ever since the Middle Ages, we have known that some infections have the capacity of passing from person to person. Therefore, the wise medic will take measures to protect themselves from becoming the next victim.

This especially makes sense from a survival standpoint: In a collapse, there will be few medically trained individuals to serve a group or community. The medic, therefore, is a valuable resource whose loss would be a calamity to those who depend on them.

Even before we knew there were such things as viruses and bacteria, efforts to protect healthcare providers were made by the use of masks. Around the year 1900, masks began to be used routinely during surgery to prevent microbes from contaminating the operative field. Masks also protected the wearer from blood spatter and other infectious fluids.

The basic surgical mask hasn't changed much in general appearance in the last century. No doubt, you've seen photos of people wearing them in epidemic zones. In Asia, especially, it is considered socially responsible to wear a face mask if you have a cold or flu and are going out in public.

Face masks have the added advantage of reminding people to keep their hands away from their nose and mouth. Many absentmindedly touch their faces with contaminated fingers repeatedly over the course of the day, a major cause of the spread of infectious disease.

Therefore, a good supply of masks is important to stockpile in your medical storage. Without these items, an infectious disease could affect your entire family or group.

Medical masks are evaluated based upon their ability to serve as a barrier to very small particles (fractions of microns) that might contain bacteria or viruses. These are tested at an air flow rate that approximates human breathing, coughing, and sneezing. Masks are also tested for their ability to tightly fit the average human face.

The most commonly available face masks use ear loops or ties to fix them in place. Higher-quality masks are now fabricated of "melt-blown" coated fabric, providing better protection than woven cotton or gauze.

It should be mentioned that medical masks are not all created equal. They have a wide range of protection based on fit. A tight fit is imperative in providing a barrier to infectious droplets. Mask thickness is also a factor: 3-ply masks (the most common version) are more "breathable"; but 6-ply masks present more of a barrier.

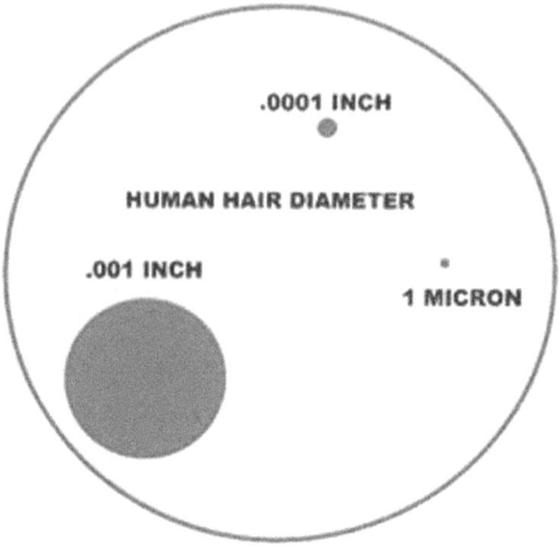

Comparing 1 Micron to the Width of a Human Hair

The upgrade to the basic mask is the **N95 respirator** mask. N95 medical masks are a class of disposable respirators that are impermeable to at least 95% of particulates greater than 0.3 microns in size. These masks protect against many contaminants but are not 100% protective, although N99 masks (99%) and N100 masks (99.7%) are also available. The N95 stands for non-oil resistant; there are also R95 (oil resistant) and P95 (oil proof) masks. These are mostly for industrial and agricultural use.

Many of these masks have a square or round "exhalation valve" in the middle, which helps with breathability. None of these masks, however, cover the eyes unless they have a built-in face shield. As such, most masks will not prevent splatter from getting in your eyes. They also aren't protective against toxic gases such as chlorine. For this, you would need a "gas mask", discussed in the section on biological warfare.

So what would be a reasonable strategy? You'll need both standard and N95 masks as part of your medical supplies. We would recommend a significant number of each as the masks will be contaminated once worn and should be discarded.

There are no absolute standards with regards to who wears what in the sick room. We would recommend using the standard surgical masks for those who are ill, to prevent contagion from coughing or sneezing, and the N95 masks for caregivers. Consider adding a supply of face shields for highly contagious infections. In this fashion, you will give maximum protection to the medical personnel.

Remember, your highest priority is to protect yourself and the healthy members of your group. Isolate those that might be contagious, have plenty of masks, as well as gloves, gowns, aprons, face shields, and antiseptics. Most importantly, pay careful attention to hand and respiratory hygiene. Your survival may depend on it.

FOOD AND WATER-BORNE ILLNESS

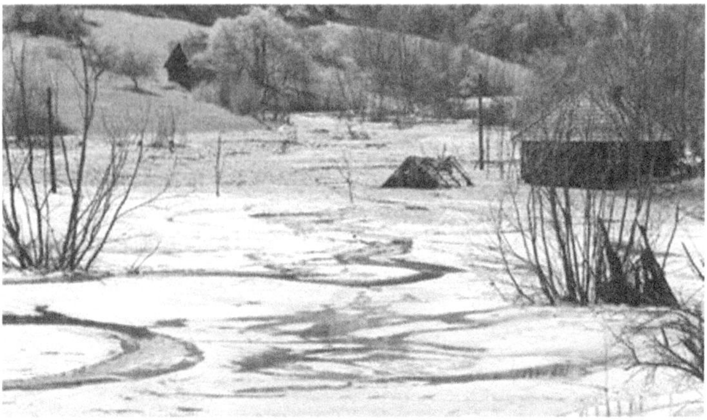

Food and water is a lot safer than in the past due to modern treatment practices. So safe, in fact, that it is taken for granted. Contaminated food and water was the source of many deaths in olden times, and still causes epidemics of infectious disease in underdeveloped countries.

Therefore, we can expect sanitation issues in the aftermath of a disaster. Aquifers may be contaminated by damage to levees or, more likely, by pollution caused by careless or uninformed citizens. Food will be difficult to cook evenly at temperatures high enough to kill germs.

Any water source that hasn't been sterilized or any food that hasn't been properly cleaned and cooked could place an entire community at risk. As the designated medic, your duty as Chief Sanitation Officer will be to assure that water is drinkable and that food preparation areas are disinfected.

Sterilizing Water

Water can be contaminated by floods, disruptions in water service, and a number of other random events. A dead raccoon upstream from where you collect your water supplies could be a source of deadly bacteria.

Even the clearest mountain brook could harbor parasites, called protozoa, which can cause disease. A parasite is an organism that, once it enters your body, takes nutrients from you without giving any benefit in return. Common parasites in backcountry waters include Giardia and Entamoeba, which can cause debilitating diarrheal disease. These microbes may affect hikers in the deepest wilderness settings.

If you're starting with cloudy water, it is because there are many small particles of debris in it. There are many excellent commercial filters of various sizes on the market that deal with this effectively. Large filters like the Berkey brand or small, portable ones like the Lifestraw brand will serve your needs at your retreat or on the trail.

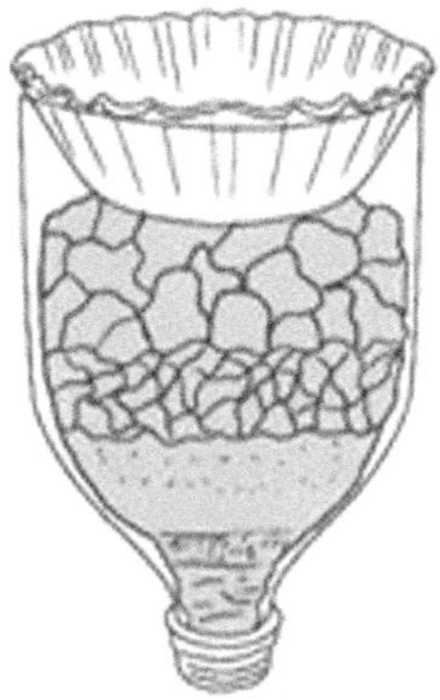

Improvised Water Filter

You could also make your own particulate filter by using a length of 4 inch wide PVC pipe and inserting 2 or 3 layers of graded-size gravel, sand, zeolite, and/or activated charcoal, with each layer separated by pieces of cloth or cotton. Once flushed out and ready to go, you can run cloudy water through it and see clear water coming out the other side.

This type of filter will get rid of particulate matter but will not kill bacteria and other pathogens (disease-causing organisms). It's important to have several ways available to sterilize your water so that it is safe to drink. This can be accomplished by several methods:

- **Boiling:** Use a heat source to get your water to a roiling boil for at least a minute, then let cool. There are bacteria that may survive the high heat, but they are in the minority.

- **Chlorine:** Household bleach sold for use in laundering clothes is a 3-8% solution of sodium hypochlorite. A 12% solution is widely used in waterworks for the chlorination of water; 15% is often used for disinfection of waste water in treatment plants.

  Household bleach has an excellent track record of eliminating bacteria and 8-12 drops in a gallon of water will do the trick. If you're used to city-treated water, you probably won't notice any difference in taste. Wait 30 minutes before you drink. Be aware that bleach in liquid form will lose potency after 6-12 months.

  Calcium Hypochlorite (68% or more) granules as used for pool chlorination can be used to make a bleach solution. A small amount of this storable product could make enough bleach to sterilize thousands of gallons of water.

  To make a bleach solution, dissolve a teaspoon of Calcium Hypochlorite in 2 gallons of water. Use this to make drinking water. Add one part of the mixture to 100 parts of water. This translates to 1 pint of bleach solution to 12 ½ gallons of water or ½ liter of bleach to every 50 liters of water. You can help eliminate the chlorine taste by pouring the water from one container to another. Wait 30 minutes before drinking.
- 2% **Tincture of Iodine:** About 12 drops per gallon of water will be effective. An eyedropper is a useful item to have as part of your supplies. Running water from a stream may need less iodine than still water from a lake. Wait 30 minutes before you drink.
- **Ultraviolet Radiation:** Exposure to ultraviolet radiation from sunlight will kill bacteria. Add water to a clear 2-liter or other bottle up to 90% full and shake vigorously for 20 seconds. Leave out in full sunlight for 6-8 hours. Oxygen released from the water molecules will help the process along and even improves the taste.

It should be noted that cloudy water will interfere with the action of ultraviolet light. Use a filter first if there are a lot of particulates in the water.

Sterilizing Food

Eating food that has been left out for too long is a recipe for regret. It doesn't take long for bacterial colonization to cause illness. Appropriate food storage, proper preparation of food, and disinfection of counter surfaces are keys to preventing disease.

An important thing to realize is that your hands are a food preparation surface. Always wash your hands thoroughly prior to cooking meals or eating. Other surfaces like counter tops, cutting boards, dishes, and utensils should also be cleaned with hot water and soap or a dilute bleach solution before using them. Soap may not always kill germs, but it helps to dislodge them from surfaces.

If you have a good supply, use paper towels to clean surfaces. Cloth kitchen towels, especially if kept damp, accumulate bacteria. If you reach a point when paper towels are no longer available, boil your towels before using them.

Wash your fruits and vegetables under running water before eating. Food that comes from plants that grow in soil may have disease-causing organisms, and that's without taking into account fertilizers like manure. You're not protected if the fruit has a rind; the organisms on the rind get on your hand and are transferred to the fruit when you peel it.

Juices from aw meats are notorious contaminants. Prepare meats separately from your fruits and vegetables. A useful item to make certain that meats are cooked safely is a meat thermometer. Assure that meats reach an appropriate safe temperature and remain consistently at that temperature. The exact temperature required varies by the type of meat:

- Beef: 145 degrees F
- Pork: 150 degrees F
- Lamb: 160 degrees F
- Poultry: 165 degrees F
- Ground Meats: 160 degrees F
- Sauces and Gravy: 165 degrees F
- Soups with Meat: 165 degrees F
- Fish: 145 degrees F

Water And Food Contamination

Epidemics caused by organisms that cause **diarrhea** and **dehydration** have been a part of the human experience since before recorded history. Cholera is an example of one particularly dangerous epidemic disease caused by poor sanitary conditions in the past. It may, once again, be an issue in the uncertain future. Many other diseases have diarrhea as a main symptom, such as the following:

Cholera: Caused by the marine and freshwater bacterium *Vibrio cholerae,* Cholera toxins produce a rapid onset of diarrhea and vomiting within a few hours to 2 days of infection. Victims often complain of leg cramps. The body water loss with untreated cholera is associated with a sixty per cent death rate. Aggressive efforts to rehydrate the patient, however, drops the death rate to only one per cent. Antibiotic therapy with doxycycline or tetracycline seems to shorten the duration of illness.

Typhus: A complex of diseases caused by bacteria in the *Rickettsia* family, it is transmitted by fleas and ticks to humans in unsanitary surroundings.

Although it rarely causes severe diarrhea, Typhus can cause severe dehydration due to high fevers and other flu-like symptoms. Five to nine days after infection, a rash begins on the torso and spreads to the extremities, sparing the face, palm, and soles. Doxycycline is the drug of choice for this disease.

Typhoid: *Salmonella typhi* is a bacteria that is found in contaminated and undercooked food. The illness it causes is called "Typh-oid fever" because it often confused with Typhus. Contamination with Salmonella in food occurs more often than with any other bacteria in the United States.

In Typhoid fever, there is a gradual onset of high fevers over the course of several days. Abdominal pain, intestinal hemorrhage, weakness, headaches, constipation, and bloody diarrhea may occur. A number of people develop a spotty, rose-colored rash. Ciprofloxacin is the antibiotic of choice but most victims improve with rehydration therapy.

Dysentery: An intestinal inflammation in the large intestine that presents with fever, abdominal pain, and severe bloody or watery mucus diarrhea. Symptoms usually begin one to three days after exposure. Dysentery, a major cause of death among Civil War soldiers, is a classic example of a disease that can be prevented with strict hand hygiene after bowel movements.

The most common form of dysentery in North America and Europe is caused by the bacteria *Shigella* and is called "bacillary dysentery". It is spread through contaminated food and water, and crowded unsanitary conditions. Ciprofloxacin and Sulfa drugs, in conjunction with oral rehydration, are effective therapies.

Another type is caused by an organism you may have read about in science class: the amoeba, a protozoan known as *Entamoeba histolytica.* Amoebic dysentery is more commonly seen in warmer climates. Metronidazole is the antibiotic of choice.

Traveler's Diarrhea: An inflammation of the small intestine most commonly caused by the Bacterium *Escherichia coli,* commonly known as E. coli. Most strains of this bacteria are normal inhabitants of the human intestinal tract, but one (E. coli O157:H7) produces a toxin (the "Shiga" toxin) that can cause severe "food poisoning". The Shiga toxin has been classified as a bioterror agent.

In this illness, sudden onset of watery diarrhea, often with blood, develops within one to three days of exposure accompanied by fever, gas, and abdominal cramping. Rapid rehydration and treatment with antibiotics such as Azithromycin and Ciprofloxacin is helpful. The CDC no longer recommends taking antibiotics in advance of a journey, but does suggest that Pepto-Bismol or Kaopectate (Bismuth Subsalicylate), two tablets four times a day, may decrease the likelihood of Traveler's Diarrhea.

Campylobacter: The second most common cause of foodborne illness in the U.S. after Salmonella, this bacteria resides in the intestinal tract of chickens and causes sickness when meat is undercooked or improperly processed. It's thought that a significant percentage of retail poultry products contain colonies of one variety, *Campylobacter Jejuni.* It is characterized as bloody diarrhea, fever, nausea, and cramping which begins two to five days after exposure. Although controversial, Erythromycin may decrease the duration of illness if taken early.

Trichinosis: Trichinosis is caused by the parasitic roundworm Trichinella in undercooked meat, mostly from domesticated pigs. Trichinosis causes diarrhea and other intestinal symptoms one to two days after exposure. Fever, headache, itchiness, muscle pains, and swelling around the eyes occur 2 weeks later. Recovery is usually slow, even with treatment with the anti-helminthic drugs Mebendazole and Albendazole (Albenza).

Giardiasis: The most common disease-causing parasite in the world is the protozoa Giardia Lamblia. It has even been found in back-country waters in many national parks in the U.S. Symptoms may present as early as one day after exposure, although it more commonly presents in one to two weeks. Patients complain of watery diarrhea, abdominal cramping, violent (often called "projectile") vomiting, and gas. Metronidazole is the drug of choice in conjunction with oral rehydration.

There are many other pathogens that can cause life-threatening dehydration if untreated. Although we have listed antibiotics in this section, most of the above will resolve on their own over time with strict attention to oral (or intravenous) rehydration. Also, some of these illnesses may be mimicked by viruses that are unaffected by antibiotics, so employ them only when absolutely necessary.

DIARRHEAL DISEASE AND DEHYDRATION

With worsening sanitation and hygiene, there will likely be an increase in infectious disease, none of which will be more common than diarrhea. **Diarrhea** is defined as an increased frequency of loose bowel movements.

If a person has 3 liquid stools in a row, it is a red flag that tells you to watch for signs of dehydration. **Dehydration** is the loss of water from the body. If severe, it can cause a series of chemical imbalances that can threaten your life. Over 80,000 soldiers perished in the Civil War, not from bullets, but from dehydration related to diarrheal disease.

Diarrhea is a common ailment and usually goes away on its own or simply by restricting your patient to clear fluids and avoiding solid food for 8-12 hours. However, there are some symptoms that may present in association with diarrhea that can be a sign of something more serious. Those symptoms are:

- Fever equal to or greater than 101 degrees Fahrenheit
- Blood or mucus in the stool
- Black or grey-white stool
- Severe vomiting
- Major abdominal distension and pain
- Moderate to severe dehydration
- Diarrhea lasting more than 3 days

All of the above may be signs of serious infection, intestinal bleeding, liver dysfunction, or even surgical conditions such as appendicitis. All of these conditions can become life-threatening if not addressed.

Dehydration

Poor sterilization technique leads to infectious diseases due to contaminated food and water. The end result (and most common cause of death) of untreated diarrheal illness is dehydration.

75% of the body's weight is made up of water. The average adult requires 3 liters of fluid per day to remain in balance. Some of that water intake comes from the liquid content of food.

Children become dehydrated more easily than adults: 4 million children die every year in underdeveloped countries from dehydration due to diarrhea and other causes.

The severity of dehydration depends on the percent of water that is lost from the body. The thirst mechanism is activated when you lose just 1% of your total body water content. You are still functioning normally but if you fail to replace the fluids, you will begin to feel ill. As the percentage of water lost increases, additional symptoms develop.

Dehydration is often classified as mild, moderate, and severe:

- **Mild dehydration:** 2% of water content lost (5% of body weight). Symptoms include anxiety, loss of appetite and decreased work efficiency. Urine is more concentrated and appears darker. Pulse rate and respiration rate may begin to increase.
- **Moderate dehydration:** 4% of water content lost (10% of body weight). In addition to the above symptoms, the patient experiences nausea and vomiting (even if they didn't before), dizziness, fatigue, and mood swings. Decreased urine output is noted. Pulse rate and respirations rise and blood pressure drops.
- **Severe dehydration:** 6% of water content lost (more than 10% body weight). In addition to the above symptoms, the patient experiences loss of coordination and becomes incoherent and delirious. Little or no urine output. Vitals signs worsen.

In severe dehydration, you will notice changes in the skin elasticity, also known as "**turgor**". To determine skin turgor, pick up the skin on the lower arm or torso between two fingers so that it is "tented" up. The skin is held for a few seconds and then released. If turgor is normal, the skin will snap back to its normal position. Skin with decreased turgor remains elevated or returns slowly to normal in a severely dehydrated individual.

Once a person is severely dehydrated, continued water loss causes the inability to regulate body temperature. As well, chemical imbalances begin to occur that just replacing water cannot repair. Organs will begin to malfunction and shock ensues. Once they reach approximately 20% water loss, the patient may slip into a coma and die.

Rehydration

Fluid replacement is the treatment for dehydration. Oral rehydration is the first line of treatment, but if this fails, intravenous fluid (IV) may be needed, which requires special skills to administer.

A person that is dehydrated is often nauseous. Always start therapy by giving your patient small amounts of clear fluids. Clear fluids are more easily tolerated than solid food and include water, clear broth, gelatin, Gatorade, and Pedialyte.

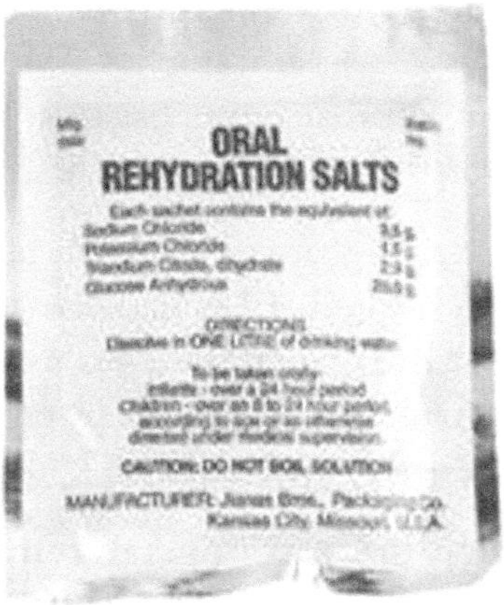

Oral rehydration packets are commercially available, but you can produce your own homemade rehydration fluid very easily: To a liter of water (2 liters for children), add:

- 6-8 teaspoons of sugar (sucrose)
- 1 teaspoon of salt (sodium chloride)
- ½ teaspoon of salt substitute (potassium chloride)
- A pinch of baking soda (sodium bicarbonate)

As the patient shows an ability to tolerate these fluids, their diet can be advanced to puddings and thin cereals like grits or farina (cream of wheat). It's wise to avoid milk as some are lactose intolerant. Once the patient keeps down bland cereals, you can slowly advance them to solid food.

A popular strategy for rapid recovery from dehydration is the **BRAT** diet, used commonly in children. This diet consists of:

- **B**ananas
- **R**ice
- **A**pplesauce
- **P**lain **T**oast (or crackers)

The advantage of this strategy is that these food items are very bland, easily tolerated, and slow down intestinal motility (the rapidity of movement of food and fluids through your system). This will slow down diarrhea and, as a result, water loss. In a collapse, you will probably not be in an area that grows bananas, but hopefully you can bake bread or have stored rice, applesauce, and crackers.

In a disaster, it's possible that you might encounter a person in shock who is desperately in need of fluids. IV hydration is certainly the best method of delivery in these cases. Although IV start sets are commercially available, buying Normal Saline solution and others are by prescription only. As such, they are difficult for the average person to stockpile in quantity.

A method out of the past, **Rectal rehydration**, also called **Proctoclysis**, may be an alternative in situations where IV therapy is unavailable. The large intestine functions to absorb water, electrolytes, and vitamins (but not nutrients), leaving solid waste. It stands to reason that, if the colon can absorb fluid introduced from "above", it should be able to absorb it from "below". This technique was used in World War I but fell out of favor once intravenous therapies were developed.

The benefit of rectal rehydration is the fact that sterilized water or oral rehydration solutions may be used effectively via the rectum to improve fluid status. This provides an inexpensive and readily available avenue when intravenous therapy isn't possible.

To perform proctoclysis on a patient, you'll need the following:

- Sterilized Water/Normal Saline/Oral Rehydration Salt solution.
- #22 Nasogastric (NG) Tube; alternatively, a #14 Foley Urinary Catheter with a 10 ml. syringe may be employed.

- A reservoir container for the fluids to be given.
- Tubing to connect the reservoir container to the NG or Foley Catheter.
- Gloves (wash your hands!) and lubricant.
- A way to monitor the rate of infusion (250 cc/hour or more).
- A way to secure the tube in place.
- A "stand" to place the reservoir at a level higher than the patient.
- Equipment to monitor vital signs (blood pressure, pulse, respiration rate).

From my perspective, points to consider include:

- The fluids used should be warmed to normal body temperature to prevent hypothermia (excessive lowering of body temperature).
- The patient should be placed on their left side; this might decrease leakage.
- Closely monitor vital signs throughout the procedure.
- The nasogastric tube can be inserted further into the large intestine than the Foley catheter, which might result in improved absorption. The Foley catheter, however, will prevent much of the leakage that you may find with the NG tube (Foleys have an inflatable balloon that can act as a "plug"). In the cases cited, the NG was inserted about 15 inches, while the Foley was inserted about 5-8 inches and then pulled back gently until the balloon met resistance.
- An enema effect may be observed if high volumes of fluids are given too quickly. If this is observed, stop proctoclysis (the patient is losing fluids).

It's important to know that proctoclysis is not for "feeding" and has even been used as a method of torture in the past. Never try this procedure if there is modern medical help available. The practice of medicine is illegal and punishable by law, so keep this method of rehydration in reserve only for post-apocalyptic, austere, or remote settings.

Treatment of diarrhea with drugs and natural remedies

Of course, there are medicines that can help and you should stockpile these in quantity. Over-the-counter Pepto-Bismol or Kaopectate (Bismuth Subsalicylate) will help diarrhea. So will Imodium (Loperamide). These drugs don't cure infections, but they will help slow down the number of bowel movements and conserve water. In tablet form, these medicines will last for years if properly stored.

A good prescription medicine for vomiting is Zofran (Ondansetron). Doctors will usually have no qualms about writing this prescription, especially if you are traveling out of the country or anywhere that the water supply is questionable.

Of course, ibuprofen or acetaminophen is helpful to treat fevers. The higher the fever, the more water is lost. Therefore, a fever reducer will help keep a person hydrated.

Various natural substances have also been reported to be helpful. Herbal remedies that are thought to "dry up" the mucous membranes in the intestine include:

- Blackberry leaf
- Raspberry leaf
- Peppermint

Make a tea with the leaves and drink a cup every 2-3 hours.

Half a clove of crushed garlic and 1 teaspoon of raw honey 4 times a day is thought to exert an antibacterial effect in some cases of diarrhea. Ginger or chamomile tea will help with abdominal cramps.

As a last resort to treat dehydration from diarrhea (especially if there is also a high fever), you can try antibiotics or anti-parasitic drugs. Clindamycin, Doxycycline, and Metronidazole or their veterinary equivalents are good choices until the stools are less watery. Dosages are discussed later in this book. These medicines should be used only as a last resort, as the main side effect of many antibiotics is...diarrhea!

DEALING WITH SEWAGE ISSUES

When our infrastructure is working, we are able to provide clean water for drinking and food safe to eat. We also have ways to easily flush waste from our immediate surroundings. When that infrastructure is damaged, however, we become easy prey for infectious disease. You only have to look back a few years to the earthquakes in Haiti and the subsequent Cholera epidemic there to know this is true.

Despite the interest that some have in becoming prepared for disasters, few have given much thought as to how they will maintain a sanitary environment for their family in times of trouble. This is despite daily news reports of hundreds or even thousands of deaths due to poor conditions in many underdeveloped countries. If you can safely dispose of waste, you will have best chance to stay healthy.

When electrical power is lost due to a storm, water utilities cannot operate the pumps that maintain water pressure in the pipes of your home. This pressure is one way that water utilities ensure that your water is free from harmful bacteria.

When the pressure is lost, a "boil water" order is established by the local authorities. Harsh lessons have been learned as a result of disasters that .led to the outfitting of waste treatment facilities with generators. Generator power is helpful, but only while you have fuel.

Therefore, we must realize that human sewage will be a big problem in the aftermath of a storm or a collapse. If the water isn't running, a community without a ready supply will have a nightmare on their hands after as little as three days.

There are various examples of this in the recent past. In the grand majority, people were clueless as to how a flush toilet worked. After filling whatever porcelain options they had, they proceeded to pick rooms where they would defecate and, as a result, their homes were uninhabitable in less than a week.

Here's where some simple planning pays off. If you have access to water (even water unfit to drink), you can have a working toilet by filling the tank with water before flushing, or by pouring a couple of gallons directly into the toilet bowl. This will trigger the siphoning action of the plumbing and send your excrement on its way. This would also work with septic tanks, but not forever.

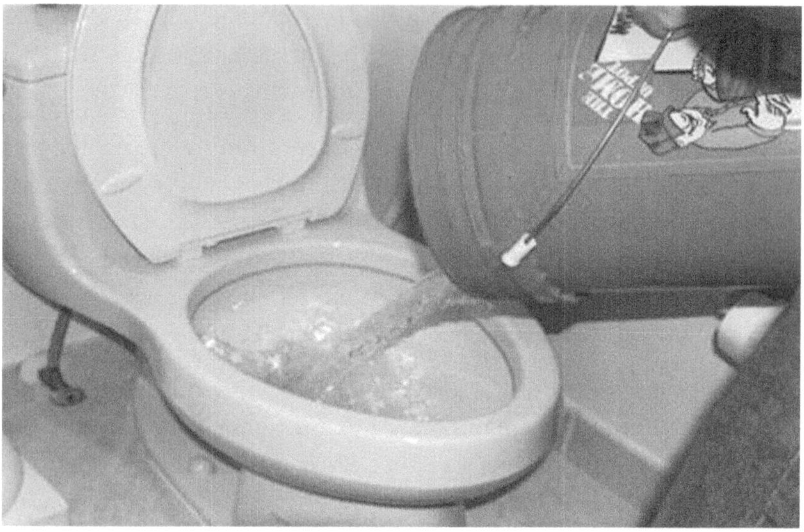

Manual Flush

If you have municipal sewer lines, you have a line known as a "lateral" that goes from your home to the sewer main. In a disaster, it's good to know if the sewer main is down. If the main line is functioning, you can use the processes in the above paragraph.

If the sewer main is down or blocked, the act of flushing the toilet will eventually back up sewage into the rest of your plumbing (known as backflow). There are backflow prevention valves that can be installed if they are not already there; try to find out if your home has them.

So what if you have no water to spare to flush a toilet? If you are in your home, empty your toilet as much as possible; then, place two layers of garbage bags (the sturdier the better) inside and lower the lid to hold them in place. Have some sand and bleach solution to pour over the waste for deodorization. If you're a cat person, you have a head start; you've probably stored away some kitty litter to use. Otherwise, consider some of the commercially produced powders that are on the market. After several uses, it will be clear that it's time to dispose of the waste, which you already have conveniently bagged.

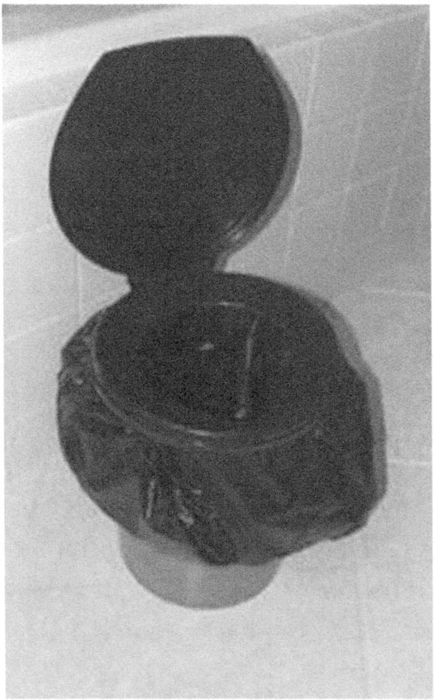

5 Gallon Bucket With "Luggable Loo" Toilet Lid

It might be even wiser to move this bodily function outdoors, as our ancestors did. Here's where a 5 gallon bucket from Home Depot or Lowe's comes in handy. Line it with the same 2 garbage bags (essential items to store in quantity) and place your toilet seat, a couple of short length 2 x 4s, or even a commercially produced plastic attachment made for that purpose on top, and you're good to "go". Use sand, dirt, kitty litter, or even quicklime along with some bleach solution until the bag is half full or so.

If you can afford them, there are even self-composting toilets that are manufactured especially for power-down scenarios.

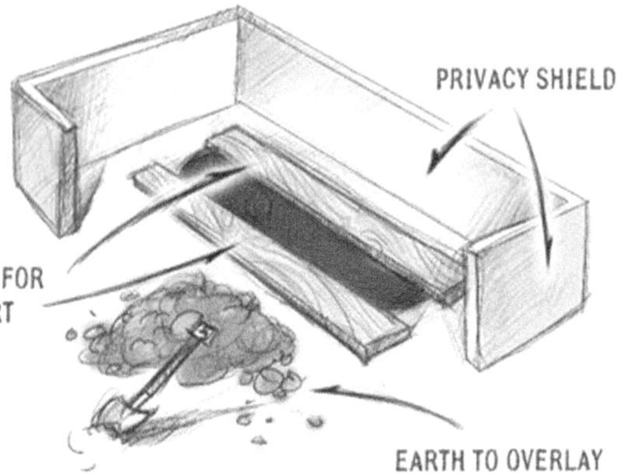

LATRINE

Of course, there is the outdoor latrine for either individual or community use. For those on the move, a single hole dug when the need arises will work if covered effectively and some important rules are followed (see below). For the long term, you will want to dig a trench latrine A trench latrine is basically just that, a trench dedicated to waste that can be utilized multiple times.

The dimensions of the latrine will depend on the length of time it is needed and the number of people in your group. For a small group, make it 18 inches wide, at least 24 inches deep and at least several feet long. Consider a longer trench and some kind of partition sheet if your group is big enough to have more than one person utilizing it at a time.

Keep the dirt from the trench in a pile next to it with a shovel, and make sure you cover up the waste after each use.

A main concern about any latrine or waste deposited in a hole is contamination of the local water supply. Follow these waste disposal rules diligently:

- Don't place a latrine anywhere near your water supply (at least 200 feet away is best)

- Disperse single holes over as wide an area as possible (again, at least 200 feet away from water)
- Don't place latrines anywhere near where rainwater runoff occurs
- Don't place latrines near food preparation or eating areas
- Avoid digging single use holes where others are likely to step
- Dig holes in raised areas; they will be less likely to cause leaching into the water supply
- Consider areas in sunlight; which heats up the soil and speeds decomposition

Finally, always be certain to wash your hands after visiting the latrine. We rarely pay enough attention to hand hygiene, and pay the penalty for this by contracting all sorts of illnesses, many of which were discussed in the last chapter. Remember that many of these germs stay alive on your hands for hours.

RODENTS AS DISEASE VECTORS

Rats, mice, and other rodents are rampant in areas with poor sanitary conditions and are vectors of many diseases you may see off-grid, such as Plague. Besides Plague, rats may pass hemorrhagic fevers, salmonella, Hantavirus, and more. A vector carries a disease to its target while not necessarily being ill itself. Rodent-proofing a retreat may be difficult, but it is necessary to maintain the health of your people.

Rats and mice are thought to have originated in Asia, but wherever these animals are introduced, they cause a significant amount of environmental and economic damage. Indeed, they are some of the world's most invasive species: Every year, a percentage of the world's food supply is contaminated by their droppings, urine, and hair.

You won't have much difficulty telling if you have rats or mice:

- There will be partially-eaten food, gnawed containers, or nesting material, often in the back of pantries.
- Mice and rats defecate 50 times a day, so there should be clear evidence of droppings, especially in attics and basements.
- The culprits may appear at night scurrying along bases of walls, they favorite route of travel.

Once rats and mice invade your home, they are very difficult to remove. Therefore, it makes sense to take measures to rodent-proof your home. You should carefully evaluate the house for points of entry from the level of the foundation to the roofline. This includes sewer lines, bathroom vents, pipes, gutters, doors, and windows.

Some rodent-proofing techniques for homes include:

- Sealing cracks in building foundations, walls, siding, and roof joints. Rodents only need a ¼ inch opening to gnaw their way into your home. Metal mesh scouring pads or galvanized window screening (not steel wool, which quickly deteriorates) may be stuffed into crevices as a temporary solution.
- Installing vent guards in bathroom or washer/dryer vents.

- Placing barriers to prevent climbing rodents from going up pipes or gutters.
- Trimming trees so that branches don't come close to the roof.
- Preventing rodents, especially rats, from tunneling under the foundation by placing flat concrete pavers or gravel extending at least 3 feet from the base of the retreat.

Rodent-proofing also involves careful attention to both indoor and outdoor sanitation.

Suggestions for inside:

- Never leave food or water out overnight. Keep your countertops, sinks, and kitchen appliances clean and disinfected. Breadboxes may seem old-fashioned, but they are there for a reason: To keep the bread away from rats and mice.
- Never leave pet food out at night and clean all bowls daily. Rodents love to eat dog and cat food. Store dry human or pet foods, in sealed containers at least 18 inches off the floor.
- Keep toilet lids down until needed.

Suggestions for outside:

- Store firewood away from your home and at least 18 inches off the ground. Keep the side and back yards free of debris that might serve as shelters.
- Trim all vegetation that abuts the house until the ground is easily inspected. Eliminate tree branches that make eaves and gutters accessible. Remove ivy or other climbing plants from exterior walls that may hide points of entry.
- Construct barriers around birdhouses and bird-feeders to prevent seed from being accessible to rodents. Remove any unused fruits or vegetables from the garden.
- Keep garbage can lids tightly closed. Deny access to water by fixing leaky faucets.
- Avoid putting animal products in your compost bin.

If rats and mice currently live in your home, you may need some traps. Your standard mousetrap is a "snap trap". Snap traps should always be placed in perpendicular fashion with the bait side against the wall. Never use just one: Place a number of them several feet apart in the rodent's usual path. Traps can also be fastened to pipes with wire or thick rubber bands if your rodent visitors are climbing to upper levels.

Another option is the glue trap. They are effective, especially against mice, but they leave you with a live animal to kill. Throw the trap and animal into a bucket of water or strike with a stick several times just behind the head.

We find rat poisons to be problematic. There is always a risk that something (or someone) that you *don't* want to kill, like a household pet or a child, might accidentally ingest it. If that's not enough to convince you, poisons may leave you with a bunch of dead, rotting animals inside your walls.

FOOD POISONING

Food poisoning may occur due to contamination of water and food supplies with toxic bacteria or viruses. Most food poisoning is actually due to eggs, dairy products and meat that have been contaminated by some type of bacteria. A virulent strain of E. coli has been implicated as the culprit in many cases.

Despite this, most animal meat is not toxic by itself (puffer fish and barracuda are exceptions that come to mind), but there are plenty of plants that have toxins that could seriously harm you. Eating apple seeds in quantity, for example, can make you sick due to cyanide-like compounds within them. Knowing what plants (or parts of plants) are safe will be important, as well as whether they must be cooked or can be eaten raw.

It's likely that everyone won't have a survival garden up and running after a major catastrophe. People will be looking to their environment for edible wild plants. Unfortunately, we'll be less than perfect in our choice of tasty greens and could easily become ill soon afterwards. Signs of food poisoning include nausea and vomiting, dizziness, vision disturbances, confusion and palpitations.

You should perform some research on what plants grow naturally in your area that have potential for use as food., as well as medicine. If there are some that you find useful, you might practice what is called "guerilla gardening": That is, planting seeds of fruits, vegetables, and herbs in areas not normally considered farmland. Once, for example, we came across a squash patch on the forest's edge while on a hike in the Great Smoky Mountains.

Not all plants are safe to eat, however, and some send up red flags that tell you to beware. Extreme caution should be taken, for example, with mushrooms and any berries that are white or red unless you have eaten them before without ill effect.

A survival edibility test can be performed to test whether an unknown plant is safe or not. This test, honestly, is controversial, so proceed with caution; experts recommend both for and against it. It basically involves a stepwise process in which you would first rub the plant against your skin to see if you are allergic to it. Then, you would place it on your lips, in your mouth, and then swallow it in increments. If you decide to try this technique, wait a period of time between one step and the next. If done properly, the whole process takes about 16 hours. That's not counting the testing of every part of the plant, such as roots, leaves, flower, and stems.

When you suspect that you have been poisoned by something you ate, wash your mouth out immediately to make sure that you don't have any material still to be ingested. Then make yourself vomit, whether it is by pressing down on the back of your tongue with two fingers or by using a preparation like Syrup of Ipecac. Most poison control centers will advise against using this product because it may be difficult to figure out exactly how much will work. The answer is to use the smallest amount of the concoction that will make you vomit. Drink clear fluids to dilute the toxin and help flush it out of your system.

Activated charcoal is another product that is used to treat poisoning. Activated charcoal in your stomach and intestines causes toxins to bind to it, therefore keeping them from entering your system. Some poison control centers don't want you to use this either, due to dosing issues and the fact that it could give you constipation. You may consider taking a laxative when you ingest the charcoal to help move things along. For dosing concerns, there are various pre-measured charcoal products that you can use in liquid or capsule form. Some brand names are SuperChar, Actidote, Liqui-char, InstaChar, and Charcodote.

The best way to prevent food poisoning is by being sure about what you're eating. The wise medic has a good edible plant guide for the area in which they live. Look for one with plenty of photos. A description of which parts are edible and which may be toxic is important. If you have access to modern medical care, get to an emergency room as soon as possible.

In mild cases, you could consider this home remedy: Squeeze four lemons and add sugar or honey to sweeten. Take this mixture and drink it twice daily. The idea behind this remedy is to kill any offending bacteria with the acidic juice. Along that same line of thinking, a remedy using four tablespoons of apple cider vinegar in a large glass of water is another option.

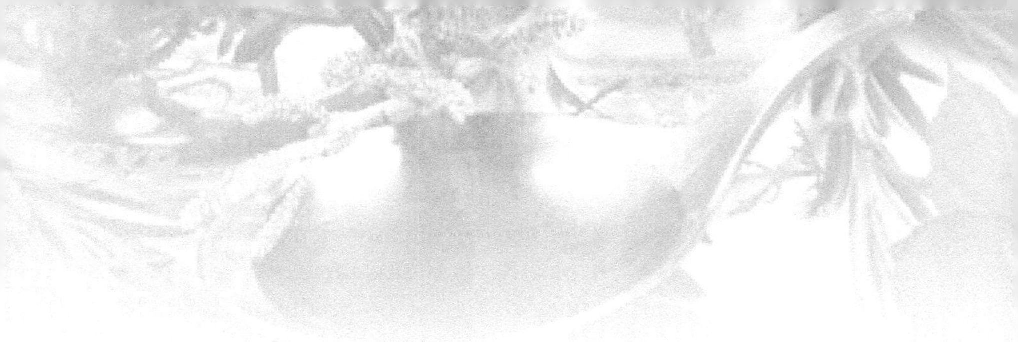

SECTION 4

✚ ✚ ✚

OTHER INFECTIONS

In the last section, we discussed some infections that are caused by poor sanitation and hygiene, such as food and water-borne illness. There are many other bacterial, viral, and parasitic diseases that may not necessarily have sanitation and hygiene as a factor. Appendicitis, for example, can occur in anyone regardless of their cleanliness or the conditions at their retreat. A simple ingrown hair may lead to a boil or abscess.

Our bodies' natural ability to fight illness is truly impressive. There are, however, no organs that are immune to infections. The ability to recognize and treat these illnesses early is essential for the successful survival caregiver. This section will discuss different types of germs, basic aspects of immunity, and some of the more common infections that you might see in your role as medic.

GERMS THAT CAUSE DISEASE

Officially, an infection is defined as the invasion of the body by microscopic organisms. A **pathogen** is any agent that can cause a disease. Pathogens cause injury to tissues by producing toxins that cause damage in various ways. Not every microbe is a pathogen. In fact, some are beneficial or even necessary for human life, such as many intestinal bacteria.

Pathogens are often carried by "vectors", from the Latin word *vectus*, or *"one who carries"*. These are humans, animals, or microbes that carry and transmit a pathogen to others. A vector does not have to be ill to carry a disease: A mosquito, for example, carries the organism that causes malaria in humans but doesn't experience the disease. "Typhoid Mary" was a domestic servant that carried Typhoid fever to many other people without feeling sick herself. The elimination of a vector from the environment (terminating Mary's employment, for example) usually ends the epidemic.

There are a number of different pathogens that cause infectious disease:

- Bacteria
- Viruses
- Protozoa
- Fungi

Bacteria

Perhaps the pathogen we hear most about it is bacteria (singular: bacterium). Bacteria were among the first life forms on Earth and present everywhere from the soil to the bottom of the ocean to the inside of your body. They may even exist on Mars. If you took the entire population of bacteria on the planet, they would have a mass exceeding the plant and animal population combined.

Bacteria have a number of shapes, ranging from spheres to rods to spirals. When bacteria reach a certain size, they reproduce by splitting in two, a process called binary fission.

Most bacteria are good guys; you wouldn't be able to digest food without them. Some, however, are pathogens and cause infectious diseases, including cholera, syphilis, anthrax, leprosy, and bubonic plague. The most common fatal bacterial diseases affect the lungs, with tuberculosis alone killing about 2 million people a year, mostly in underdeveloped countries.

Although many bacteria have become resistant, they can usually be killed with antibiotics.

There are many different types of bacteria. Most bacteria don't need to enter the host's cells to reproduce. A subgroup called *Rickettsia,* however, depends on entry, growth, and reproduction within a host cell.

Rickettsiae are the cause of typhus, Rocky Mountain spotted fever, and a number of other infectious diseases. *Rickettsia* do not, however, cause rickets, a deformity of long bones which is a result of vitamin D deficiency.

Viruses

Viruses are microscopic infectious agents that can reproduce only inside the living cells of other organisms. Viral particles without a host are known as "**virions**". Virions only act as a living organism when they enter a host cell. Viruses can infect all types of life forms, from animals and plants all the way down to bacteria.

Examples of common human diseases caused by viruses include the common cold, influenza, chickenpox, rabies, hepatitis, and herpes. Many serious viral diseases such as Ebola, AIDS, Zika, and MERS are caused by viruses.

Viruses can be spread by:

- Mosquitoes and other vectors
- Airborne droplets in coughs or sneezes
- Contact with blood or other bodily fluids
- Oral-fecal contamination
- Ingestion of contaminated food or water

Viral infections provoke an immune response in your body that usually kills the infecting virus. Immune responses to viruses can also be produced by **vaccines**, which confer an immunity to the specific viral infection. However, some viruses evade these immune responses and result in chronic infections, such as AIDs or Hepatitis C. There are antiviral drugs, but antibiotics have no effect.

Protozoa

Protozoa are one-celled microbes with animal-like behavior, such as the ability to move. They are restricted to moist or aquatic environments. Transmission is mostly by drinking or using contaminated water, but some are transmitted by animal vectors.

Protozoa cause infectious diseases in humans such as malaria, giardia, dysentery, sleeping sickness, and amoebiasis. A common vaginal infection is caused by a protozoan called trichomonas.

Protozoa are mostly susceptible to treatment with certain antibiotics, such as metronidazole (also known as Fish-Zole).

Fungi

Fungi (singular: Fungus) include microorganisms such as yeasts and molds. Fungal infections most commonly affect skin and mucous membranes like the oral cavity and vagina, but can invade other areas in individuals with weakened immune systems. They are treated with anti-fungal medications in topical or oral form.

How Infections Spread

An infectious disease, if it affects only one person, is usually within the ability of a community to handle. If it spreads, however, it can run rampant and cause real damage. It's important for you, the medic, to understand the mechanisms by which a community-wide outbreak can occur.

Ingestion - Eating infected animals is a common way for pathogens to spread among humans. Bats and monkeys are part of the diet of many people in Africa, and are known carriers of the Ebola or Lassa fever virus. Poultry is thought to be the reason that humans get the bird flu.

Inhalation – Airborne spread, that is, breathing in droplets from the infected, which can contain germ-laden blood splatter, phlegm, or saliva. Bodily fluids usually have a great deal of bacteria or viruses and some of them can be aerosolized into the air. Influenza is a typical example. Air droplets or blood splatter can easily enter your mouth, nose, eyes, or an open sore.

Injection – Transmission can occur from needle sticks or other medical items. Hepatitis and HIV are commonly passed this way. Mosquitoes also "inject" pathogens into humans with their bite.

Absorption - Touching secretions from the infected and then touching mouth, eyes, or open sores. You won't believe how often this happens. Just look at the average person for a while and count the number of times they touch their face. The West African practice of family members washing the body of deceased Ebola victims is probably responsible for entire families wiped out by the disease.

Sexual – A number of infections are transmitted from the semen and bodily secretions of infected persons. Syphilis and gonorrhea are typical examples. Ebola can be transmitted sexually for weeks after a patient has recovered from the disease.

Pregnancy – Passed from mother to fetus – HIV, Syphilis, and Zika virus are just some of the diseases that can be passed this way.

Complacency – Lack of attention to infection control is probably the biggest reason for the spread of pandemic diseases.

ABDOMINAL INFECTIONS

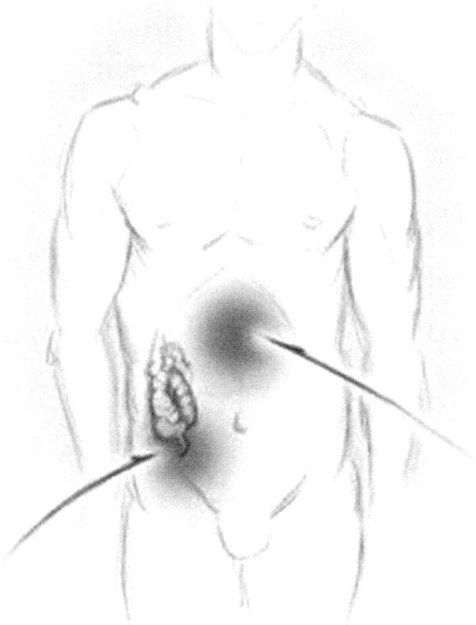

PAIN AREAS LIKELY
IN APPENDICITIS

There are various infections that can cause abdominal pain, some of which are treated medically and others which are treated surgically. In the last section of this book, we discussed a number of them that are related to poor sanitary conditions. They are, however, just some of the infections that you may encounter in the abdomen.

Appendicitis

One relatively common issue in young people that could be life-threatening in survival settings is appendicitis. 300,000 people have their appendix removed surgically every year in the United States

Appendicitis can occur in anyone, but most likely affects people under 40 years of age. The appendix is a tubular worm-shaped piece of tissue 2-4 inches long which opens into the intestine at the lower right side of the abdomen. The appendix was once an important organ, and still is in some animals (for example, horses). It is shrunken and nonfunctional, however, in modern humans. This is an example of a "vestigial" organ, which means that it exists but serves little useful purpose.

The hollow inside of the appendix has a tendency to become blocked by bits of hard excrement. This allows bacteria to multiply inside and cause inflammation and infection. If the problem is not treated, the appendix can fill up with pus and burst, spilling infected matter into the abdominal cavity. This causes a condition called "**peritonitis**" where the lining of the abdomen becomes inflamed. Before the development of antibiotics, it was not unusual to die from appendicitis; one well-known victim was the silent film star Rudolph Valentino.

Some believe that a diet rich in seeds causes appendicitis. Others believe that a lack of fiber is responsible. Although these are (rare) possibilities, most cases have no obvious cause.

Appendicitis first presents with vague discomfort in the area of the belly button, but moves down to the lower right quadrant of the abdomen after 12-24 hours. This area, also known as "**McBurney's Point**", is located about two thirds of the way down from the belly button to the top of the right pelvic bone.

Other likely symptoms may include:

- Nausea and Vomiting
- Loss of appetite
- Fever and Chills
- Abdominal Swelling
- Pain worsening with coughs or walking
- Difficulty passing gas
- Constipation or Diarrhea
- Nausea and vomiting
- Reluctance to move lower extremities, which triggers movement of abdominal muscles

To diagnose this condition, press down on the lower right of the abdomen. Your patient will probably find it painful. Pressing on the *left* lower quadrant may elicit pain in the lower right quadrant, as well. A sign of a possible ruptured appendix may be "**rebound tenderness**". Pressing down on the right lower quadrant will cause pain, but it will be even more painful when the hand is removed.

As soon as you make the diagnosis, restrict the patient to small amounts of clear liquids. Surgical removal of the appendix is curative here, but will be difficult to carry out without adequate anesthesia.

If modern surgical care is unavailable, consider giving the patient antibiotics by mouth in the hope of eliminating an early infection. Intravenous antibiotics, such as Cefoxitin, are more effective than related oral antibiotics, such as Cephalexin (Keflex, Fish-Flex), but will be less available in disaster settings. Some studies achieved success with intravenous antibiotics in uncomplicated cases of appendicitis if used early.

A combination of Ciprofloxacin (veterinary equivalent: FISH-CIN) and Metronidazole (FISH-ZOLE) is an option if intravenous antibiotics and surgical intervention are not available. It is also acceptable in those allergic to Penicillin. Recovery, although slow, may still be possible if treatment is begun early. Antibiotics are discussed in detail later in this book.

Can surgery be performed in situations where general anesthesia is unavailable? The answer is: Not without difficulty. Having said that, surgeons in third world countries have, when needed, performed appendectomies under local anesthesia. Video resources for you to view one such surgery are listed at the end of this book.

Before surgery is contemplated to deal with an inflamed appendix, you must be certain that you are dealing with that exact problem. Sometimes, different medical problems present with similar symptoms, and you will have to do some detective work to differentiate one from another. This is called the "**differential diagnosis**".

There are various conditions, some related to infection and some not, which may mimic appendicitis. The following are just a few:

Diverticulitis

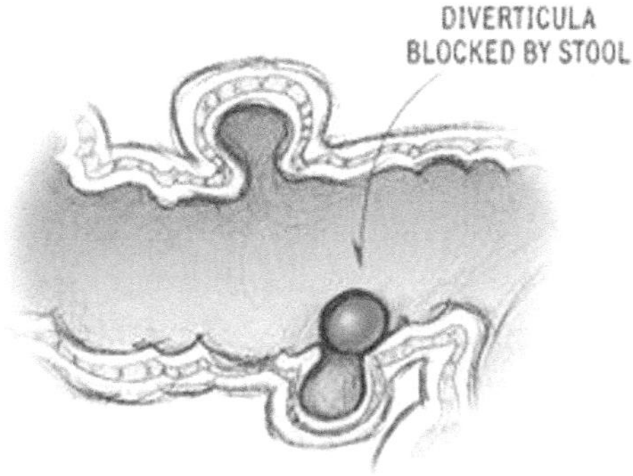

DIVERTICULITIS

Diverticulitis, unlike appendicitis, is seen mostly in older patients. Diverticula are small pouches in the large bowel that resemble an inner tube peeking out of a defect in an old-timey car tire. These areas may become blocked just like the appendix might. The symptoms are very similar, but most diverticulitis patients will complain of pain in the lower *left* quadrant instead of the right.

Diverticulitis is treated with restriction to liquid diet and antibiotics. A combination of Metronidazole 500 mg four times a day orally plus Ciprofloxacin (Cipro, Fish-Flox) 750 mg twice daily or Trimethoprim Sulfa 160 mg/Sulfamethoxazole 800mg (Bactrim, Bird Sulfa) twice daily is acceptable therapy.

Other inflammatory conditions in the bowel, such as Crohn's Disease or Ulcerative Colitis, may present with pelvic pain that mimics diverticulitis or appendicitis. These are commonly treated with steroids but may require surgery.

Pelvic Inflammatory Disease

A female pelvic infection is usually caused by sexually transmitted diseases such as gonorrhea or chlamydia. Pelvic Inflammatory Disease (also called "PID") may mimic the pain of appendicitis but is more often felt on both sides of the lower abdomen. PID will also present with fever and a foul vaginal discharge.

Pelvic Inflammatory Disease can cause major damage to internal female anatomy. Scarring ensues as the body tries to heal, sometimes causing infertility and chronic pelvic pain. Serious female infections involving the pelvis are best treated with antibiotics such as Doxycycline, sometimes in combination with Metronidazole twice a day for a week. It is important to treat sexual partners as well.

Tubal Pregnancy

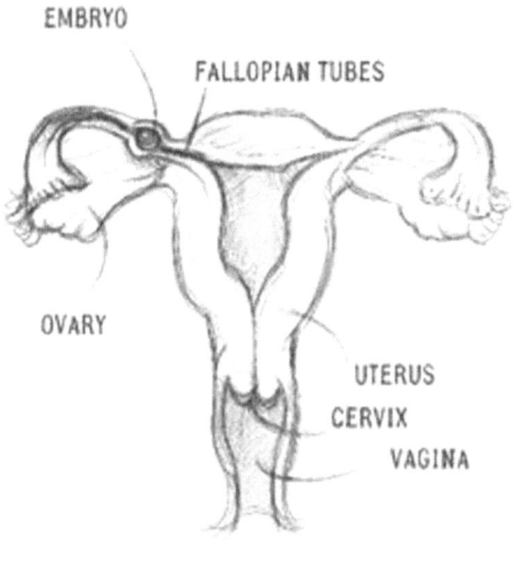

TUBAL ECTOPIC PREGNANCY

In women of childbearing age, a tubal (also called "ectopic") pregnancy should be ruled out. This is a condition that occurs in 1 in every 125 pregnancies. A **tubal pregnancy** occurs when a fertilized egg fails to implant in the normal location (the uterine wall) and implants in the Fallopian tube instead. It grows in this tiny canal until it reaches a size that bursts the tube. This will cause pain and internal bleeding that could be life-threatening. If the fallopian tube on the right side is involved, it can present similarly to appendicitis.

In this case, the pain is due to the presence of blood rather than infection. If you have women of childbearing age in your family or survival group, make sure to have some pregnancy tests in your medical supplies. A woman with a missed period, positive pregnancy test, and severe pain on one side of the lower abdomen has a tubal pregnancy until proven otherwise. If the abdomen becomes filled with blood and vital signs become unstable, surgical intervention would be the only option.

Ovarian Cysts

Other female issues in the pelvis, such as large or ruptured ovarian cysts, could also cause pain due to pressure or bleeding. An ovarian cyst is an accumulation of walled-off fluid. Many arise from egg follicles. Most are benign but some can be cancerous, especially in older women.

Most cysts cause pain by pressing against other internal structures. When they rupture, however, they cause a painful irritation of the abdominal lining or an episode of internal bleeding. Sometimes, ovarian cysts resolve spontaneously, but a ruptured cyst that is actively bleeding will require surgery. A right-sided ruptured cyst could appear similar to appendicitis as the pain is in a similar location.

The diagnosis of appendicitis or other causes of abdominal pain without modern diagnostic equipment will be challenging. Despite this, we have to remember that, in the past, healthcare providers had only physical signs and symptoms to help them reach a diagnosis.

Hopefully, we will never be placed in a situation where modern medical care is not available. Many of the conditions described above will represent a possibly fatal result without the ability to perform surgery or give intravenous medications.

Hepatitis

The largest internal organ in the abdomen is the liver. This organ is extremely important for survival, and any impairment in its function is dangerous. The liver has many duties, including:

- Production of bile to help digestion
- Filtration of toxins from the blood (for example, alcohol)
- Storage of certain vitamins and minerals
- Production of amino acids for protein synthesis
- Maintenance of normal levels of glucose (sugar) in the blood
- Conversion of glucose to glycogen for energy storage
- Production of cholesterol (yes, you need cholesterol)
- Production of urea (main component in urine)
- Processing of old red blood cells
- Production of certain hormones

Hepatitis is the term used for inflammation of the liver. Mostly caused by viruses, this condition causes the inability of the body to process toxins and perform the other functions listed above, and can be life-threatening.

Hepatitis may be caused by oral/fecal contamination: This is a form of disease transmission in which pathogens in fecal particles pass from one host into the oral cavity into the same or other host. As such, we were in a quandary regarding whether to put this in the hygiene and sanitation section or here. We decided to place it here as some common types of liver damage are not hygiene-related, such as those caused by alcohol abuse and drug reactions. Hepatitis can also be spread by sexual contact.

Types of Hepatitis

There are various types of Hepatitis. The most frequently seen ones are Hepatitis A, Hepatitis B, and Hepatitis C. Hepatitis B and C can become chronic inflammations with long-lasting ill effects. Acute symptoms include muscle and joint aches, fever, nausea, vomiting, diarrhea, and headache. The liver, which can be found on the right side of the abdomen just below the lowest rib, becomes enlarged and tender.

Long term effects of chronic inflammation include weakness, general ill feeling (called "malaise"), permanent enlargement of the liver, and much more.

The hallmark sign of hepatitis, however, is "**jaundice**". You will find that your patient's skin and the whites of their eyes will turn yellow. Their urine becomes darker and their stools turn grey. There is also a sensation of itchiness that is felt all over the body. Add to this a feeling of extreme fatigue, weight loss, vague nausea, and sometimes fever.

In some circumstances, people with hepatitis may have no symptoms at all and still have the ability to pass the illness to others.

Hepatitis A: The hepatitis A virus is found in the bowel movements of an infected individual. When a person eats food or drinks water that is contaminated with the virus, they develop a flu-like syndrome that can quickly become serious. It can also be passed sexually. You are thought to be contagious for some time before symptoms appear. Hepatitis A usually resolves on its own in about 2 weeks.

The risk of hepatitis A exists in normal times as well as post-catastrophe. If a restaurant employee with hepatitis A doesn't wash his hands after using the bathroom, everyone that eats there may get sick.

Hepatitis B: This type can be spread by exposure to infected blood products, semen, and vaginal fluids. Symptoms are usually indistinguishable from Hepatitis A, although they may lead to a chronic condition known as "**cirrhosis**" that leads to permanent liver dysfunction. Long-term alcohol or drug abuse can also lead to this condition.

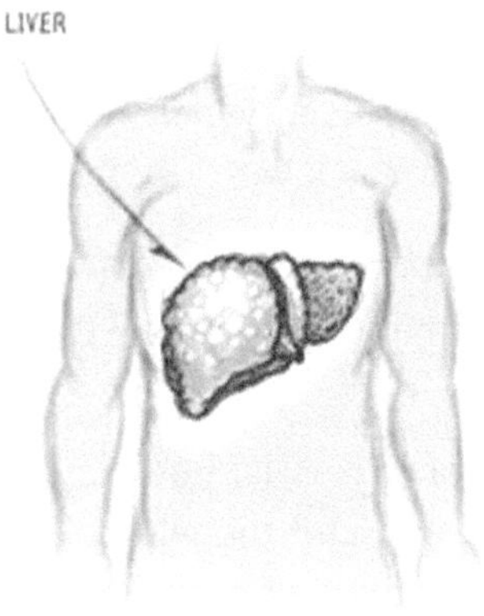

CIRRHOSIS

In cirrhosis, the functioning cells of the liver are replaced by nodules that do nothing to help metabolism. Possible signs and symptoms include:

- **Ascites:** Accumulation of fluid resulting in a swollen abdomen.
- **Varicose veins**: Enlarged veins, especially in the stomach and esophagus
- **Jaundice:** Yellowing of the skin and eyes
- **Swollen ankles and legs**

Hepatitis C: About 200 million people are chronically infected with hepatitis C virus throughout the world. It is a blood-borne virus contracted by intravenous drug use, transfusion, and unsafe sexual practices. A percentage of these patients will progress to cirrhosis over time and, sometimes, liver failure over time.

Treatment of Hepatitis

Other than making your patient comfortable, there isn't very much that you will be able to do in an austere setting regarding this condition.

The drugs used for this condition will simply be unavailable. Most cases of Hepatitis, however, are self-limited, which means that they will resolve on their own after a period of time. Expect at least 2 – 6 weeks of down time. There is a vaccine available for Hepatitis B.

You can, however, practice good preventive medicine by encouraging the following policies for your family or community:

- Wash hands after using the bathroom and before preparing food.
- Wash dishes with soap in hot water.
- Avoid eating or drinking anything that may not be properly cooked or filtered.
- Make sure children don't put objects in their mouths.

Natural support for the liver

There are a few "detoxifying" and anti-inflammatory herbal remedies that may help support a liver afflicted with hepatitis. Some of these supplements include:

- Milk Thistle
- Artichoke
- Dandelion
- Turmeric
- Licorice
- Red Clover
- Green Tea

Remember these are not cures, but may assist your other efforts by having a restorative effect.

Nutritional strategies that may help:

- Avoid fatty foods and alcohol
- Increase zinc intake
- Decrease protein intake
- Improve hydration status, especially with herbal teas, vegetable broths and diluted vegetable juices.

URINARY TRACT INFECTIONS

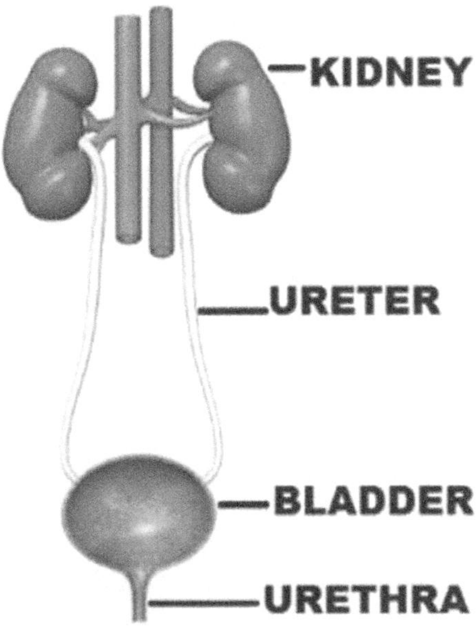

URINARY TRACT

Solid waste is eliminated through the bowels. Liquid waste is excreted through the urinary tract. The urinary tract includes the kidneys, ureters, bladder, and urethra. It is, essentially, the body's plumbing.

You might find it interesting to know that urine, although a waste product, is normally sterile. Despite this, most women have experienced a urinary tract infection, or "UTI" at some point in their lives. An infection of the bladder, also known as "**cystitis**", usually affects the **urethra** (the tube from the bladder to the outside) as well.

Although men are not immune to urinary tract infection, they are much less susceptible to them. The male urethra is much longer than its female counterpart; micro-organisms must travel a longer distance to reach the bladder.

Various different organisms may cause urinary tract infections: E. coli is the most common. Some bacteria that cause UTIs, such as gonorrhea, are sexually transmitted. In men, painful urination (also called "**dysuria**") is very common with urinary tract infections, while most women might only note a yellowish discharge from the vagina.

Although painful urination is not uncommon in cystitis, the most common symptom is frequent trips to the restroom ("**frequency**"). Some people notice that the stream of urine is somewhat hard to start ("**hesitancy**") or may feel an urgent need to go without warning ("**urgency**").

If not treated, a bladder infection may possibly ascend to the kidneys, causing an infection known as "**pyelonephritis**". Conditions relating to the kidneys are called "**renal**". Once an infection is in the kidney, your patient may experience:

- One-sided back or flank pain
- Persistent fever and chills
- Abdominal pain
- Bloody, cloudy, or foul-smelling urine
- Dysuria
- Sweating
- Mental changes (in the elderly)

Kidney infections can be diagnosed by tapping the flank lightly at the level of the lowest rib with the side of a closed first. Normally, this will elicit no response in a healthy patient but flinching from someone with an infection. Kidney stones, discussed later in this book, may also cause tenderness in this region but are less often associated with fever.

Once the infection is in the kidneys, antibiotics will be necessary. If the infection is not treated, the condition may progress to "**septicemia**" or "**sepsis**", once the infection reaches the bloodstream. These patients will show signs of shock, such as rapid breathing, decreased blood pressure, fever and chills, and impaired mental status.

Prevention and treatment of UTIs

Preventative medicine plays a large role in decreasing the likelihood of this problem. Adherence to basic hygienic methods in those at high risk, especially women, is warranted. Standard recommendations include:

- Wiping from front to back after urinating or defecating.
- Urinating right after an episode of sexual intercourse.
- Avoid postponing urination when there is a strong urge to do so.
- Drinking lots of fluids.
- Wearing cotton undergarments to allow air circulation in areas that might otherwise encourage bacterial or fungal growth.

Treatment revolves around the vigorous administration of fluids. Lots of water will help flush out the infection by decreasing the concentration of bacteria in the bladder or kidney. Applying warm compresses to the bladder region is soothing for patients with cystitis.

Antibiotics are another mainstay of therapy. The following are most often used for renal infections (brand names and veterinary equivalents in parenthesis):

- Sulfamethoxazole-trimethoprim (Bactrim, Septra, Bird-Sulfa)
- Amoxicillin (Amoxil, Fish-Mox)
- Nitrofurantoin (Macrobid)
- Ampicillin (Fish-Cillin)
- Ciprofloxacin (Cipro, Fish-Flox)

An over-the-counter medication that eliminates the painful urination seen in urinary infections is Phenazopyridine (also known as Pyridium, Uristat, Azo, etc.). Don't be alarmed if your urine turns reddish-orange; it is an effect of the drug and is temporary. Vitamin C supplements are thought to reduce the concentration of bacteria in the urine, and should also be considered.

A few natural remedies for urinary tract infections are listed below:

- Garlic
- Echinacea extract or tea.
- Goldenrod tea with 1-2 tablespoons of vinegar.

- Uva Ursi (1 tablet).
- Cranberry tablets (1 to 3 pills).
- Alka Seltzer in 2 ounces warm water (poured directly over the urethra)

Use any one of these remedies three times per day.

One more alternative that may be helpful is to perform an external massage over the bladder area with 5 drops of lavender essential oil (mixed with castor oil) for a few minutes. Then, apply a gentle heat source over the area; repeat this 3 to 4 times daily. The combination of lavender/castor oil and warmth may help decrease bladder spasms and pain.

INFECTIONS CAUSED BY YEAST

In addition to viruses and bacteria, our body may be susceptible to infections with "yeast". Yeast is a fungus that is one-celled and reproduces by budding off the parent. The human body naturally harbors certain types but can be damaged by others.

Fungal infections may be local, as in vaginal infections, "ringworm", or "athlete's foot", or systemic (throughout the entire body). Some people are affected by intestinal fungal infections that can affect digestion. Systemic fungal infections have been blamed for many illnesses, but proven cases seem to occur mostly in the very young or the elderly; those with compromised immune systems can also be affected.

Vaginal Infections

Vaginal yeast infections (also called "**Monilia**") are extremely common and are not an indication of a sexually transmitted disease. A woman with a yeast infection will complain of vaginal itchiness and have an odorless thick white discharge reminiscent of cottage cheese.

This infection is often easily treated with short courses of over-the-counter creams or vaginal suppositories such as miconazole (Monistat). Recurrent infections resistant to miconazole may be treated with prescription fluconazole (Diflucan) 150mg orally in a single dose. Repeat in 3 days if symptoms persist.

Non-yeast vaginal infections, those caused by bacteria or protozoa, also exist and are called "**bacterial vaginosis**" and "**trichomoniasis**", respectively. These tend to have gray or green discharge with a foul odor, and are treated with a prescription antibiotic/anti-parasitic medication called Metronidazole (veterinary equivalent: FISH-ZOLE), 500 mg orally twice a day for 7 days or 4 500mg once.

The time-honored vinegar and water douche, performed once a day, is very effective in eliminating minor vaginal infections.

Douche with 1 tablespoon of vinegar per quart of water. Use this method only until your patient feels better. Women who douche often are, paradoxically, *more* likely to get yeast infections. This occurs because douching disrupts the normal pH balance and allows naturally occurring organisms in the vagina to overrun their environment.

Acidophilus supplements, in powder or capsule form, may be a good oral treatment. Cranberry juice and yogurt are thought to be good foods for vaginal infections because they change the pH of the organ to a level inhospitable to yeast. To relieve itching, sit in a bath of warm water with a few drops of lavender or tea tree oil for 15 minutes. Repeat as needed.

If these aren't available, some have used garlic for its antibacterial and anti-fungal action. Inserting a clove of garlic wrapped in gauze in the vagina for short periods of time (less than eight hours) may be helpful. Make sure you leave a "tail" of gauze that you can easily reach to remove the garlic.

Oral Infections

Yeast infections may be seen in the mouth of infants and some others. This infection is known as "**Thrush**" and is identified by white patches on the inside of the cheeks, the roof of the mouth, and other areas of the oral cavity. Thrush can cause irritation and the white patches are adherent, causing bleeding if wiped off. Occasionally, the nipples of breastfeeding mothers are affected.

Oral thrush may be treated conventionally with liquid Fluconazole (Diflucan) once a day for a week. Nystatin, another antifungal, is available in a "swish-and-swallow" version for oral thrush or can be applied topically four times a day to infected nipples for approximately five to seven days.

Alternative remedies reported to be effective for oral yeast infections include:

- Swabbing the oral cavity with yogurt.
- Applying acidophilus to nipples or other items likely to go in an infant's mouth.
- Applying white vinegar (distilled) or very dilute baking soda solutions (1 teaspoon to 8 ounces of water) to nipples.
- Swabbing the oral area with virgin coconut oil.

Athlete's Foot

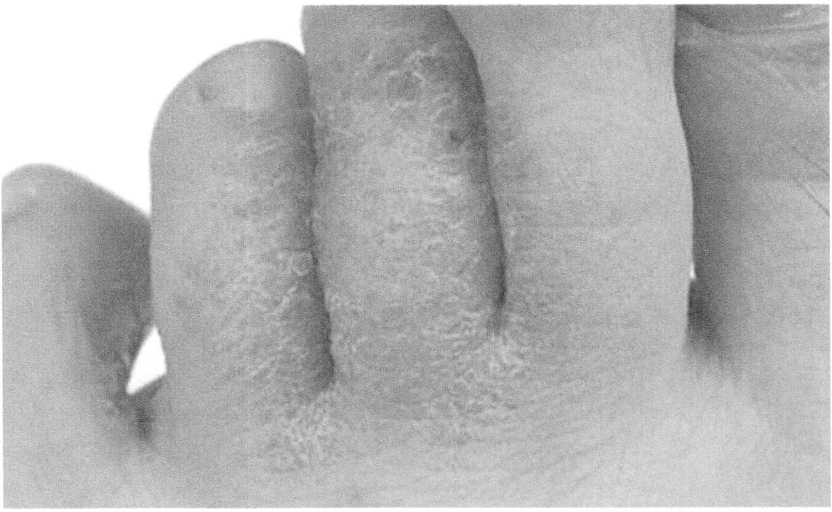

Athlete's foot (also known as "**tinea pedis**") is an infection of the skin caused by a type of fungus. This condition may, if not treated, last for years. Although usually seen between the toes, you might see it also on other parts of the feet or even on the hands between the fingers.

Athlete's foot is contagious. It can be passed by sharing shoes or socks with, or even by simply walking on the same wet surfaces, as those who have the infection.

Any fungal infection is made worse by moist conditions. People who are prone to Athlete's foot commonly:

- Spend long hours in closed shoes
- Keep their feet wet for prolonged periods
- Have a tendency to get cuts on feet and hands
- Perspire a lot

To make the diagnosis, look for:

- Flaking of skin between the toes or fingers.
- Itching and burning of affected areas

- Reddened skin
- Discolored nails
- Fluid drainage from surfaces traumatized by repeated scratching

If the condition is mild, keeping your feet clean and dry may be enough to allow slow improvement of the condition. Oftentimes, however, topical antifungal ointments or powders such as miconazole or clotrimazole (Lotrimin) are required for elimination of the condition. In the worst cases, oral prescription antifungals such as fluconazole (Diflucan) are needed. Don't use anti-itching creams very often; they keep the area moist and may delay healing.

A favorite home remedy for Athlete's Foot involves placing Tea Tree Oil liberally to a foot bath and soak for 20 minutes or so. Dry the feet well and then apply a few drops onto the affected area. Repeat this process twice daily. Try to keep the area as dry as possible between treatments.

For prevention of future outbreaks of Athlete's Foot, apply tea tree oil once a week before putting on socks and shoes.

One method that does *not* work is urinating on your feet in the shower. Although there is ammonia in urine that might kill germs, it's not strong enough to kill the Athlete's foot fungus.

Ringworm

Ringworm is a fungal infection on the surface of the skin. Tinea, the fungus that causes Athlete's foot, is just as likely to affect any other area of the skin. Often, it will appear as a raised, itchy patch that is darker on the outside. As such, it may resemble a sharply-defined ring, and is called "Ringworm". Ringworm has nothing to do with worms.

If Ringworm occurs in a hairy area, it will likely cause bald patches. Consistent scratching at the patches will cause blistering and oozing. Treatment, both conventional and natural, follows a similar process as that described for Athlete's Foot.

Make sure to:

- Keep skin as dry as possible.
- Use Antifungal (Miconazole, Clotrimazole) or drying powders or creams.
- Avoid tight-fitting clothing on irritated areas
- Wash regularly.
- Wash sheets daily.

CELLULITIS

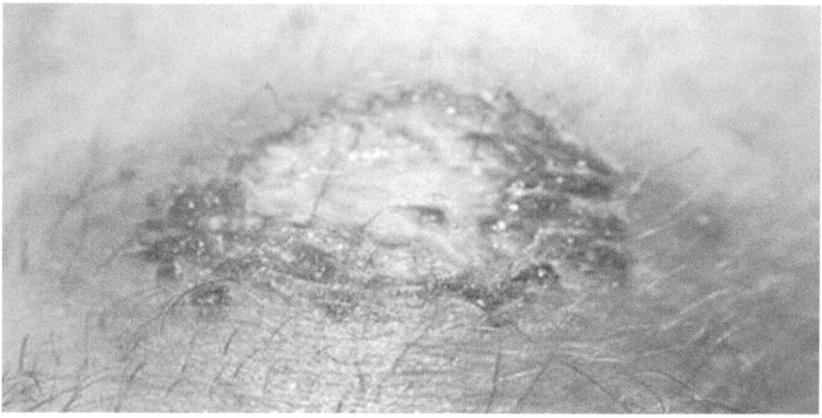

Any soft tissue injury carries with it a degree of risk when it comes to infection. Due to the availability of antibiotics, infections from minor wounds or insect bites are relatively easy to treat today. Without them, even small wound infections may enter the circulation and become life-threatening.

In a survival situation, antibiotics will be precious commodities. You, as medic, should dispense them only when absolutely necessary. The misuse of antibiotics, along with their excessive use in livestock, is part of the reason that we're seeing an epidemic of antibiotic resistance in this country. 80% of all the antibiotics in use today are given to livestock, not to treat infection, but to speed up growth and get meat to market sooner. It is not known how antibiotics work to accelerate maturation.

Despite your best efforts to care for a wound, there is always a chance that an infection will occur. Infection in the soft tissues below the superficial level of the skin (the "**epidermis**") is referred to as "**cellulitis**". Below the epidermis, the main layers of soft tissue are the "**dermis**" (you've seen this area when you scraped your knee as a kid) the subcutaneous fat, the muscle layers, and their attendant blood vessels and nerves.

Cellulitis is easy to deal with in normal times, but it will be an epidemic in the aftermath of a major disaster. The sheer number of cuts, scrapes, and burns incurred from performing activities of daily survival will make it one of the most prevalent medical problems. In unsanitary conditions, these wounds are more likely to become infected.

The end result might be a whole body (also referred to as "**systemic**" infection known as "**sepsis**". Once sepsis develops, inflammation of the spinal cord ("**meningitis**") or bony structures ("**osteomyelitis**") can further complicate the situation. In the past, people who became septic often died.

The bacteria that can cause cellulitis are on your skin right now. Normal inhabitants of the surface of your skin include Staphylococcus and Group A Streptococcus. They do no harm until the skin is broken and they enter deeper tissues. As they don't belong there, they start causing inflammation. A resistant bacteria called MRSA (Methicillin-Resistant Staphylococcus Aureus) may be found on skin and cause cellulitis. The usual antibiotics are ineffective in MRSA cases.

As an aside, Cellulitis has nothing to do with the dimpling on the skin called cellulite. The suffix "-itis" simply means "inflammation", so cellul-itis simply means "inflammation of the cells", appendicitis means "inflammation of the appendix", and so on…

Conditions that might cause cellulitis include:

- Any injury that causes a break in the skin, including insect bites and stings, animal (or human) bites, knife or bullet wounds, surgical incisions, and more
- Ulcers from chronic illness, such as diabetes
- Varicose veins due to poor circulation
- Use of steroids or other medications that affect the immune system
- Intravenous drug use

The symptoms and signs of cellulitis are:

- Discomfort in the area of infection
- Fever and Chills
- Exhaustion (**fatigue**)
- General ill feeling (**malaise**)

- Muscle aches (**myalgia**)
- Heat in the area of the infection compared to non-affected areas
- Redness, usually spreading towards torso
- Swelling in the area of infection (causing a sensation of tightness)
- Drainage of pus/cloudy fluid from the area of the infection
- Foul odor coming from the area of infection

Other, less common, symptoms that can occur with this disease:

- Hair loss at the site of infection
- Joint stiffness caused by swelling of the tissue over it
- Nausea and vomiting

Although the body can sometimes resolve cellulitis on its own, treatment usually includes the use of antibiotics; these can be topical, oral or intravenous. Most cellulitis will improve and disappear after a 10 – 14 day course of therapy with medications in the Penicillin, Erythromycin, or Cephalosporin (Keflex) families. Amoxicillin and Ampicillin are particularly popular. MRSA cellulitis can be treated with clindamycin and the sulfa drug combination trimethoprim-sulfamethoxazole.

If the cellulitis is in an extremity, it is helpful to keep the limb elevated. It would be wise to complete the full course of antibiotics to prevent recurrences.

Other helpful strategies include warm compresses or soaks to the affected area, and the use of ibuprofen (Advil) or acetaminophen (Tylenol) to decrease pain, discomfort, and fever.

ABSCESSES

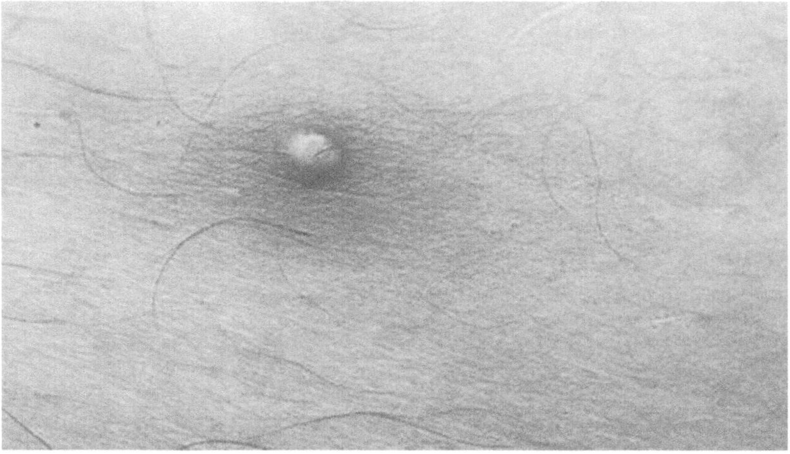

An **abscess** is a collection of pus. Pus is the debris left over from your body's attempt to eliminate an infection; it consists of white and red blood cells, live and dead microbes, and inflammatory fluid. When associated with the skin, an abscess is called a "boil".

If the abscess was not caused by an infected wound or diseased tooth, it is possible that it originated in a "**cyst**", which is a hollow, walled-off structure filled with fluid. There are various types that can become infected and form skin abscesses:

Sebaceous cysts: skin glands often associated with hair follicles, they are concentrated on the face and trunk. These cysts produce oily material known as "sebum".

Inclusion cysts: These occur when skin lining is trapped in deeper layers as a result of trauma. They continue to produce skin cells and grow.

Pilonidal cysts: These cysts are located over the area of the tail-bone, and are due to a malformation during fetal development. They easily become infected and require intervention.

The body's attempt to cure an infection is a good thing. However, abscesses or boils have a tendency to be walled off as a result, which also makes it hard for medications like antibiotics to penetrate. As such, you may have to intervene by performing a procedure.

To deal with an abscess, an avenue must be made to evacuate the pus. The easiest way to do this is to place warm moist compresses over the area, also known as "ripening the abscess". Apply the compress over the area for 15 minutes or so every couple of hours during the day. This will help bring the infection to the surface of the skin, where it will form a "head" and, hopefully, drain spontaneously. The abscess will go from firm to soft as it ripens; it'll develop a "whitehead" pimple at the likely point of exit.

You'll be tempted to squeeze the boil in an effort to relieve the pressure discomfort. Doing this, however, may make the infection worse. Patience is important for a few days to give the abscess a chance to resolve on its own.

If a few days go by without spontaneous drainage, it may become clear that a boil or abscess will not respond to lesser treatment and needs surgical intervention. This is called "**lancing a boil**" or, in medical-ese, "**incision and drainage**". Always wash your hands and put on gloves before attempting this or, really, any other medical procedure.

Clean the area with an antiseptic and apply a numbing agent (even ice will do). You'll need a sharp sterile instrument such as a scalpel (a #11 blade is best). If you don't have a sterile instrument, you can put a thin blade over a fire until it becomes red hot, then let cool.

Using the tip of the scalpel, pierce the skin over the abscess perpendicular to the surface of the skin. The pus should drain freely, and your patient will probably experience immediate relief from the release of pressure. Sometimes a small Kelly clamp is useful to break up little compartments in the abscess called "**loculations**", Have some extra gauze handy, as a large boil can be messy to treat.

Irrigate the wound with lots of saline solution or clean water. A thin gauze moistened with Betadine is then placed in the abscess cavity, commercially available as "iodoform packing". Finally, apply an antibiotic ointment like Bactroban or raw, unprocessed honey to the skin surrounding the incision and cover with a clean bandage. Change the packing twice daily until the abscess cavity fills in. If the abscess returns, the walls may need removal in a more extensive procedure.

Oral antibiotics are a useful additional tool to treat boils, whether or not you decide to lance them. Amoxicillin, Cephalexin, or Erythromycin are options that are available in veterinary equivalents (Fish-Mox, Fish-Flex, and Fish-Mycin, respectively).

Incision and drainage may be helpful for dental abscesses as well, but may not save nearby teeth. Information about how to extract a tooth may be found in the dental section of this book. Other abscesses may occur in organs like the liver or the ovary; these can be life-threatening but require major surgical intervention to treat, not an option in survival settings.

TETANUS

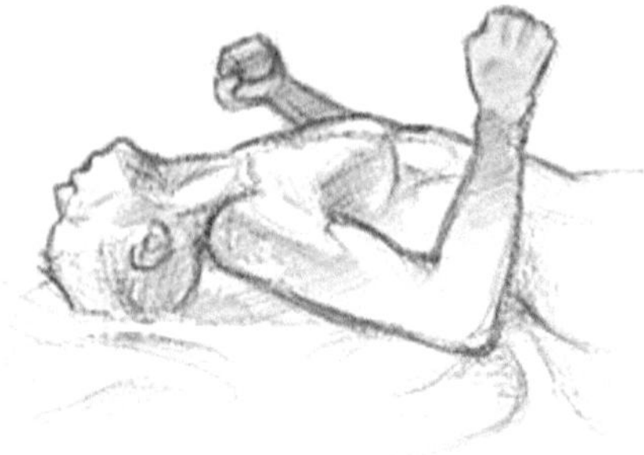

TETANUS

Most of us have dutifully gone to get a tetanus shot when we stepped on a rusty nail, but few have any real concept of what tetanus is and why it is dangerous. The role of the survival medic is to know the answers to these questions. Knowledge of risks, prevention, and treatment will be the armor plate in your medical defense.

Tetanus (from the Greek word tetanos, meaning tight) is an infection caused by a bacteria called Clostridium tetani. The bacteria produces spores (inactive bacteria-to-be) that primarily live in the soil or the feces of animals. These spores are capable of living for years and are resistant to extremes in temperature.

Tetanus is relatively rare in the United States, with about 50 reported cases a year. Worldwide, however, there are more than 500,000 cases a year. Today, most victims are found in developing countries. After a disaster, however, tetanus cases can occur anywhere. The medic must know how to recognize and treat it.

Most tetanus infections occur when a person experiences a break in the skin. The most common cause is some type of puncture wound, such as an insect or animal bite, a splinter, or even that rusty nail. The skin is the most important barrier to infection, and any chink in the armor leaves you vulnerable.

When a wound becomes contaminated with Tetanus spores, the dormant spore becomes activated as a full-fledged bacterium and reproduces rapidly. Damage to the victim comes as a result of a strong toxin excreted by the organism known as Tetanospasmin. This toxin specifically targets nerves that serve muscle tissue.

Tetanospasmin binds to motor nerves, causing "misfires" that lead to involuntary contraction of the affected areas. This neural damage could be in one area or can affect the entire body. You would possibly see the classical symptom of "**Lockjaw**", where the jaw muscle is constantly clenched. Any muscle group, however, is susceptible to the contractions if affected by the toxin. This includes the respiratory musculature, which can inhibit normal breathing and cause damage due to lack of oxygen.

The most severe cases seem to occur at extremes of age, with newborns and those over 65 most likely to succumb to the disease. Death rates from generalized Tetanus hover around 25-50%, higher in newborns.

Initial symptoms may not present themselves for up to 2 weeks. You should be on the lookout for the following:

- Sore muscles (especially near the site of injury)
- Weakness
- Irritability
- Difficulty swallowing
- Lockjaw (also called "Trismus"; facial muscles are often the first affected)

As the disease progresses, you may see:

- Progressively worsening muscle spasms (may start locally and become generalized over time)
- Involuntary arching of the back (sometimes so strong that bones may break or dislocations may occur!)
- Fever
- Respiratory distress
- High blood pressure
- Irregular heartbeats

The first thing that the survival medic should understand is that, although an infectious disease, Tetanus is not contagious. You can feel confident treating a Tetanus victim safely, as long as you wear gloves and observe standard clean technique. Begin by washing your hands and putting on your gloves. Then, wash the wound thoroughly with soap and water, using an irrigation syringe to flush out any debris. This will, hopefully, limit growth of the bacteria and, as a result, decrease toxin production.

You will want to administer antibiotics to kill off the rest of the bacteria in the system. Metronidazole (veterinary equivalent: Fish-Zole) 375-500mg twice a day or Doxycycline (Bird-Biotic) 100 mg twice a day are known to be effective. The earlier you begin antibiotic therapy, the less toxin will be produced. IV rehydration, if you have the ability to administer it, is also helpful. The patient will be more comfortable in an environment with dim lights and reduced noise.

Late stage Tetanus is difficult to treat without modern technology. Ventilators, Tetanus Antitoxin, and muscle relaxants/sedatives such as Valium are used to treat severe cases but will be unlikely to be available in a long term survival situation. For this reason, it is extraordinarily important for the survival medic to watch anyone who has sustained a wound for the early symptoms listed above.

As medic, you must obtain a detailed medical history from anyone that you might be responsible for in times of trouble. This includes immunization histories where possible. Has the injured individual been immunized against Tetanus? Most people born in the U.S. will have gone through a series of immunizations against Diphtheria, Tetanus, and Whooping Cough early in their childhood. If not, encourage them to get up to date with their immunizations against this dangerous disease as soon as possible. Booster injections are usually given every 10 years.

Tetanus vaccine is not without its risks, but severe complications such as seizures or brain damage occur is less than one in a million cases. Milder side effects are more common, such as fatigue, fever, nausea, headache, and inflammation in the injection site.

Given the life-threatening nature of the disease, this is one vaccine that you should encourage your people to receive, regardless of your feelings about vaccines in general. If not caught early, there may be little you can do to treat your patient in an austere setting.

MOSQUITO-BORNE ILLNESSES

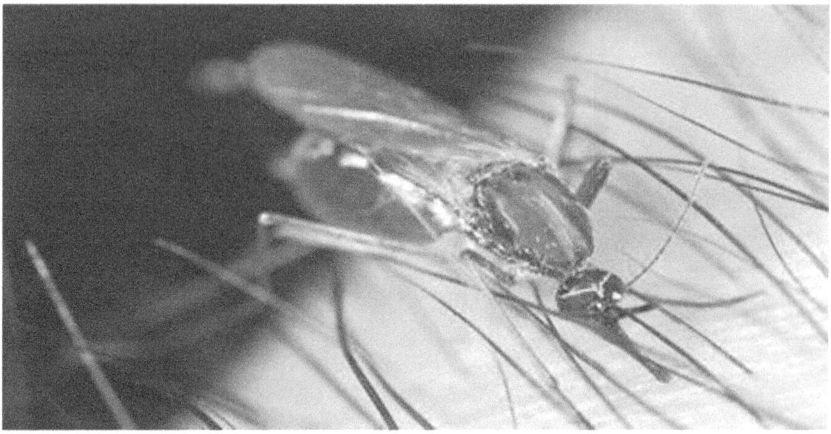

Although the stings of bees or wasps may cause allergic reactions, mosquito bites are much more likely to transmit infectious disease. The increased amount of time you'll spend outside in a survival situation will increase the chances of exposure to one or more mosquito-borne illnesses.

Malaria

One of the most notorious diseases caused by mosquito vectors is Malaria. Malaria is caused by a microscopic organism called a protozoan. When female mosquitoes (only females bite humans) of the *anopheles* species obtain a meal by biting you, they inject these microbes into your system. Once in the body, they colonize your liver. From there, they go to your blood cells and other organs.

Symptoms of Malaria appear flu-like, and classically present as periodic chills, fever, and sweats. The patient becomes anemic as blood cells are damaged by the protozoa. With time, periods between episodes become shorter and permanent organ damage may occur.

Diagnosis of malaria cannot be confirmed without a microscope, but anyone experiencing relapsing fevers with severe chills and sweating should be considered candidates for treatment. The medications used for Malaria are Chloroquine, Quinine, and Quinidine, among others.

Sometimes, an antibiotic such as Doxycycline or Clindamycin is used in combination with the above. Physicians are usually sympathetic towards prescribing these medications to those who are contemplating trips to places where mosquitoes are rampant, such as some underdeveloped countries. They are also available in veterinary equivalents (discussed later)

Zika Virus

A little-known virus of equatorial Africa and Asia, the Zika virus has crossed the Atlantic and has wreaked havoc in South America, especially among pregnant women and their newborns. Zika is transmitted by Aedes mosquitoes.

Most people with symptoms experience a mild flu-like syndrome, but an infection during a pregnancy can yield a newborn with a specific birth defect called microcephaly. Microcephaly is an abnormally small head (smaller than 98% of newborns) with correspondingly smaller brain. It can lead to mild disability in some cases, but could be incompatible with life in others.

Zika virus has no treatment or vaccine at the time of this writing, although researchers are working on options. Efforts to combat the virus and its complications, therefore, center on mosquito control.

Chikungunya

This disease, transmitted by the *Aedes* family of mosquito, affected more than a million in the Western Hemisphere when it arrived from Africa two years ago. Chikungunya (an African term meaning "that which bends up") is a viral illness that is not fatal but causes fever as well as excruciating pain in joints. The pain is reminiscent of severe arthritis and can last for weeks, months, or even years.

Other symptoms, besides joint pain and fever, include:

- Headache
- Nausea and vomiting
- Red eyes

- Sensitivity to light
- Leg swelling

There is no known cure or treatment other than pain relief and fever control through medications like Acetaminophen (Tylenol). The disease is prevented by good mosquito control. Areas where air-conditioning is widely available seem to be less affected.

Dengue Fever

Another viral disease transmitted by the same mosquito species that transmit Chikungunya and Zika is Dengue Fever. The patient experiences flu-like syndromes and joint pains similar to Chikungunya except that Dengue fever causes a measles-like skin rash. In severe cases, blood clotting mechanisms are impaired, and spontaneous bleeding from orifices may occur. Dengue fever is increasingly being diagnosed in deep Southern regions of the United States.

Yellow Fever

Yellow fever is a viral mosquito-borne infection that was responsible for many deaths during the building of the Panama Canal. It has also been the cause of community-wide outbreaks in places like New Orleans.

Symptoms include fever, chills, nausea, and muscle pains which usually goes away in about five days. After a day or so of improvement, the fever might come back and abdominal pain occurs as the liver becomes affected, causing jaundice (a yellowing of the skin and eyes) as in hepatitis. Organ damage and bleeding ensue.

West Nile Virus

Originally from Africa, West Nile Virus is another disease spread by *Aedes* mosquitoes. It has spread throughout the world in the last twenty years, including the United States. Symptoms include a flu-like presentation, vomiting, and rashes. Severe cases affect the nervous system, especially in the very young, the very old, and those with weakened immune systems. Inflammation of the brain (**encephalitis**) or the spinal cord lining (**meningitis**) may occur. West Nile Virus and a number of other mosquito-borne illnesses may also be seen in horses.

Other mosquito-borne viral diseases include Eastern Equine Encephalitis, St. Louis Encephalitis, and Western Equine Encephalitis. Although many of these are tropical diseases, a number of cases of each are reported each year in the United States.

Although some of the viral diseases described above have vaccines, they are rarely prescribed unless you are going into an area where the risk is high. Treatment is mostly aimed at relieving the symptoms. For example, ibuprofen for joint aches or acetaminophen for fever.

Mosquito Control

The fewer mosquitoes near your retreat, the less likely you will fall victim to one of these diseases. You can decrease the population of mosquitoes in your area and improve the likelihood of preventing illness by:

- Looking for areas of standing water that could serve as mosquito breeding grounds. Drain all water that you do not depend on for survival.
- Monitoring the screens on your retreat windows and doors and repairing any holes or defects.
- Being careful to avoid outside activities at dusk or dawn. This is the time that most mosquitoes are most active. *Aedes* mosquitoes, however, bite all day long.
- Wear long pants and shirts whenever you venture outside.
- Have a good stockpile of insect repellants. If you are going to use sunscreen, apply it first and then apply the insect repellant.

Some insect repellants are meant to be applied to clothing only, such as Permethrin. DEET is acceptable for skin. Avoid placing DEET on skin, however, that will be covered with clothing. DEET is acceptable for use by pregnant and breastfeeding women to prevent Zika virus.

If you are reluctant to use chemical repellants, you may consider natural remedies. Plants that contain Citronella may be rubbed on your skin to discourage bites. Lemon balm has been recommended in the past, but, despite having a fragrance similar to citronella, does not have the same bug-repelling properties.

When you use an essential oil to repel insects, re-apply frequently and feel free to combine oils as needed. Besides Citronella oil, you could use:

- Lemon Eucalyptus oil
- Cinnamon oil
- Peppermint oil
- Geranium oil
- Clove oil
- Rosemary oil

PANDEMICS

In modern times, we have become highly dependent on the high technology that has, in many cases, eliminated the scourge of infectious disease. Antibiotic and antiviral medications are now available in their 3rd or 4th generation versions, and physicians aren't reluctant to use them despite the threat of antibiotic resistance.

Most are reluctant to consider the possibility that a major disaster may wipe out the ability to manufacture these drugs. Significant restrictions exist which put antibiotics and antivirals out of reach of the common man. This hard reality will place us at the mercy of infectious diseases, and some of these have the potential to kill millions on a global scale.

Diseases that cause widespread outbreaks may be endemic, epidemic, or pandemic:

- An **Endemic** disease is one regularly found among particular people or in a certain area. Malaria, for example, is endemic in many tropical countries.
- An **Epidemic** disease is a rapid widespread occurrence of an infectious disease in a community that is not "endemic". Influenza is epidemic, as it isn't always raging in a particular area, but arrives suddenly or periodically.
- A **Pandemic** occurs when an infectious disease runs rampant throughout different regions or, in the case of the Spanish Flu pandemic of 1918, the whole world.

The World Health Organization rates its level of concern about a disease entering a new area with Phase alerts. These go as follows:

- **Phase 1**: A virus is found in animals; no known infections in humans.
- **Phase 2**: The disease has caused proven infection in humans.
- **Phase 3**: Small clusters of disease occur in humans but do not affect entire communities.

- **Phase** 4: The disease now affects entire communities. The disease qualifies as an epidemic, but the risk for a pandemic, although greatly increased, is not certain.
- **Phase** 5: Spread of disease between humans is occurring in more than one country in a region. The Ebola outbreak of 2014 is an example of this phase, with cases in communities in several different West African countries.
- **Phase** 6: Community-level outbreaks are in at least one additional country in a different region. The Zika virus, with millions of cases in Africa, Asia, Polynesia, and now, the Western Hemisphere, is the latest example of a full pandemic.

Diseases That Cause Pandemics

Pandemics of varying severities occur about three or four times per century. Some are particularly noteworthy, such as the Spanish Flu of 100 years ago or the Black Death of the middle ages. Although infectious disease is still with us, modern medicine has greatly decreased its effect on society, and even eradicated it in some cases (smallpox). It is still important, however, to know how to recognize and treat them.

We have already discussed a number of possible epidemic or pandemic diseases, such as Cholera, Influenza, Chikungunya, Zika, Malaria, and others. Here are some other infections that have been pandemics or are candidates for the next one.

Tuberculosis: An infection of the lungs and other organs caused by mycobacteria, Tuberculosis (TB) is so common in certain regions that it is considered endemic. Lately, a number of variants are appearing that are completely resistant to currently available antibiotics.

A chronic cough and bloody phlegm are typically seen, but TB can affect more than the lungs. It can damage various organs, including the female pelvic organs. Even mild tuberculosis requires combination antibiotic therapy for a period of months, something that would exhaust the typical survival medicine cabinet.

Plague: The Plague, once called "The Black Death", is another disease commonly associated with the word "pandemic". Plague is caused by the bacteria *Yersinia Pestis*. It is found in fleas that infest rats and other rodents. Different forms of plague can be spread in the air, by direct contact, or by contaminated water or food.

The symptoms of plague depend on the type:

- **Bubonic plague**: Bubonic plague, the most common type, causes flu-like symptoms and infects lymph nodes. An accumulation of bacteria, blood, and pus in these structures gives rise to lumps called **buboes.** Buboes are blackish in color and are seen in the armpits and groin.
- **Pneumonic plague**: Pneumonic plague infects the lungs. The patient begins to vomit or cough up blood (also known as "**hemoptysis**"). The patient develops shortness of breath and, if untreated, death occurs in less than 48 hours.
- **Septicemic plague:** Bacteria may pass from buboes into the bloodstream, or may directly enter the body through an open wound. Besides fever and other general symptoms, a blood abnormality called DIC (**disseminated intravascular coagulation**) occurs. In DIC, events lead to a depletion of the blood clotting factors. This causes spontaneous and unstoppable bleeding into the skin, lungs, kidneys, and other organs.

Of the various types of plague, pneumonic plague does damage the fastest and kills almost all infected in one or two days if untreated. In modern times, Plague is treatable with antibiotics such as Doxycycline, Tetracycline, or Ciprofloxacin (if detected very early). Prevention is through rodent-proofing, a topic discussed elsewhere in this book.

SARS (Sudden Acute Respiratory Syndrome) in Asia and **MERS** (Middle East Respiratory Syndrome), a virus in the same family, have caused respiratory illnesses rapidly leading to the need for intensive care. Thought to arise from animal reservoirs, the existence of these viruses in the coronavirus family (and the high death rate associated with them) is the reason why many in those areas wear face masks in public.

Ebola: The cause of a major epidemic in West Africa in 2014, Ebola is a viral hemorrhagic fever. Probably transmitted by consuming natural reservoirs of the disease, such as bats, flu-like symptoms begin 2-21 days after exposure.

As the disease progresses, it causes bleeding which affects organs and leaks out the ears, nose, and eyes. Bruising is seen on the skin. Bloody diarrhea and vomit, as well as other bodily fluids, are highly contagious.

The virus can live on surfaces for a number of days unless those surfaces have been cleaned with soap and water or Chlorine bleach. Although there is no cure, promising new treatments and vaccines have been developed.

Leprosy: Now called "Hansen's Disease", Leprosy is a chronic condition caused by the bacterium *Mycobacterium leprae*. It is the second most common infectious disease caused by mycobacteria after tuberculosis.

Despite victims being cast out from society in the past, leprosy is actually not that contagious. You can catch it only if you come into frequent contact with air droplets from coughs and sneezes from an infected person.

Leprosy primarily affects the skin, but it also affects nerves and organs. Loss of sensation, muscle weakness, and paralysis may occur. Damage leads to striking skin deformities and the loss of fingers, toes, nose, and other parts.

Leprosy is treated with long-term antibiotic combinations. This isn't an easy proposition, as it would bankrupt the medical supplies of a group. In survival settings, we may again see those with Hansen's disease cast out from society.

Measles: Measles is a contagious airborne viral disease that was once so common it was considered a childhood rite of passage. The disease was almost eradicated in the U.S. in the 2000's but has experienced a resurgence significant enough to be worth knowing how to identify and treat. In long-term survival settings, we can expect it to be even more common as the number of unvaccinated children increase.

Measles is so highly contagious that, if you haven't been vaccinated and are exposed, you have a 90% chance of catching the disease. Also known as **Rubeola**, Measles shouldn't be confused with **Rubella** (German Measles) or **Roseola**, a milder viral illness also seen in childhood.

Measles patients present with a fever as high as 104 degrees Fahrenheit. 2-3 days later, a red patchy rash appears, usually starting on the head and face and then working its way downward. So many "spots" develop that the patches coalesce into even bigger blotches as times goes on. Other symptoms often resemble respiratory and eye infections. Remember the "**three C's**" of measles:

- Cough
- Coryza (head cold symptoms like nasal congestion, etc.)
- Conjunctivitis (red eyes)

Many also manifest white spots on the inside of the mouth called "Koplik's Spots". In severe cases, patients may develop diarrhea, pneumonia, ear infections, and convulsions. Treatment revolves around the treatment of symptoms.

Smallpox: Caused by infection with the *variola* virus, the smallpox victim has high fever and a rash where many small uniform blisters or pimples cause pustules cover the body. It is related to Chickenpox, where the pustules are variable in size. Scarring commonly occurs.

The airborne virus is deadly and spreads quickly, especially affecting populations that haven't been previously exposed. Death rates, for example, among Native Americans were high when they were first exposed to European settlers. Worldwide vaccination programs have all but eradicated this disease from the modern world. The last recorded naturally-occurring case was reported in 1977.

Human Immunodeficiency Virus (HIV): A viruses now mostly seen in certain subgroups in developed countries, HIV and AIDS (Acquired ImmunoDeficiency Syndrome) is currently epidemic in Africa and other parts of the world. It reached pandemic status until drugs were developed that led to effective treatments.

THE SURVIVAL SICK ROOM

In good times, we have the luxury of modern medical facilities and advanced techniques to isolate a sick patient from healthy people. If we ever find ourselves in a grid-down scenario, most of these advantages will go the way of the dinosaur, and we will be placed in, essentially, the same medical environment we experienced in the 19th century.

We do have the benefit of modern knowledge. We are aware of how contagious diseases are spread and we know how to sterilize supplies, so we have a head start on our ancestors. Using this knowledge, it should be possible for the medically prepared to put together a "sick room" or "hospital tent" that will minimize the chance of infectious disease running rampant through your community. It's important to care effectively for the sick while keeping the healthy out of the reach of contagion.

In the face of a looming catastrophe, quickly make the decision to stay in place or get out of Dodge. If you're staying in place, choose a room where the sick will be cared for. That room should:

- Be far from common areas like the kitchen.
- Have good ventilation and light.
- Have a door that can be closed.

If you're leaving the area, choose a hospital tent and place it on the periphery of your camp. Making these decisions before things go bad is important, or you will inevitably be kicking someone out of their room or tent. As such, you can expect resentment at a time when everyone needs to pull together to survive.

Makeshift Sick Rooms

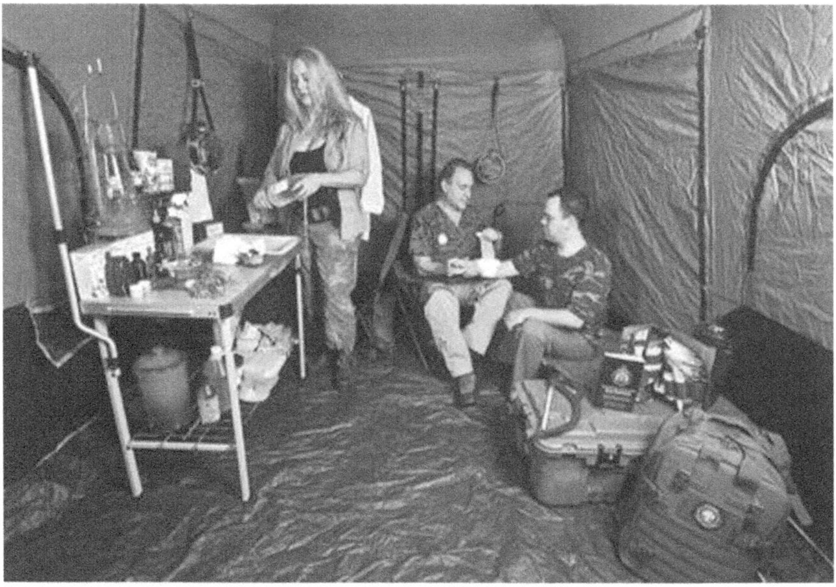

If you don't have a spare room or tent, you'll have to raise a makeshift barrier, such as a sheet of plastic, to separate the sick from the healthy. Even if you have a dedicated sick room, you'll want to keep injured group members separate from those with infectious diseases such as influenza. Although wounds will sometimes become infected, they won't likely be contagious in an otherwise healthy person.

If you're staying in place, your sick room's air conditioning ducts will be close to useless in a power-down scenario, and could actually pose a major risk to the rest of your group. Cover them with duct tape. Keep windows or vent flaps open, however, except in particularly inclement weather.

Furnishings should be minimal, with a work surface, an exam area, and bed spaces. Cloth surfaces, such as upholstered furniture and carpets, can harbor disease-causing organisms and should be avoided if possible. Even bedding for the contagious might best be covered in plastic. The more areas that can be wiped down/disinfected easily, the better.

It's important to have a way to eliminate waste products from your bedridden patients, even if it's just a 5 gallon bucket and some bleach. Have closed containers like hampers available to put used sick room items that need to be cleaned.

A station near the entrance of the room or tent for masks, gloves, gowns, and aprons would be very helpful. You'll should also have a basin with water, soap, or other disinfectant kept for exclusive use by the caregiver. There should only be one person involved in caring for those with contagious illnesses. Thermometers should be dipped in alcohol.

For supplies, get plenty of masks and gloves; gowns can be commercially-made plastic coveralls, full body aprons, or even dry cleaning clothes covers. Many people consider medical supplies to consist of gauze, tourniquets, and battle dressings, but you must also dedicate sets of sheets, towels, pillows, and other items to be used in the sick room. Keep these items separate from the bedding, bathing, and eating materials of the healthy members of your family or group.

The above may seem excessive to you, but you can never have enough dedicated medical supplies. You may save the life of a loved one or even your entire group if you are diligent in putting together your medical stores.

Cleaning supplies should also be considered medical preparedness items. You'll want to clean the sick room thoroughly on a daily basis. Clean hard surfaces that may have germs on them with soap and water, or use other disinfectants such as a 1:10 bleach solution. Pay attention to doorknobs, tables, sinks, toilets, counters, and even toys.

Wash bed sheets and towels frequently; boil them if you have no other way to clean them. They should be considered infected, so wash your hands right after touching them. The same goes for plates, cups, etc. Any equipment brought into the sick room should stay there.

One additional item that will be important to your sick room patients: Give them a noisemaker of some sort that will allow them to alert you when they need help. This will decrease anxiety and give them confidence that you will know when they are in trouble.

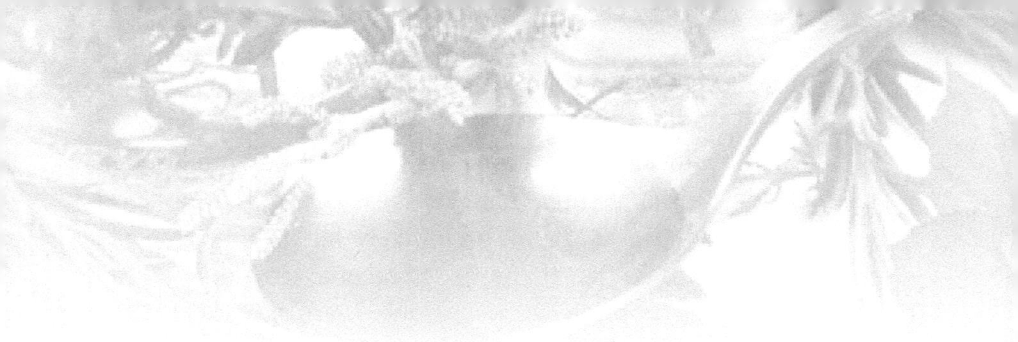

SECTION 5

✚ ✚ ✚

NATURAL DISASTERS AND ENVIRONMENTAL ISSUES

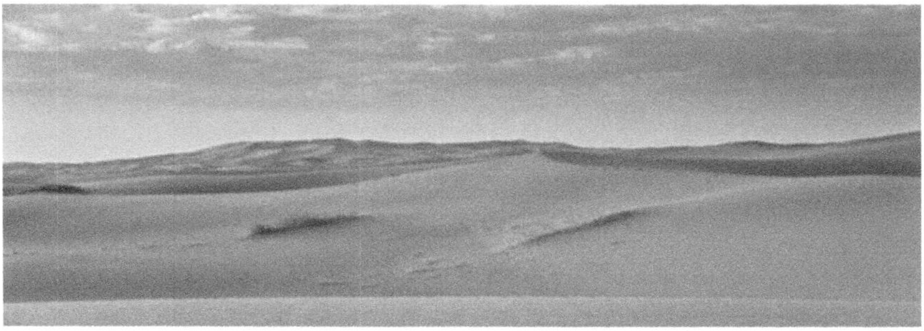

A creature's habitat is the place where it lives. This could be a forest, a lake, the branches of a tree, or the underside of a leaf. If you're a human being, your habitat is likely a town; few humans can call the wilderness their home. When you are in an environment that is not your own, careful planning is necessary to avoid running afoul of the elements.

The focus of your medical training should be general, but also take into account the type of environment that you expect to live in if a collapse occurs. If you live in Miami, it's unlikely you'll be treating a lot of people with hypothermia. If you live in Siberia, it's unlikely you'll be treating a lot of people with heat stroke. Learn how to treat the likely medical issues for the area in which you live.

Dealing with the environment also means being prepared for natural disasters which may occur in your area. If, for example, you live in the part of the United States known as Tornado Alley, you must have access to solid shelter and be ready to handle traumatic injuries. If you do not prepare for disasters, you have made your environment an enemy, and it is a formidable one, indeed.

Temperature-Related Medical Issues

One major environmental risk is the effect of ambient temperature. Humans tolerate a very narrow range and are susceptible to damage as a result of being too cold or too hot. Your body has various methods it uses to control its internal "core" temperature, either raising it or lowering it to appropriate levels. The body core refers to the major internal organ systems that are necessary to maintain life, such as your brain, heart, liver, and others. The remainder (your skin, muscles and extremities) is referred to as the "periphery".

Your body regulates its core temperature in various ways:

- **Vasoconstriction** – blood vessels tighten to decrease flow to periphery, thereby decreasing heat loss.
- **Vasodilation** – blood vessels expand to increase flow, thereby increasing heat loss.
- **Perspiration** – sweat evaporates, causing a cooling effect.
- **Shivering** – muscles produce heat by movements which create warmth.
- **Exertion** – increasing work levels produce heat, decreasing work levels decrease heat.

Your body also regulates its temperature by common sense, adding or subtracting layers of clothing to match the environment.

Illness related to exposure to extreme cold is referred to as "**Hypothermia**". Illness related to exposure to excessive heat is called "**Hyperthermia**", but is better known by the terms "Heat Exhaustion" and "Heat Stroke".

Many environmental causes of illness are preventable with some planning. If you are in a hot environment, don't schedule major outdoor work sessions in the middle of the day. If you absolutely must work in the heat, provide a canopy, hats, sunscreens, and other protection. Be certain that everyone arrives well-hydrated and gets plenty of water throughout. Expect each person to require a pint of water an hour while working in the heat. Failure to take precautions could lead to dehydration (discussed in the section on diarrheal disease), sunburns, and increased likelihood of work injury.

Likewise, those in cold environments should take the weather into account when planning outdoor activities in order to avoid hypothermia issues, such as frostbite. Youngsters especially will run out into the cold without paying much attention to dressing warmly. Adults will often ignore the wind chill factor. Likewise, if someone has had too much to drink, impaired judgment may put them in jeopardy of suffering a cold-related event.

Part of the healthcare provider's role is to educate each and every member of their family or group on proper planning for outdoor activities. Monitor weather conditions as well as the people you're sending out into the heat or cold; otherwise, your people are at significant risk.

HYPERTHERMIA (HEAT-RELATED ISSUES)

In the aftermath of storms or in the wilderness, you may find yourself without shelter to protect you from the elements. In the heat of summer, a common condition you'll encounter might be heat stroke, otherwise known as **hyperthermia**. Even in cold weather, significant physical exertion in an over-clothed and under-hydrated individual could lead to heat injuries. The elderly are particularly prone to issues relating to overheating, and must be watched closely if exposed to the sun.

Heat Exhaustion And Heat Stroke

The ill effects due to overheating are called "**heat exhaustion**" if mild to moderate; if severe, these effects are referred to as "**heat stroke**". Heat exhaustion usually does not result in permanent damage, but heat stroke does; indeed, it can permanently disable or even kill its victim. It is a medical emergency that must be diagnosed and treated promptly.

The risk of heat stroke correlates strongly to the "heat index", a measurement of the effects of air temperature combined with high humidity. Above 60% relative humidity, loss of heat by perspiration is impaired, increasing the chances of heat-related illness. Exposure to full sun increases the reported heat index by as much as 10-15 degrees F. In other words, it is the equivalent of being out in much hotter weather than you would anticipate.

Simply having muscle cramps or a fainting spell does not necessarily signify a major heat-related medical event. You will see "heat cramps" often in children that have been running around on a hot day. Getting them out of the sun, massaging the affected muscles, and providing hydration will usually resolve the problem.

To make the diagnosis of heat exhaustion, a significant rise in the body's core temperature is required. As many heat-related symptoms may mimic other conditions, a thermometer should be a component of your medical supplies.

In addition to muscle cramps and/or fainting, heat exhaustion is characterized by:

- Confusion
- Rapid pulse
- Flushing
- Sweating
- Nausea and Vomiting
- Headache
- Temperature elevation up to 105 degrees F

If no action is taken to cool the victim, heat stroke may ensue. Heat stroke, in addition to all the possible signs and symptoms of heat exhaustion, will manifest as loss of consciousness, seizures or even bleeding (seen in the urine or vomit). Breathing becomes rapid and shallow.

If not dealt with quickly, shock and organ malfunction may ensue, leading to your patient's demise. The skin is likely to be hot to the touch but, unlike heat exhaustion, sweating might be absent. The body makes efforts to cool itself down until it hits a temperature of 106 degrees or so. At that point, thermoregulation breaks down and the body's ability to use sweating as a natural temperature regulator fails. In heat stroke, the body core can rise to 110 degrees Fahrenheit or more.

You'll notice that the skin becomes red, not because it is burned, but because the blood vessels are dilating in an effort to dissipate some of the heat.

In some circumstances, the patient's skin may actually seem cool. It is important to realize that it is the body *core* temperature that is elevated. A person in shock may feel "cold and clammy" to the touch. This finding could mislead you, but simply taking a reading with your thermometer will reveal the patient's true status.

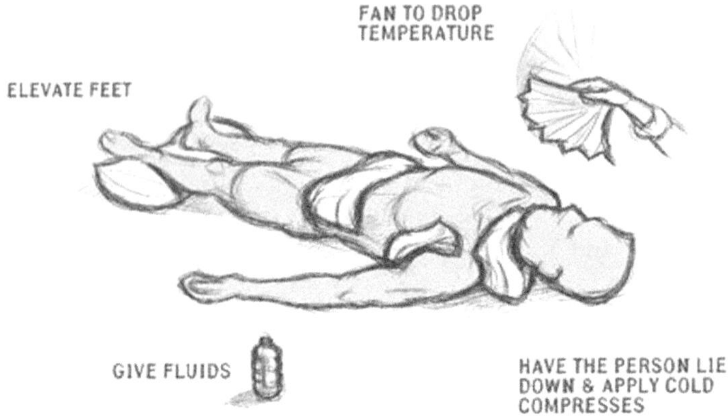

HYPERTHERMIA

Treating Heat Stroke

When overheated patients are no longer able to cool themselves, it is up to their rescuers to do the job. If hyperthermia is suspected, the victim should immediately:

- Be removed from the heat source (for example, the sun).
- Have their clothing removed.
- Be drenched with cool water (or ice, if available).
- Have their legs elevated above the level of their heart (the shock position).
- Be fanned or otherwise ventilated to help with heat evaporation.
- Have moist cold compresses placed in the neck, armpit and groin areas.

Why the neck, armpit and groin? Major blood vessels pass close to the skin in these areas, and you will more efficiently cool the body core. In the wilderness, immersion in a cold stream may be all you have in terms of a cooling strategy. This is a worthwhile option as long as you are closely monitoring your patient.

Oral rehydration is useful to replace fluids lost, but only if the patient is awake and alert. If your patient has altered mental status, fluids may enter their airways; this causes damage to the lungs.

You might think that acetaminophen or ibuprofen could help to lower temperatures, but this is actually not the case. These medications are meant to lower fevers caused by an infection, and they don't work as well if the fever was not caused by one.

Wear clothing appropriate for the weather. Tightly swaddling an infant with blankets, simply because that is "what's done" with a baby, is a recipe for disaster in hot weather. Have everyone wear a head covering. A bandanna soaked in water, for example, would be effective against the heat. Much of the sweating we do comes from our face and head, so towel off frequently to aid in heat evaporation.

If you can avoid dehydration, you will likely avoid heat exhaustion or heat stroke. Work or exercise in hot weather (especially by someone in poor physical condition) will easily cause a person to lose body water content.

A loss of just 1% of your total water initiates the thirst mechanism. You'll need a pint of water an hour to stay hydrated. If thirst is not quenched, as little as 2% water loss begin to affect work efficiency, mood, and other parameters. At 6%, you're as delirious and uncoordinated as if you've been crawling for miles through Death Valley. At 10-20%, organs fail and your patient goes into a coma and may die.

Carefully planning your outdoor work in the summer heat and keeping up with fluids will be a major step in keeping healthy and avoiding heat-related illness. Monitor the workload (and the workers) and you'll stay out of trouble.

HYPOTHERMIA (COLD-RELATED ISSUES)

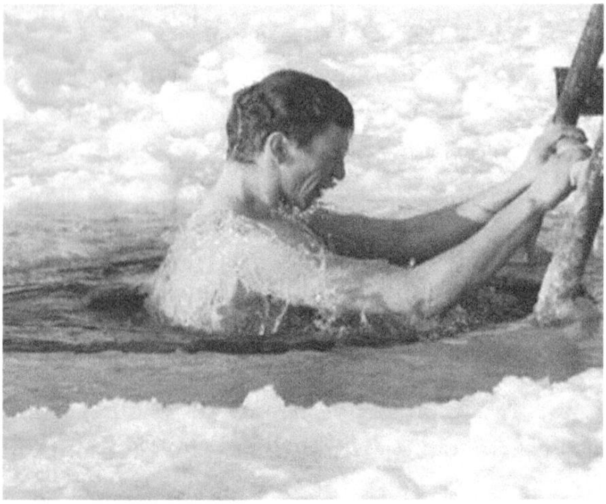

Hypothermia

Hypothermia is a condition in which body core temperature drops below the temperature necessary for normal body function and metabolism. The normal body core temperature is defined as between 97.5-99.5 degrees Fahrenheit (36.0-37.5 degrees Celsius). Cold-related illness occurs once the core temperature dips below 95 degrees (35 degrees Celsius).

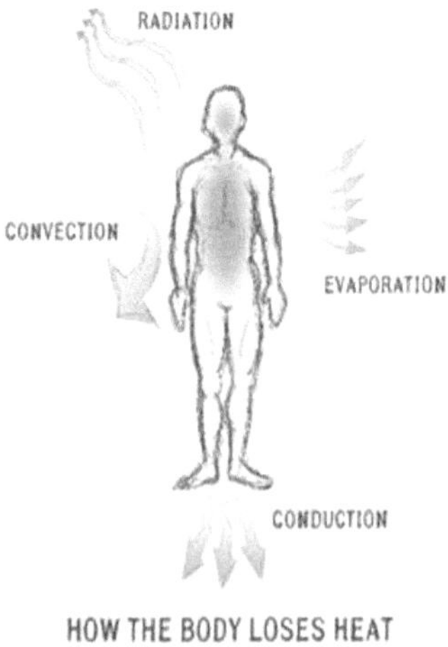

HOW THE BODY LOSES HEAT

The body loses heat in various ways:

Evaporation – the body perspires (sweats), which releases heat from the core.

Radiation – the body loses heat to the environment anytime that the ambient (surrounding) temperature is below the core temperature (say, 98.6 degrees Fahrenheit). For example, you lose more heat if exposed to an outside temperature of 20 degrees F than if exposed to 80 degrees F.

Conduction – The body loses heat when its surface is in direct contact with cold temperatures, as in the case of someone falling from a boat into frigid water. Water, being denser than air, removes heat from the body much faster.

Convection – Heat loss where, for instance, a cooler object is in motion against the body core. The air next to the skin is heated and then removed, which requires the body to use energy to re-heat. **Wind Chill** is one example of air convection: If the ambient temperature is 32 degrees F but the wind chill factor is at 5 degrees F, you lose heat from your body as if it were actually 5 degrees F.

Most heat is lost from the head area, due to its large surface area and tendency to be uncovered. Direct contact with anything cold, especially over a large area of your body, will cause rapid cooling of your body core temperature. The classic example of this would be a fall into cold water. When the Titanic sank in 1912, hundreds of people fell into near-freezing water. Within 15 minutes, they were probably beyond medical help.

The body, when it is exposed to cold, kicks into action to produce heat once the core cools down below 95 degrees Fahrenheit (35 degrees Celsius). The main mechanism to produce heat is shivering. Muscles shiver to produce heat, and this will be the first symptom you're likely to see. As hypothermia worsens, more symptoms will become apparent if the patient is not warmed.

Aside from shivering, the most noticeable symptoms of hypothermia will be related to mental status. The person may appear confused, uncoordinated, and lethargic. As the condition worsens, speech may become slurred; the patient will appear apathetic and uninterested in helping themselves, and may fall asleep. This occurs due to the effect of cooling temperatures on the brain; the colder the body core gets, the slower the brain works. Brain function is supposed to cease at about 68 degrees Fahrenheit, although there have been exceptional cases where people (usually children) survived even lower temperatures.

Prevention of Hypothermia

An ounce of prevention is worth a pound of cure. To prevent hypothermia, you must anticipate the climate that you will be traveling through, including wind conditions and wet weather. Condition yourself physically to be fit for the challenge. Travel with a partner if at all possible, and have enough food and water available for the entire trip.

It may be useful to remember the simple acronym C.O.L.D. This stands for: Cover, Overexertion, Layering, and Dry:

- Cover. Protect your head by wearing a hat. This will prevent body heat from escaping from your head. Instead of using gloves to cover your hands, use mittens. Mittens are more helpful than gloves because they keep your fingers in contact with one another. This conserves heat.
- Overexertion. Avoid activities that cause you to sweat a lot. Cold weather causes you to lose body heat quickly; wet, sweaty clothing accelerates the process. Rest when necessary; use rest periods to self-assess for cold-related changes. Pay careful attention to the status of your elderly or juvenile group members. Diabetics are also at high risk.
- Layering. Loose-fitting, lightweight clothing in layers do the best job of insulating you against the cold. Use tightly woven, water-repellent material for wind protection. Wool or silk inner layers hold body heat better than cotton does. Some synthetic materials, like Gore-Tex, work well also. Especially cover the head, neck, hands and feet.
- Dry. Keep as dry as you can. Get out of wet clothing as soon as possible. It's very easy for snow to get into gloves and boots, so pay particular attention to your hands and feet.

One factor that most people don't take into account is the use of alcohol. Alcohol may give you a "warm" feeling, but it actually causes your blood vessels to expand; this results in more rapid heat loss from the surface of your body. The body reacts to cold by constricting the blood vessels, so expansion from alcohol would negate the body's efforts to stay warm.

Alcohol and recreational drugs also cause impaired judgment. Those under the influence might choose clothing that would not protect them in cold weather.

The diagnosis of hypothermia may be difficult to make with a standard glass thermometer because it doesn't register below 94 degrees Fahrenheit. Unless you have a thermometer that can measure low ranges, it may be difficult to know for certain that you're dealing with this problem. However, if you encounter a person who is unconscious, confused, or lethargic in cold weather and who temperature does not register, assume they are hypothermic until proven otherwise.

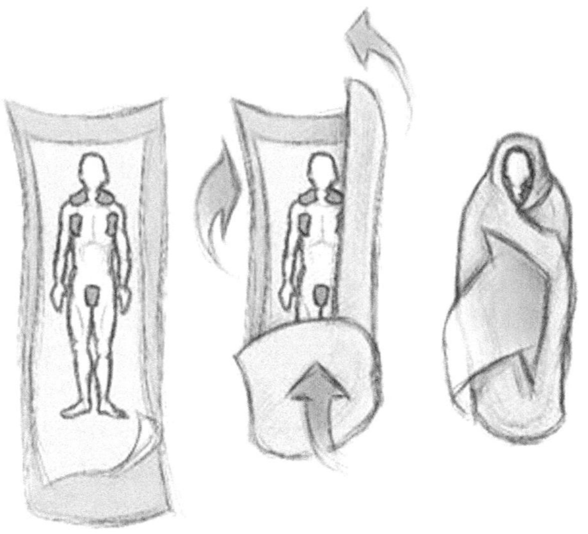

HYPOTHERMIA WRAP

Treating Hypothermia

Immediate action must be taken to reverse the ill effects of hypothermia. Important measures to take are:

- **Get the person out of the cold.** Transport to a warm, dry location. If you're unable to move the person out of the cold, shield them as much as possible. Be sure to place a barrier between them and the cold ground.
- **Monitor breathing.** A person with severe hypothermia may be unconscious. Verify that the patient is breathing and check for a pulse. Begin CPR if necessary.
- **Take off wet clothing.** If the person is wearing wet clothing, remove them gently. Cover them with layers of dry blankets, including the head, but leave the face clear.
- **Share body heat.** To warm the person's body, remove your clothing and lie next to the person, making skin-to-skin contact. Then cover both of your bodies with blankets. Some people may cringe at this notion, but it's important to remember that you are trying to save a life. Gentle massage or rubbing may be helpful, but vigorous movements may be traumatic.
- **Give warm oral fluids**. If the affected person is alert and able to swallow, provide a warm, nonalcoholic, non-caffeinated beverage to help warm the body. Remember, alcohol does not warm you up!
- **Use warm, dry compresses**. Use a first-aid warm compress (a fluid-filled bag that warms up when squeezed), or a makeshift compress of warm (not hot) water in a plastic bottle. Apply a compress only to the neck, chest wall or groin. These areas will spread the heat much better than putting warm compresses on the extremities, which sometimes worsens the condition.
- **Avoid applying direct heat.** Don't use hot water, a heating pad or a heating lamp directly on the person. The extreme heat can damage the skin, cause strain on the heart, or even lead to cardiac arrest.

If left untreated, hypothermia leads to complete failure of various organ systems and death. People who develop hypothermia due to cold exposure are also vulnerable to other cold-related injuries, such as frostbite and immersion foot.

Blizzard Survival

Winter storms occur every year in the United States, and cause fatalities among the unprepared. 70% of deaths occur due to traffic accidents and 25% from being caught outside during the blizzard. If a disaster takes you off the grid but you're still in your home, keep everyone in one room, preferably without windows; the heat from their bodies will make a small room warmer. If you use some form of alternative heat, however, make certain that there is reasonable ventilation.

Winter conditions don't just affect people; they affect cars as well. Cold affects rubber and metal; it even decreases the battery's efficiency. Tires become stiff and flat for the first few hundred yards. Your oil and other lubricants become thicker at cold temperatures. This makes the engine work harder.

Therefore, vehicles that will be doing duty in extreme cold should be "winterized". This involves switching to a lighter viscosity oil, changing to snow tires, and choosing the right (anti-freeze) ratio of coolant to water. Gas tanks should never be less than half full.

Outside

You're not a bear, so you can't hibernate through the cold weather; you'll have to take measures to avoid getting stranded out in the cold. Many deaths from exposure are avoidable if simple precautions are taken

The first thing that you should do before planning a day outdoors in snowy weather is consult your weather radio for the forecast. If a storm is on the way, postpone your outing until the weather improves.

Dress appropriately and in layers. Each successive layer of clothing traps warm air near your body. Wool is the best material for staying warm. Unlike cotton, wool will stay warm even if somewhat wet, and wicks perspiration away from the skin. Wet clothing will cause you to lose body core temperature faster, so have an extra outfit in your backpack.

If you're in the wilderness, seek some form of shelter immediately to get out of the wind. There are more types of shelters than are within the scope of this book, but one can be made in a "tree well". A tree well is the sunken area around the trunk in very deep snow. This area is relatively easy to excavate and, if the tree has low-hanging branches, should provide some protection from falling snow. Look for natural barriers nearby that may serve as windbreaks, but beware of slopes where you may be exposed to drifting snow or avalanches.

The space you dig out should be small, as small shelters take less effort to keep warm than large ones. Pack your snow "walls" well, so that they can retain heat better and support a makeshift roof. Place evergreen boughs and debris on the floor to protect you from the cold ground. Then add some on top to make a roof. Tarps or solar blankets may be used for this purpose, but winds might easily blow them off. Tie rocks to the corners as weights.

If a tree well is not an option, digging a "cave" out of deep snow can serve to insulate you from the wind (think igloo). If you make a fire, be sure to have ventilation holes in your shelter. Entrances and ventilation holes should open at a 90 degree angle to the prevailing winds.

Stay hydrated but don't eat snow. Your body must first melt it and loses heat as a result. If you don't have fire to melt snow, put a container with it in your clothes, but not next to the skin. Hypothermia and other cold-related medical issues are covered elsewhere in this book.

Stranded In The Car

The first question you should ask before you get in the car in cold weather is "Is this trip necessary?". If you don't have to leave the house in a snowstorm, don't. Period. If you do, drive as if your life depended on it, because it does. Don't speed, tailgate, or weave from lane to lane. Make turns slowly and deliberately, and be careful to avoid quick stops and starts.

Let's say that, despite your best efforts, you're stuck on the road in a blizzard. Help may be on the way, but what if it isn't? The first thing to do is to stay calm and don't leave the car. It's warmer there than outside and, at least, you're protected from the wind. Having adequate shelter is one of the keys to survival in the wilderness or on a snow-covered highway.

Wet snow can block up your exhaust system and cause carbon monoxide gas to enter the passenger compartment. You'll need fresh air, but don't crack a window on the side where the wind is coming from. If you're in a group, huddle together as best you can to create a warm pocket in the car. Rub your hands, put them in your armpits, or otherwise keep moving to make your muscles produce heat.

Maybe you can dig yourself out, but beware of overexertion in extreme cold. You'll sweat, and wet clothes are a main cause of hypothermia. If you have flares, use them to let others know you need help.

The Winter Survival Car Kit

There are a number of items that you should always have in your car, especially in cold weather. These are meant to keep you safe if the unthinkable happens and you're stranded without hope of rescue. This is the minimum that the winter survival car kit should contain:

- Wool blankets (for warmth; wool can stay warm even if wet)
- Spare sets of dry clothes, especially socks, hats, and mittens.
- Hard warmers or other instant heat packs (activated by shaking, they'll last for hours)
- Matches, lighters, and fire starters to manufacture heat
- Flashlights and candles (keep batteries in backwards until you need them to extend life).
- Small multi-tool with blade, screwdrivers, pliers, etc.
- Larger combination tool like a foldable Chinese Army shovel (acts as a shovel but also an axe, saw, etc.)
- Sand or rock salt (to give traction where needed)
- Tow chain or rope
- Flares
- Starter cables (for jump starts)
- Water and food (energy bars, MREs, dehydrated soups, candies)
- Baby wipes (for hygiene purposes)

- A medical kit and medications
- Tarp and duct tape (brightly colored ones will be more visible and aid rescue)
- Metal cup or thermos (to melt snow, make soup, etc.)
- Noisemaker (whistle) to signal for help
- Cell phone and charger, weather radio

Of course, a full set of camping supplies would be useful to keep if you have space in your car. The items above will give you a head start in keeping safe and sound even if stranded. With a plan of action, a few supplies, and a little luck, you'll survive even in the worst blizzard.

Frostbite and Immersion (trench) Foot

Frostbite, or freezing of body tissues, usually occurs in the extremities, but sometimes affects the ears and nose. Initial symptoms include a "pins and needles" sensation and numbness. Skin color changes from red at first, then become white and waxy as the condition progresses. As tissues continue to lose circulation, they turn blue. If the color then changes to black, a condition known as "**gangrene**" has set in. Gangrene is the death of tissue resulting from loss of circulation. Once this happens, amputation may be required to eliminate the non-viable parts.

Immersion foot (formerly known as Trench Foot) causes damage to nerves and small blood vessels due to prolonged immersion in water. When seen in areas other than the feet, this condition is referred to as "chilblains". Immersion foot appears similar to frostbite, but might have a more generally swollen appearance.

Frostbite or Immersion Foot is treated with a warm water (no more than 104 degrees F/39 degrees C) soak of the affected extremity for 30-60 minutes or the skin returns to red. Also, 81mg of aspirin or 400-600 mg of ibuprofen can be given for pain and to prevent clots in damaged blood vessels. Follow these treatment tips:

1. Don't allow thawed tissue to freeze again. The more often tissue freezes and thaws, the deeper the damage (think about what happens to a steak that goes from the freezer to outside and back again). If you can't prevent your patient from being exposed to freezing temperatures again, you should wait before treating, but not more than a day.
2. Don't rub or massage frostbitten areas. Rubbing frostbitten tissue will result in damage to already injured tissues.
3. Don't use heat lamps or fires to treat frostbite. Your patient is numb and cannot feel the frostbitten tissue. Significant burns can ensue.
4. You can use body heat to thaw mild frostbite. Put mildly frostbitten fingers under your arm, for example, to warm them up.

Cold Water Safety

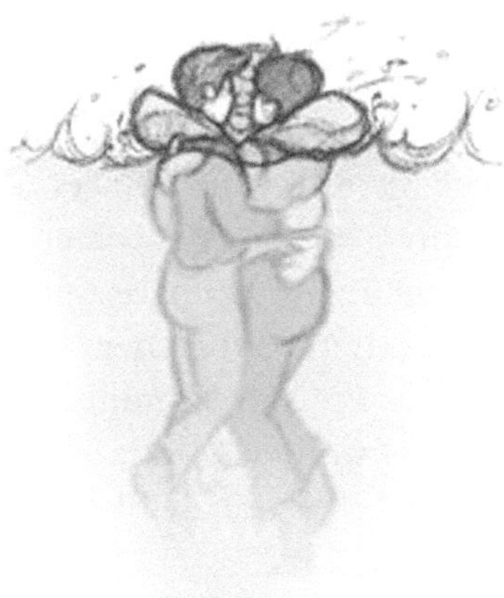

THE HUDDLE

Water doesn't have to be cold to cause hypothermia. Any water that's cooler than normal body temperature will cause heat loss. You could die of hypothermia off a tropical coast if immersed long enough.

In the event that you find yourself in cold water, you'll need to have a strategy that will keep you alive until you're rescued. First, we'll talk about falling into the water when your boat capsizes, and then we'll talk about falling through the ice during a winter hike.

To increase your chances of survival in cold water:

- **Wear a life jacket.** Whenever you're on a boat, wear a life jacket. A life jacket can help you stay alive longer by enabling you to float without using a lot of energy and by providing some insulation. Jackets with built-in whistles are best, so you can signal that you're in distress.
- **Keep your clothes on.** While you're in the water, don't remove your clothing. Button or zip up. Cover your head if at all possible. The layer of water between your clothing and your body is slightly warmer and will help insulate you from the cold. Remove your clothing only after you're safely out of the water and then do whatever you can to get dry and warm.
- **Get out of the water, even if only partially.** The less percentage of your body exposed to cold, the less heat you will lose. Climbing onto a capsized boat or grabbing onto a floating object will increase your chances of survival, even if you can only partially get out of the water. However, don't use up energy swimming unless you have a dry place to swim to.
- **Position your body to lessen heat loss.** Use a body position known as the Heat Escape Lessening Position (think H.E.L.P.) to reduce heat loss while you wait for help to arrive. Just hold your knees to your chest; this will help protect your torso (the body core) from heat loss.
- **Huddle together.** If you've fallen into cold water with others, keep warm by facing each other in a tight circle and holding on to each other.

Falling Through The Ice

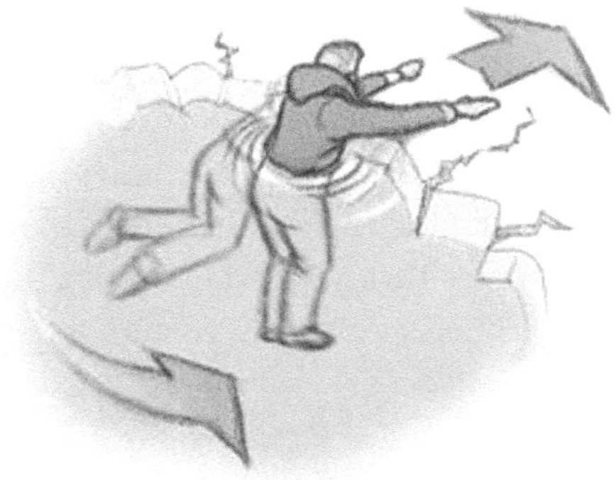

FALL THROUGH THE ICE

What if you're hiking in the wilderness and that snow field turns out to be the icy surface of a lake? Whenever you're out in the wild, it makes sense to take a change of clothes in a waterproof container. This way, you'll have something dry to wear if you get wet. Also, have a fire starter that will work even when wet.

Ice can handle the weight of an average human if four or more inches thick. This "safe" thickness may be undermined, however, by flowing water just below the surface, which weakens the underside of the ice. When it comes to walking on ice, safety is never guaranteed.

Knowing the above, you might be able to identify weaker areas in the ice. Is the ice on the edge of the water body firm? If it's slushy or cracked, it's unlikely to be safe. Slushy ice is deteriorating and not a reliable walking surface. The safest ice to be on is clear blue in color due to higher density, although testing for thickness with an ice pick or auger is prudent.

Thinner areas of ice tend to be darker in color. Ice that thaws and refreezes in layers might be white in color, but is questionable due to air pockets. Areas of contrasting colors indicate an uneven thickness and should be avoided.

If you run afoul of thin ice, you will fall through. Your body will react to a sudden immersion in cold water by an increased pulse rate, blood pressure, and respirations. Although it won't be easy, make every effort to keep calm. You have a few minutes to get out before you succumb to the effects of the cold. Panic is your enemy.

Get your head out of the water by breathing in and bending backward. Tread water and quickly get rid of any heavy objects that are weighing you down. Keep your clothing on, though. It has air pockets that are helping you stay buoyant. Turn your body in the direction of where you came from; you know the ice was strong enough to hold you there.

Now, try to lift up out of the ice using your hands and arms. Keep them spread in front of you. Kick with your feet to give some forward momentum. At the same time, try to get more of your body out of the water. An ice pick in each hand will help gain a handhold, and should be carried by anyone who expects to be traveling on ice.

Lift a leg onto the ice and then lift and roll out onto the firmer surface. Do not stand up! Keep rolling in the direction that you were walking before you fell through. This will spread your weight out, instead of concentrating it on your feet. Then crawl away until you are sure that you're safe. Start working to get warm immediately.

Avalanche Preparedness

Snow slides are part and parcel of the winter wilderness experience, and it pays to know what to do if you're caught in one. This is not just good advice for skiers or backcountry campers; anyone driving on mountain roads in winter or bugging out to a remote location could get caught in an avalanche if not prepared.

Besides general hypothermia, there are a variety of ways that you can die as a victim of a snow slide.

- Trauma: serious injury is not uncommon in an avalanche, and not just due to the weight of the snow. Debris, such as rocks, branches, and even entire trees, can be carried along in the cascade.
- Suffocation: it isn't unusual to die due to asphyxiation when buried in the snow. Densely packed snow is like concrete, and

many victims may find themselves immobilized and unable to help themselves.

Hypothermia is, surprisingly, the cause of death in only a small percentage of avalanche victims. It's much more likely that they will perish due to traumatic injury or suffocation before they freeze to death. Factors involved in deciding your fate include the density of the snowpack, air pockets for breathing, position of the body in the snow, injuries sustained, and whether you brought rescue equipment along.

On any wilderness trek, it makes sense to go in a group. That goes for avalanche country as well, except for one thing: Space your party out far enough so that there's not too much weight on any one area of snow.

Besides cold weather clothing, specialized gear for the mountaineer would include:

- **An avalanche beacon:** A device that emits a pulsed radio signal. Everyone in the group carries one. If a member gets buried in an avalanche, the rest of the party picks up the signal from under the snow. The receivers interpret the signal into a display that aids the search.
- **An avalanche shovel:** Short aluminum shovels that fit inside your backpack and help chop and remove snow and debris over a buried hiker. These shovels usually have telescoping shafts. Shovels with "D-shaped" grips may be advisable, as they can be used with mittens.
- **An avalanche probe**: Essentially, a stick 2 meters in length or more that helps you pinpoint the exact location of an avalanche victim. You can use it to tell a victim under the snow from the ground: The victim will feel softer than the surrounding terrain.
- **A helmet:** Many fatalities occur due to head trauma from rocks and debris flung around by the snow. A helmet is a wise choice for any mountain hiker, skier, or snowboarder.
- **Skier's Air Bags:** Relatively new, these brightly colored air bags auto-inflate with a trigger. They work like a life jacket to keep you buoyant and, therefore, closer to the surface of the snow. An excellent new addition to your backpack, it will also help you stay buoyant in a fall through the ice.

As the avalanche begins

90% of avalanches are triggered by the victim. To survive, rapid action will be needed:

Yell: Let everyone in your group know that you're in trouble. At the very start of the slide, wave your arms and shout as loud as you can to alert as many people as possible to your location.

Move: If you started the avalanche, you may notice a crevice forming in the snow. Jump uphill of it quickly and you might not get carried off. If this isn't an option, run sideways as fast as you can away from the center_of the event. That's where the snow will be moving fastest and with the most force.

Get Lighter: Heavier objects sink in snow, so jettison a non-airbag backpack and unnecessary heavy equipment so that you'll be closer to the surface. Throwing off something light isn't a bad idea either: A loose glove or hat on top of the snow could signal rescuers to your general location and save precious time. Deploy your avalanche air bag if you have one.

Hug a tree (or rock): If the avalanche is relatively small, you could grab the nearest immobile object and hold on for dear life. In a very large avalanche, trees and rocks may not be safe anchors; trees can be uprooted by the sheer force of the snow slide.

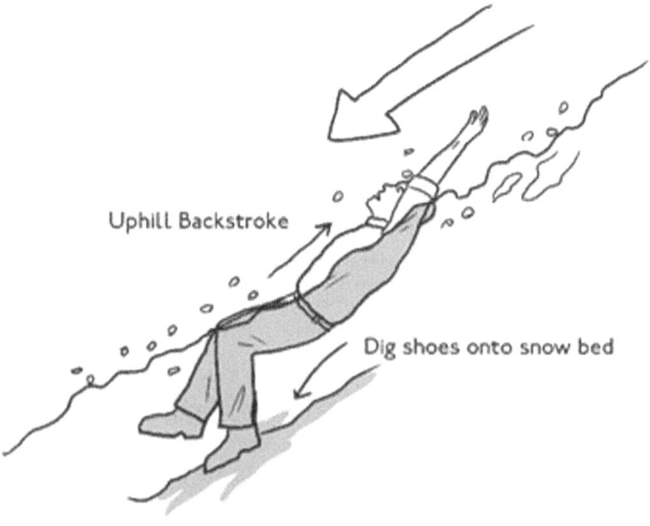

Swim! The key is to stay as close to the top of the snow as possible. Increase your surface area by spreading your legs (feet downhill) and raising your hands. While in this position, swing your arms while trying to stay on your back (easier to breathe if face up), similar to swimming backstroke. Try to keep your foot on top of the moving snow bed. With any luck, this strategy will keep you towards the surface of the snow.

Buried in the snow

You did your best, but still got completely buried in the snow. You've got little more than 15 minutes, on average, before you suffocate. Snow may be porous, but warm breath melts the snow which then refreezes as solid ice. This makes breathing difficult.

As the snow slows: The larger the air pocket you have, the longer you'll survive. As the avalanche slows to a stop, put one arm in front of your face in such a way as to form a space that will give you the most air. If possible, raise the other arm straight up toward the avalanche surface. Your glove might signal your location to rescuers. Expand your chest by breathing deeply; this will give you more room to breathe once the snow has settled.

Once buried: Once you are completely buried, the snowpack may be so dense as to prevent you from moving. Stay calm, in order to use up less oxygen. If you're not sure which way is up, spit. The spit will go towards the ground due to gravity. If you can move, work to make a bigger air pocket towards the direction of the surface.

You'll only have a second or two to act to avoid most avalanches. Rapid action, and some basic rescue equipment, may prevent you from being the harsh winter's latest victim.

ALTITUDE SICKNESS

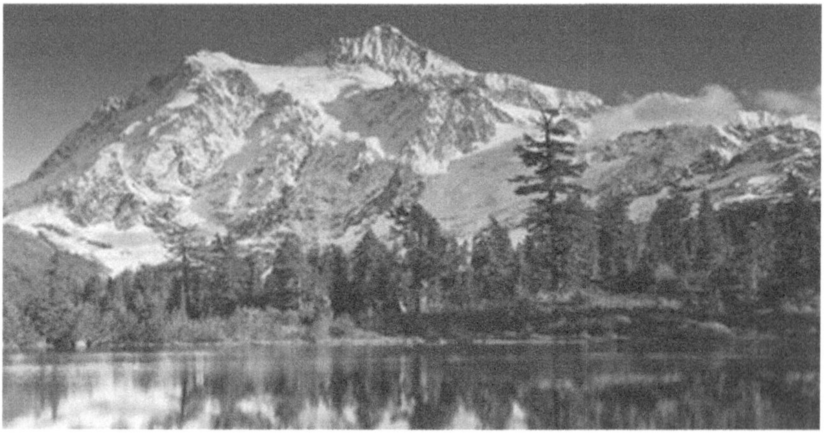

In any survival situation, we might find ourselves having to relocate from a home at sea level to a "bug-out" location in the mountains. When this becomes necessary, it's likely that you will be moving fast. The rapid change in elevation will, for some, cause a condition known as **Altitude Sickness** or Acute Mountain Sickness (AMS). This occurs as a result of entering an area with lower oxygen availability and reduced air pressures without first acclimating oneself. Altitude sickness occurs most commonly at elevations approaching 8,000 feet above sea level. It is aggravated by exertion, something you certainly will have to do if you're traveling by foot.

Although Altitude Sickness is usually a temporary condition, some patients may develop complications in the form of "**edema**" of certain organs. Edema is the accumulation of fluid. In altitude sickness, it may occur in the lungs ("pulmonary edema") or brain ("cerebral edema"). Either of these conditions can be life-threatening.

Like many illnesses, the best strategy against altitude sickness is prevention. Choose your route to your retreat so that the ascent is as gradual as possible. Do not attempt more than 2,000 feet of ascent per day. Ensure that your personnel do not become dehydrated as they ascend, and, especially, avoid the consumption of alcohol.

Some normal people may be susceptible to AMS at lower elevations than others. If you have no choice but to make a rapid ascent, close monitoring of every member of your party will be important. You will usually see patients present to you with symptoms similar to a hangover or influenza (minus the fever). If mild, you will commonly see:

- Fatigue
- Insomnia
- Dizziness
- Headaches
- Nausea and Vomiting
- Lack of appetite
- Tachycardia (fast heart rate)
- "Pins and Needles" sensations
- Shortness of breath

Those who will have major complications of altitude sickness will present with the following:

- Severe shortness of breath
- Confused and apathetic behavior
- Cough and chest congestion (not nasal)
- Cyanosis (blue or gray appearance of the skin, especially the fingertips and lips)
- Loss of coordination
- Dehydration
- Hemoptysis (coughing up blood)
- Loss of consciousness

Treating altitude sickness requires rest, if only to stop further ascent and allow more time to acclimate. It may be wisest to go back down to a lower elevation. If available, a portable oxygen tank will be useful upon onset of symptoms. A diet high in carbohydrates is thought to reduce ill effects.

A medication commonly used for both prevention and treatment is the prescription drug Acetazolamide (Diamox). It has a "**diuretic**" effect, which means that it speeds the elimination of excess fluid from the body by urination. Therefore, it will help prevent the accumulation of fluid in the lungs or brain.

Acetazolamide is superior to many other diuretics in that it also forces the kidneys to excrete bicarbonate. By increasing the amount of bicarbonate excreted, the blood becomes more acidic. Acidifying the blood stimulates ventilation, which increases the amount of oxygen in the body. This effect may not be immediate, but will speed up recovery.

Usual dosages of Acetazolamide are 125 to 1,000 mg daily, preferably starting a couple of days before the planned ascent. The medicine can serve to prevent as well as to treat altitude sickness.

Other medicines known to have a beneficial effect include the blood pressure medication Nifedipine and the steroid Decadron, especially in those with edema in the lungs and brain.

When you visit your physician, notify him that you are planning a trip into high elevations and would like to avoid altitude sickness. Usually, you will be given an Acetazolamide prescription in case of emergency. The other medications mentioned will be more difficult to obtain, however, and may have more side effects.

There is some evidence that Gingko Biloba may be helpful in the natural prevention of altitude sickness. A small amount of an extract of this substance has been shown to allow the brain to tolerate lower oxygen levels.

WILDFIRE PREPAREDNESS

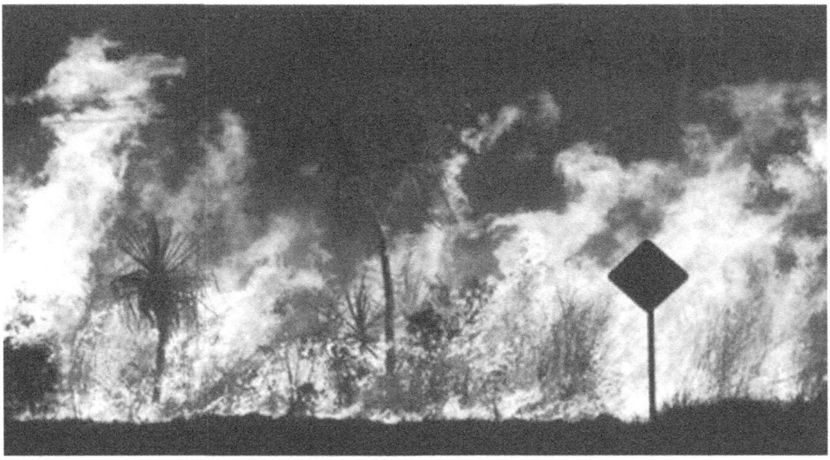

Many in the preparedness community either already have or are planning to have a rural retreat. This means that, if you expect to live or at least spend time in a remote location, you'll have the responsibility to defend it from acts of nature such as the occasional wildfire.

Fire is one of nature's ways to renew the land. Some seeds, such as those of the lodgepole pine, actually require fire to help them germinate. Despite the long-term beneficial effect to the forest, fire is an issue that presents a danger to the humans in it. Although wildfires may occur at any time of year, summertime in drought-prone areas is particularly dangerous.

Once you are in your homestead or long-term retreat, you'll have to take a look around to evaluate the risk level of natural as well as man-made catastrophes. A basic strategy is what we call "vegetation management". Your goal is to direct fires away from your shelter.

There are a few ways to accomplish this. One is to eliminate potential fuel by cleaning up dead wood from the ground close to the building and off the roof. Another is to situate your woodpile away from other structures.

Also, you'll have to remove some of the living vegetation from around your home. This is counter to some advice you'll get regarding keeping your home invisible, and it means that you'd have to remove those thorny bushes you've planted under your windows for defense purposes. This can be a tough decision, but you just might have to make a choice between fire protection and privacy.

Another factor to consider is the material that your retreat is made of. How much fire resistance does your structure have? A wood frame home with wooden shingles will go up like a match in a wildfire. If you are constructing a place to live in times of trouble, you should try to build as much flame resistance into your home as possible.

Defensible Spaces

So, let's create a **defensible space**. A defensible space is an area around a structure where wood and vegetation are treated, cleared, or reduced to slow the spread of wildfire towards a structure. Having a defensible space will also provide room to work for those fighting the fire.

The amount of defensible space you'll need depends on whether you're on flat land or on a steep slope. Flatland fires spread more slowly than a fire on a slope because hot air and flames rise. A fire on a steep slope with wind blowing uphill will spread quickly and produces "**spot fires**". These are small fires that ignite vegetation ahead of the main burn, due to small bits of burning debris in the air.

Some landscaping may be necessary to decrease the chance of fire spreading in your direction. You'll want to thin out those thick canopied trees near your house. Any nearby tree within 50 feet on flat land, or 200 feet downhill from your retreat on top of the mountain, needs to be thinned. You should prune branches below 10-12 feet high, and separate trees by at least 10-20 feet. Also, eliminate all shrubs at the base of the trunks.

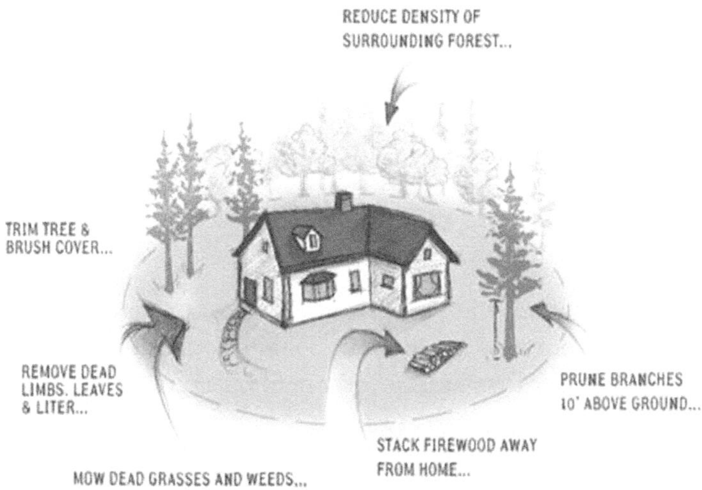

WILD FIRE SAFETY

Of course, once you have a defensible space, the natural inclination is to want to defend it, even against a forest fire. Unfortunately, you have to remember that you'll be in the middle of a lot of heat and smoke. Unless you're a 22 year old Navy Seal in full fire gear and mask, you're probably not going to be able to function effectively.

Even if you *are* a 22 year old Navy Seal, you'll have to take the others under your care into account. The safest option for all involved would be to hit the road if there's a way out. It's a personal decision, but it should also be a realistic one.

If you're leaving, have your supplies already in the car, as well as any important papers you might need to take (don't forget some cash). If you have electricity, make sure you shut off any air conditioning system that draws air into the house from outside. Turn off all your appliances, close all your windows and lock all your doors. Like any other emergency, you should have some form of communication open with your loved ones so that you can contact each other.

If you find yourself in the middle of a fire, make sure you're dressed in long pants and sleeves and heavy boots. A wool blanket is very helpful as an additional outside layer because wool is relatively fire-resistant. If you don't have wool blankets, this is a good time to add some to your storage; keep some in your car.

If you're in a building, stay on the side of the building farthest from the fire outside. Choose a room with the least number of windows (windows transfer heat to the inside). Stay there until you have to leave due to smoke or the building catching fire.

If that's the case and you have to leave, wrap yourself in a blanket, leaving only your eyes uncovered. Some people think it's a good idea to wet the blanket first; it isn't. Wet materials transfer heat much faster than dry materials and can cause severe burns.

If you're having trouble breathing because of the smoke, stay low. Crawl out of the building if you have to. There's less smoke and heat the lower you go. Keep your face down towards the floor to protect your airways. Make sure to have some eye wash in your medical kit, as smoke is a major irritant.

If you ever encounter a person that is actually on fire, you have to act quickly. In circumstances where a person's clothes are on fire, remember the old adage "**Stop, Drop, and Roll**".

- **Stop:** Your patient will be panicked and likely running around trying to put out the flames. This generates wind which will fan the flames. Stop the patient from running away.
- **Drop:** Knock the patient to the ground and wrap tightly with a wool blanket. Heavy fabrics are best.
- **Roll:** Roll the patient on the floor until the flames are extinguished. Immediately cool any burned areas of skin with copious amounts of water.

Smoke Inhalation

Other than burns, which are discussed in another part of this book, you can become seriously ill or even die simply from inhaling too much smoke. Remember, you can heal burns on your skin, but you can't heal burns in your lungs. The scars from the burns will damage the lungs' ability to absorb oxygen. Damage from smoke inhalation can occur in several ways:

- **Simple Combustion:** Combustion uses up oxygen near a fire and can kill a person simply from oxygen deficit. This is called "**hypoxia**". The larger the fire, the more oxygen it removes from the area. This is particularly dangerous in a closed space, such as a building fire.
- **Carbon Dioxide:** Some by-products of smoke may not directly kill a person, but could take up the space in the lungs that oxygen would ordinarily use.
- **Chemical irritants:** Many chemicals founds in smoke can cause injury when they come in contact with the lung. This amounts to a burn inside the lung tissue, which causes swelling and airway obstruction. Chlorine gas, used in World War I, is an example of a deadly chemical irritant.
- **Other asphyxiants:** Carbon monoxide, cyanide, and some sulfides may interfere with the body's ability to utilize oxygen.

Symptoms of smoke inhalation may include:

- Cough
- Shortness of breath
- Hoarseness
- Upper airway spasm
- Eye irritation
- Headaches
- Pale, bluish or even bright red skin
- Loss of consciousness leading to coma or death

Your evaluation of the patient with smoke inhalation may show soot around the mouth, in the throat, and in nasal passages. All of these areas may be swollen and inflamed. The victim will likely be short of breath and have a hoarse voice.

Of course, you will want to get your patient out of the smoky area and into an environment where there is clean air. This may not be as easy as it seems in a major fire. You must be very careful not to put yourself in a situation where you are likely to succumb to smoke inhalation yourself. Always consider a surgical mask or even a gas mask before entering a conflagration to rescue a victim.

It is important to have some way to deliver oxygen to your patient if needed. There are many portable commercially-available canisters which would be useful to get oxygen quickly into the lungs.

Don't expect a rapid recovery from significant smoke inhalation. Your patient will become short of breath with the slightest activity. These symptoms may go away with time, or may become permanent disabilities.

Prevention by planning escape routes and having regular drills will allow your people to get out of dangerous situations quickly. Make sure everyone knows what to do in advance.

TORNADO PREPAREDNESS

There are many natural disasters that might befall a community, but one of the most unpredictable is a tornado. Every year, hundreds of people are killed by these storms, but many injuries and deaths may be avoided with sound preparation.

A **tornado** is a violently rotating column of air that is in contact with both the surface of the earth and the thunderstorm (sometimes called a "**supercell**") that spawned it. From a distance, tornadoes usually appear in the form of a visible dark funnel with all sorts of flying debris in and around it. Because of rainfall, they may be difficult to see when close up.

A tornado (also called a "twister") may have winds of up to 300 miles per hour, and can travel for a number of kilometers or miles before petering out. They may be accompanied by hail and will emit a roaring sound that will remind you of a passing train. We have personally experienced this at our own home, and we can tell you that it is terrifying.

There are almost a thousand tornadoes in the United States every year, more than are reported in any other country. Most of these occur in "Tornado Alley", an area that encompasses areas of Texas, Oklahoma, Missouri, Kansas, Arkansas, and neighboring states. Spring and early summer are the peak seasons.

Injuries from tornadoes usually come as a result of trauma from the flying debris that is carried along with it. Strong winds can carry large objects and fling them around in a manner that is hard to believe. Indeed, there is a report that, in 1931, an 83 ton train was lifted and thrown 80 feet from the tracks.

Tornadoes are categorized as level 0-5 by the Enhanced Fujita Scale, which is based on wind speeds and the amount of damage caused:

- **F0** Light: Winds 40-72 miles per hour; smaller trees uprooted or branches broken, mild structural damage
- **F1** Moderate: winds 73–112 miles per hour; Broken windows, small tree trunks broken, overturned mobile homes, destruction of carports or toolsheds, roof tiles missing

- **F2** Considerable: winds 113–157 miles per hour; Mobile homes destroyed, major structural damage to frame homes due to flying debris, some large trees snapped in half or uprooted
- **F3** Severe: winds 158–206 miles per hour; Roofs torn from homes, small frame homes destroyed, most trees snapped and uprooted
- **F4** Devastating: winds 207–260 miles per hour; Strong-structure buildings damaged or destroyed or lifted from foundations, cars lifted and blown away, even large debris airborne
- **F5** Incredible: winds 261–318 miles per hour; Larger buildings lifted from foundations, trees snapped, uprooted and debarked, objects weighing more than a ton become airborne missiles

Although some places may have sirens or other methods of warning you of an approaching twister, it is important to plan for your family to weather the storm. Having a plan *before* a tornado touches down is the most likely way you will survive the event. Children should be taught where to find the medical kits and how to use a fire extinguisher. If appropriate, teach everyone how to safely turn off the gas and electricity.

When you are in the path of a tornado, take shelter immediately unless you live in a mobile home. These are especially vulnerable to damage from the winds. If there is time, get to the nearest building that has a tornado shelter; underground shelters are best.

If you live in Tornado Alley, consider putting together your own underground shelter. Unlike bunkers and other structures built for long-term use, a tornado shelter only has to provide safety for a short period of time. As such, it doesn't have to be very large; 8-10 square feet per person would be acceptable. Despite this, be sure to consider ventilation and the comfort or special needs of those using the shelter.

If you don't have a shelter, find the safest place in the house where family members can gather. Basements, bathrooms, closets or inside rooms without windows are the best options. Windows can easily shatter from impact due to flying debris.

For added protection, get under a heavy object such as a sturdy table. Covering your body with a sleeping bag or mattress will provide an additional shield. Discuss this plan of action with every member of your family often, so that they will know this process by heart.

If you're in a car and can drive to a shelter, do so. Although you may be hesitant to leave your vehicle, remember that they can be easily tossed around by high winds; you may be safer if there is a culvert or other area lower than the roadway. It is not safe to hide under a bridge or overpass, however, as the winds can easily reach you.

In town, leaving the car to enter a sturdy building is appropriate. If there is no other shelter, however, staying in your car will protect you from some of the flying debris. Keep your seat belt on, put your head down below the level of the windows, and cover yourself if at all possible.

If you're out hiking when the tornado hits, get away from heavily wooded areas. Torn branches and other debris become missiles, so an open field or ditch may be safer. Lying down flat in a ditch or other low spot in the ground will give you some protection. Make sure to cover your head if at all possible, even if it's just with your hands.

HURRICANE PREPAREDNESS

A hurricane is a large tropical storm with winds that reach a constant speed of 74 miles per hour or more. In the United States, hurricanes regularly ravage the Gulf and East Coasts, causing billions of dollars of damage. Even in high-risk hurricane zones, most people are completely unprepared for the severe rain, winds, flooding, and general mayhem that these storms can cause.

Certainly, these storms can be severe, but they don't have to be life-threatening. Unlike tornadoes, which can pop up suddenly, hurricanes are first identified when they are hundreds, if not thousands of miles away. We can watch their development and have a good idea of how bad the storm might get and how much time we have to get ready. Unfortunately, they can affect a lot more area than the average tornado.

Hurricanes are categorized based on wind speed. The Saffir-Simpson Hurricane Wind Scale uses "maximum sustained" winds, meaning continuously reaching up to the numbers below when the storm hits:

- Category 1: 74-95 miles per hour
- Category 2: 96-110 miles per hour
- Category 3: 111-130 miles per hour
- Category 4: 131-155 miles per hour
- Category 5: Greater than 155 miles per hour

Higher category storms may cause incredible damage and loss of life, such as occurred in Hurricane Katrina in 2005. You will have to put together an effective plan of action with regards to shelter, food, power, and other important issues. You may also have to make a decision regarding evacuation. Unlike some disaster scenarios, you can actually outrun one of these storms if you get enough of a head start.

If you live on the coast or by a river, there will be rising waters (the "storm surge") that may cause dangerous flooding. The authorities will issue an evacuation order in many cases. If you live in prefabricated housing, such as a trailer, or near the coast, it is the wisest course of action.

Cities may no longer have plans for civil defense, but they still do for hurricanes in regions at risk. Oftentimes, the municipality will assign a hurricane-resistant public building in your own community as a designated shelter.

If you do choose to leave town, plan to go as far inland as possible. Hurricanes gain strength from the warm water temperatures over the tropical ocean; they lose strength quickly as they travel over land. Despite this, Hurricane Wilma in 2005 hit Florida's West Coast and still caused damage to our home just a few miles from Florida's East Coast.

It might be a wise move to make reservations at a hotel early; there will be little room at the inn for latecomers. In any case, this is the time to check out that "bug-out bag" to make sure it's ready to go. Although most people pack for 72 hours off the grid, that number is relatively arbitrary; be prepared to at least have a week's supply of food, drinking water, clothing, and medical supplies.

Usually, you will not be ordered to evacuate except in the most extreme cases. As such, your preparations will determine how much damage you sustain. You should have an idea of what your home's weak spots are. Do you know what amount of sustained winds your structure can withstand?

Since South Florida was devastated by Hurricane Andrew in 1992, new homes there must have the strength to withstand 125 mph winds. Most homes, however, are made to handle 90 mph (minimum hurricane strength is >74 mph). If the coming storm has sustained winds over that level, you may not be able to depend on the structural integrity of your home.

If you decide to stay, make sure you designate a safe room somewhere in the interior of the house. It should be in a part of the home most downwind from the direction of the oncoming hurricane. Figure out who's coming to ride out the storm with you, and plan for any special needs they may have.

Make provisions for any animals you will be sheltering and move all outdoor furniture and potted plants either inside the house or up against the outside wall, preferably secured with chains. Don't forget to put up the hurricane shutters if you have them.

One special issue peculiar to South Florida is coconuts: They turn into cannonballs in a hurricane. Cut them off the tree before the winds come. Interestingly, the palm trees themselves, as they don't have a dense crown, seem to weather most high winds without a problem. Many other trees can't say the same; prune them to allow wind to flow through.

Indoor planning is important, as well. Communications may be out in a major storm, so have a NOAA weather radio and lots of fresh batteries. You will likely lose power, so keep your gas and propane tanks filled. Install foot and head bolts on double entry doors.

As the storm approaches, you'll want to fill up bathtubs and other containers with water. Turn your refrigerator and freezer down to their coldest settings, so that food won't spoil right away if the power fails. Make sure you know how to shut off the electricity, gas, and water, if necessary.

There's another kind of power you should be concerned about. In the aftermath of a storm, credit card verification may be down; without cash, you may have no *purchasing* power at all.

Of course, have some waterproof tarps available, in case of lost roof shingles. Roofers are going to be pretty busy after a major storm, and might not get to you right away. In South Florida after Hurricane Wilma, there were still blue tarps on roofs more than a year later.

If you've hunkered down in your home during the storm, make sure that you've got books, board games, and light sources for when the power goes down. Kids (and most adults) go stir crazy when stuck inside, especially if they don't have smartphones or computers in service. Here's where you will finally be thankful for those battery-powered hand-held gaming devices.

Take time to discuss the coming storm with your family in advance so everyone will have an idea of what to expect. This will keep fear down to a minimum. Give the kids some responsibility, as well. Give them the opportunity to pack their own bag or select games to play. Keep their minds busy and their nerves calm.

After the storm, inland flood water may be polluted. Do not walk around in, drink nor bathe in this water. Thorough sterilization is required using some of the methods discussed earlier in this book. Do not eat fresh food that has come in contact with floodwater; if cans of food have been exposed to the water, wash them off with soap and clean, hot water before opening.

Also, watch for downed power lines; they have been the cause of a number of electrocutions in the aftermath of a storm. In some cases, entire families have lost their lives jumping into electrified water to save a relative. You should never touch someone who has been electrocuted without first shutting off the power source; if you can't shut off the power, you will have to move the victim. Use a nonmetal object, such as a wooden broom handle or dry rope. If you don't, the current could pass through their body and shock you.

EARTHQUAKE PREPAREDNESS

Hurricanes are more significant for residents of the Gulf or East Coasts of the United States, but the West Coast and even some areas of the Midwest have another disaster to worry about: **Earthquakes**. Some populated areas are near "fault lines". A **fault** is a fracture in a volume of base rock. This is an area where earth movement releases energy that can cause major surface disruptions. This movement is sometimes called a "seismic wave".

The strength of an earthquake has been historically measured using the Richter scale. This measurement (from 0-10 or more) identifies the magnitude of tremors at a certain location. Quakes less than 2.0 on the Richter scale may occur every day, but are unlikely to be noticed by the average person. Each increase of 1.0 magnitude increases the strength by a factor of 10. The highest registered earthquake was The Great Chilean Earthquake of 1960 (9.5 on the Richter scale).

A newer measurement, the Moment Magnitude scale, calculates each point of magnitude as releasing more than 30 times the energy of the previous one. It is considered more accurate than the Richter scale, especially for higher magnitude earthquakes.

If the energy is released offshore, a "**tsunami**" or tidal wave may be generated. In Fukushima, Japan, a powerful earthquake (8.9 magnitude) and tsunami wreaked havoc in 2011, causing major damage, loss of life, and meltdowns in local nuclear reactors.

A major earthquake is especially dangerous due to its unpredictability. There is usually little notice given beforehand. Make sure each member of your family knows what to do no matter where they are when an earthquake occurs. Unless it happens in the dead of night, it's unlikely you will all be in the house together. Planning ahead will give you the best chance of gathering your family together and making the best of a bad situation.

To be prepared, you'll need, at the very least, the following:

- Food and water
- Power sources

- Alternative shelters
- Medical supplies
- Clothing appropriate to the weather
- Fire extinguishers
- Means of communication
- Money (don't count on credit or debit cards if the power's down)
- An adjustable wrench to turn off gas or water

Figure out where you'll meet in the event of tremors. Find out the school system's plan for earthquakes so you'll know where to find your kids. It would be appropriate to always have a "get-home" bag put together at work or in the car. Some food, liquids, and a pair of sturdy, comfortable shoes are useful items to have available.

Especially important to know is where your gas, electric, and water main shutoffs are. Make sure that everyone has an idea of how to turn them off if there is a leak or electrical short. Know where the nearest medical facility is, but be aware that you may be on your own; medical responders are going to be overwhelmed and may not get to you quickly.

Look around your house for fixtures like chandeliers and bookcases that might not be stable enough to withstand an earthquake. Flat screen TVs, especially large ones, could easily topple. Be sure to check out kitchen and pantry shelves, and the stability of anything hanging over the headboard of your bed.

What should you do when the tremors start? If you're indoors, get under a table, desk, or something else solid and hold on. If cover isn't available, stand against an inside wall. Don't try to use elevators. You should stay clear of windows, shelves, and kitchen areas.

While the building is shaking, don't try to run out; you could easily fall down stairs or get hit by falling debris. We had always thought you should stand in the doorway because of the frame's sturdiness, but it turns out that, in modern homes, doorways aren't any more solid than any other part of the structure.

Once the initial tremors are over, go outside. Once there, stay as far out in the open as possible, away from power lines, chimneys, and anything else that could fall on top of you.

You could, possibly, be in your automobile when the earthquake hits. Get out of traffic as quickly as possible; other drivers are likely to be less level-headed than you are. Don't stop your car under bridges, trees, overpasses, power lines, or light posts. Stay in your vehicle while the tremors are active.

One issue to be concerned about is gas leaks; make sure you don't use your camp stoves, lighters, or even matches until you're certain all is clear. Even a match could ignite a spark that could lead to an explosion. If you turned the gas off, you might consider letting the utility company turn it back on.

Don't count on telephone service after a natural disaster. Telephone companies only have enough lines to deal with 20% of total call volume at any one time. It's likely all lines will be occupied. Interestingly, this doesn't seem to apply to texts; you'll have a better to chance to communicate by texting than by voice due to the wavelength used.

FLOOD PREPAREDNESS

After a discussion of tornadoes, hurricanes, and earthquakes, you might be surprised to know that floods are the most likely natural disaster that can affect U.S. citizens. Just about any storm can cause a deluge of water, and this can cause a deluge in the biblical sense. Even in semi-arid Boulder, Colorado, it happened in 2013 when 6 months of rain fell during a week's time. As such, it's important to know flood preparedness.

The definition of a flood is an overflow of water that submerges land which is normally dry. Flooding may occur as an overflow of water from seacoasts, rivers, or lakes. It can be a result of water overflowing levees and sea walls. Floods may also occur due to an accumulation of rainwater on saturated ground.

Some floods develop slowly, while others (called flash floods), can develop in a very short time and affect areas where it wasn't even raining. As a result, it often catches the population downstream by surprise, causing severe damage and loss of life.

Types Of Floods

Areal Floods: Flood waters that accumulate quickly on flat areas when the ground is saturated with water. Floods related to rainfall can also occur if water falls on an impenetrable surface, such as concrete or frozen ground, and cannot be rapidly absorbed.

Riverine Floods: Floods happen in rivers when the flow rate exceeds the capacity of the river channel, particularly at bends in the waterway. These are highly dangerous, as people tend to live and work by rivers due to access to fertile soil, irrigation, and trade routes.

Coastal Floods: Flooding on the coast is commonly caused by a combination of sea tidal surges caused by winds and low barometric pressure. Coastal areas may be flooded by storm events, such as hurricanes, resulting in waves over-topping seawalls and levees.

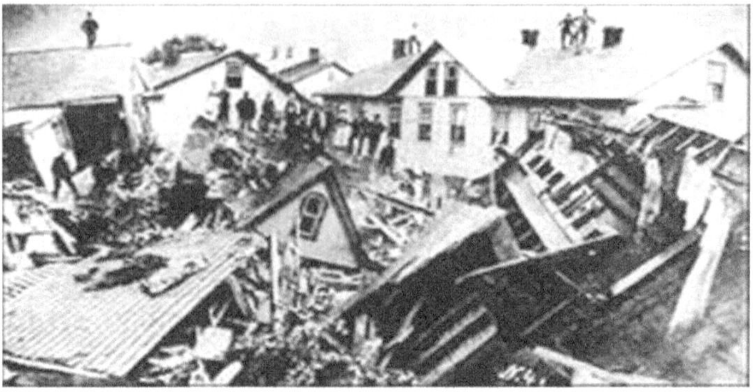

Aftermath of dam collapse in Johnstown, Pennsylvania, 1889

Consequences of Flooding

Failures of infrastructure, such as the collapse of a dam, may cause catastrophic flooding as seen in the 1889 Johnstown, Pennsylvania event that took 2,200 lives. Major flooding may also be caused by the effects of an earthquake or even a volcanic eruption. If these events often occur at sea, they may result in tidal wave ("tsunamis"). Penetration of salt water causes widespread failure of fresh water delivery systems and may make farmland infertile, sometimes for years.

Flood waters are not safe to drink due to contamination by sewage. As a result, water-borne illness such as diarrheal disease may take a major toll on the population. Cholera and Typhoid are just some of the diseases caused by contaminated water that may affect entire communities.

Other issues include the inability of aid to get to flooded areas and the inundation of farmland causing loss of the season's crops. Some industries may fail, leading to depression in the affected area. Once water and food shortage combine with the inability to receive help or make a living, economic collapse and civil unrest are likely to follow.

The scenario above is not purely hypothetical: Disasters related to flooding have sometimes caused millions of short- and long-term casualties. In both 1887 and 1931, major flooding of rivers in China ended up costing one and three million lives, respectively. If you take out war, famine, and pandemics, flooding is, undeniably, the deadliest of human tragedies.

Flood Safety

Most people have heard of hurricane or tornado watches and warnings, but the U.S. weather service also tries to warn the populace of flooding. If you live in a low-lying area, especially near a dam or river, then you should heed warnings when they are given and be prepared to evacuate quickly.

Here are some flood safety tips:

Get Out Early: Make the decision to leave for higher ground before extensive ponding occurs.

Avoid Walking Through Flowing Water: Drowning is the most common cause of death during a flood, especially a flash flood. Wilderness experts know that rapidly-moving water can knock you off your feet even if shallow.

Don't Drive Through a Flooded Area: As many people drown in their cars as anywhere else. Cars stall and roads could easily be washed out. Try to figure out if there is a "high road" to safety *before* a flood occurs.

Beware Of Downed Power Lines: current is easily conducted through water. Watch for downed power lines; you don't have to touch them to be killed, only step in the electrified water.

Turn Off The Power: If you have reason to believe that water will get into your home, turn off the electricity. Don't use appliances or motors that have gotten wet unless they have completely dried. You might have to dismantle some to clean out debris.

Watch Out For Intruders: Critters that have been flooded out of their homes may seek shelter in yours. Snakes, raccoons, and other unfriendly creatures may decide your home is now their territory. More ominously, human intruders may also become interested in your property.

Look Before You Step: After a flood, watch where you step; there is debris everywhere. The floors of your home may be covered in mud, causing a slip-and-fall hazard.

Check for Gas Leaks: Don't use candles, lanterns, stoves, or lighters unless you are sure that the gas has been turned off and the area is well-ventilated.

Exhaust Fumes Can Kill: Generators, camping stoves, or charcoal grills should only be used outside. Their fumes can be deadly.

Clean Out Saturated Items Completely: Don't use floodwater as drinking water or to cook food unless you have thoroughly sterilized and filtered it. Make sure you have food storage in waterproof containers, and wash the outside of containers that have been in the water.

Floods are just one of the many natural disasters that can endanger your family. Pay close attention to storm and flood warnings and you'll have a head start on keeping them safe.

MUDSLIDE PREPAREDNESS

A mudslide, sometimes called a "debris flow", is a landslide with a high water content. Mudslides act like a river that, if the mud is thick, has the consistency of wet concrete. Mud, rocks, trees, and other large objects are carried along and can cause homes to collapse and a huge amount of traumatic injury to residents. In the U.S., 25-50 deaths occur annually as a result of landslides.

Periods of heavy rainfall or snow melt saturate the ground and cause instability in sloping areas. Areas prone to earthquakes, hurricanes, wildfires, and other natural disasters are especially susceptible.

Humans contribute to this susceptibility with poor planning: Roads that are cut into hills and mountains make mudslides more likely. Riverside retreats at the base of a hill or mountain are also vulnerable. Before building that dream home on the mountain:

- Beware of steep slopes, natural or man-made runoff conduits, or eroded areas.
- Have the county Geological Survey specialist assess your property for possible mudslide risk.
- Consider flexible pipe fittings (installed by pros) that are less prone to gas or water leaks.
- Consider building a retaining wall in likely mudslide channels.
- Avoid areas that have experienced mudslides in the past.
- Plan out at least two evacuation routes.
- Have a battery-powered NOAA weather radio.
- Have a medical kit with items to deal with both traumatic injury and water sterilization.

Warning Signs

Mudslide prone areas will begin to show signs that trouble is on the way:

- Cracks develop in walls, flooring, paving, driveways, or foundations.
- Outside structures (for example, stairs) begin to separate from buildings

- Doors and windows start becoming jammed.
- Utility lines start breaking.
- Fences, trees, and utility poles start tilting.
- Water starts accumulating in strange places
- Roads and embankments along slopes start breaking off at the edges.
- The terrain starts to "bulge" or starts slanting at the base of the slope.

During The Event

- Turn on the NOAA radio and listen to warnings as they are reported.
- Warn your neighbors!
- If a mudslide is imminent, leave the area if at all possible, with the understanding that roads may be washed out.
- If you stay home, get to the second story if you have one.
- Watch for and avoid downed power lines.
- As the slide passes through, get under a table and curl into a ball, protecting your head.
- If you're trapped in the mud, survival rates go up if you can form an air pocket around you. You can survive without water for 3-4 days if you had to.

MARITIME SURVIVAL

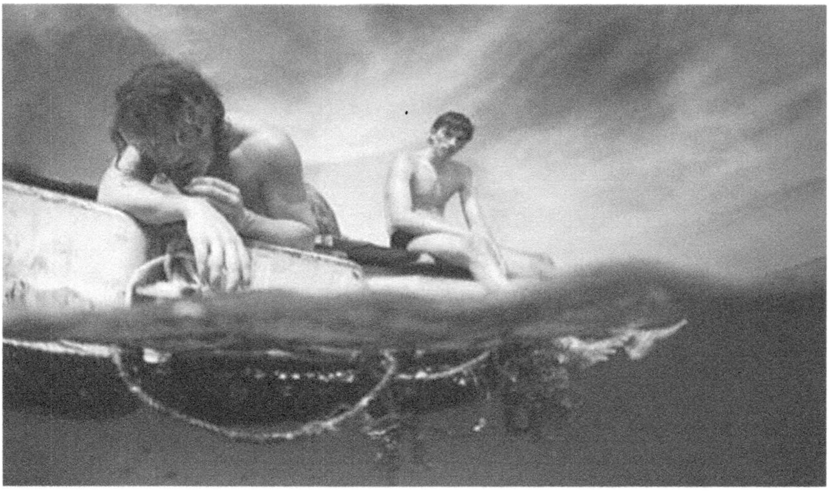

Speaking of high waters, there are various circumstances where people spend time on the open ocean. Earth is a water planet, and 70% or more of its surface covered by it. Storms and high waves capsize boats and put survivors to the ultimate test with few provisions and little equipment. It's important to have an idea of what to do if you find yourself in open water without rapid rescue.

Your survival in an ocean disaster depends on your ability to stay hydrated, obtain nourishment, and be protected against exposure to wind and temperature extremes. Before embarking on an ocean voyage, you should have a good idea of what supplies and equipment exist for use in an emergency. Your ability to access and use what's available could determine whether you live or die.

In normal times, you should file a "float plan" with the marina. Similar to an airplane's flight plan, it gives people on shore an idea of where you're going and when you are expected back. In this way, rescue operations will begin quickly when you fail to return as planned.

Water Temperature And Heat Loss

Hypothermia, discussed earlier in this book, is a major cause of death in boating mishaps. Water doesn't have to be particularly cold to cause hypothermia. Any water that's cooler than normal body temperature will cause heat loss. Average survival times decrease as the water temperature gets colder:

- 60-70 degrees Fahrenheit: 12 hours
- 50-60 degrees Fahrenheit: 6 hours
- 40-50 degrees Fahrenheit: 1 hour
- Lower than 40 degrees: Less than an hour

With A Life Jacket

In calm or rough seas, you should always wear a life jacket. Many come with whistles, beacons, and other items that might help identify your location to your crewmates. Flotation devices (life preservers) attached to a good length of rope can be thrown or a crew member sent with one to retrieve the victim.

If your boat capsizes or sinks, rapid action is necessary to increase your chances of survival. If there is time to send out a distress signal, do so. Many supply containers are meant to float; gather as many together as possible. They can help you stay above water and the supplies may save your life. If you're in waters that are used frequently by other boaters or shipping vessels (but not in view of dry land), try to stay near the area where your boat sank.

Without A Life Jacket

The above strategies work well for those with life vests, but what if you don't have one?

If you end up in the water without a life jacket, a lot more exertion is required to keep above water. At one point or another, you'll get tired. If you float on your back, it will require less energy to keep your face out of water. Arch your back and spread out your arms and legs; this should allow you to breathe with the least effort.

Another way to "rest" without a life jacket involves relaxing the body in between breaths. Inhale while treading water and then "lie" face down with arms forward. Repeat when you need another breath.

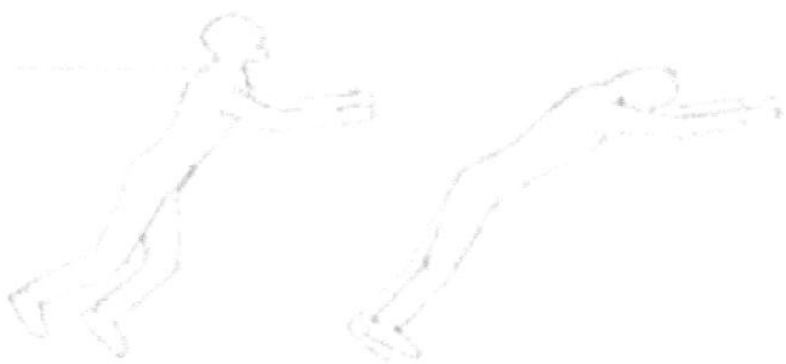

Inhale, tread water, then lie face down and relax your body

Sharks

Every sailor's nightmare is to be thrown overboard in shark-infested waters. All oceans have sharks, although only about 20 or so species are known to attack humans. Sharks are perfectly engineered to live and hunt in the sea; you aren't.

Shark skin is extremely abrasive and they often bump into potential prey before they attack. As such, you should make sure to keep your clothing on, including your shoes. Blood from abraded skin will excite them. In addition to blood, sharks are attracted to urine, feces, and thrashing movements.

If you are in the water with other swimmers, form a circle facing outward to better defend yourselves. Whether alone or in a group, slap the water with cupped hands or shout underwater if a shark approaches. Otherwise, try to kick or punch it, especially in the areas of the "snout", eyes, and gills. These strategies might deter a curious shark.

Do not "play dead", as this will not discourage them. Likewise, swimming as fast you can will only make you appear like a thrashing fish. You can't outswim a shark. Make slow, smooth strokes and keep the shark in view if possible.

In A Life Raft

A much better way to survive if stranded in the ocean is to be in a life raft, not in the water with sharks. In a raft, you can use your skills to survive longer and have a better chance of rescue.

If you find yourself in a life raft after abandoning a sinking ship, the first thing you need to do is get away from the ship itself. Sinking ships sucking down people nearby, as seen in the movie "Titanic".

Paddle into the wind in case a fire starts. This is because burning oil on the water and the toxic smoke it creates will spread downwind. Once the ship has gone to the deep and fire is no longer a risk, check the water for anything that might be useful. Anything not bolted down to the ship may rise to the surface and can be snatched up and utilized by survivors.

Many modern life rafts have survival kits and paddles built in. Another useful item for the raft is some sort of signaling device; a hand mirror can reflect the sun and be seen from a passing plane or boat. Some newer rafts come with a beacon.

Unless land is in sight, it is wise to stay as close to the last known position of the ship as possible. This is where all rescue efforts will begin, so the closer you are to where the ship sank, the more likely you will be found. This is especially useful if you are in widely traveled areas or shipping lanes.

If you're in a remote part of the ocean, the direction that birds fly may help you determine where the nearest land is. Seabirds will fly from land in the early morning and fly towards land in the evening. Water will appear lighter as it gets shallower and waves decrease in size.

The direction of the wind may help you find land. Wind usually blows towards land in the day and away at night. Why? Dry land absorbs heat from the sun faster than water. Warm air over land will rise and the cool air over the water rushes in to replace it. At night, water cools more slowly than land. The warmer air over the water rises and the cool air from the land rushes away towards the water.

If you're approaching land, try to find sandy stretches of beach. Rocks and coral below the surface may tear the bottom of your raft or cause injury if you get out. Paddle sideways in rip currents and you should make steady progress towards land.

If you're not close to land, don't exert yourself. You need to protect your body, conserve your resources, and limit your consumption. Many modern rafts have a canopy, but if you are in an open raft you'll want to erect some sort of shelter. Use anything you can, such as a tarp, part of a sail, even spare clothing. If it's hot, you can dampen your clothing with sea water to cool off, although this can cause skin irritation over time. If it's cold, put as much clothing on and utilize anything that can serve as a windbreak. There are commercially made anti-exposure suits that are made especially for this purpose.

Realize that the floor of your life raft will be colder than the walls, so don't sleep lying down if you're in cold weather. If it's hot, however, the floor might help keep you cool. Keep the inside of the raft covered and as dry as possible.

A canopy can also double as a rain catch to collect fresh water, which is going to be your biggest challenge. The first day in the raft, don't drink any water at all. Come up with a water rationing system and stick to it. The minimum amount of water necessary to stay in decent shape is 1 liter a day. It's possible to survive on as little as 2 to 5 ounces a day, although this will weaken you over time.

Water And Food

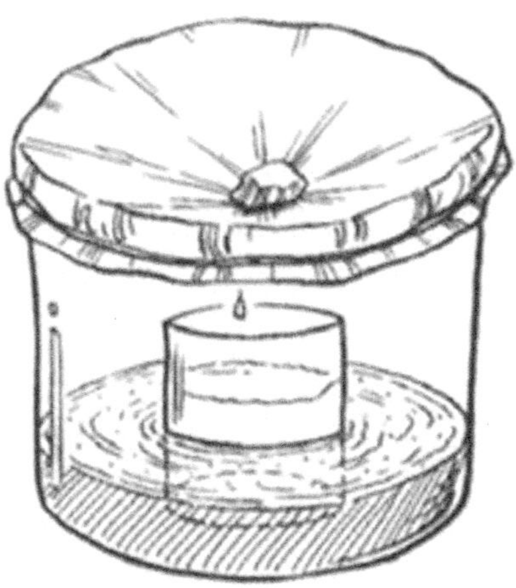

Simple Solar Still

Regardless of what you may have read, you can't drink sea water. It will dehydrate you due to the large amount of salt it contains, but you can get condensation from sea water if you have a few supplies. You'll need a pot, another smaller pot, some plastic wrap or sheeting, and 1 or 2 weights.

Fill the larger pot with sea water and put the smaller pot in the larger pot. Cover the whole thing with plastic and put a weight over the center of the smaller pot. Condensation of fresh water will occur on the inside of the plastic sheet. Because of the weight, fresh water will drip into the smaller pot, which you can drink from. They call this contraption a "solar still".

Save whatever food you have for after the first day or two. You can go a long time without food, so ration it out slowly so that it will last. You might be able to catch curious fish, sea turtles, or seabirds, which you'll just have to eat raw. Inedible parts may be used as bait. One stranded survivor said he caught fish by wiggling dirty clothes in the water and scooping them up with a fishing net. Using flashlights at night may attract fish.

Be aware that too much protein may cause you to use your body's water to digest it. We're told that fish eyes contain fluid that you can ingest safely.

Can you eat seaweed? The answer is often yes. Many seaweeds are part of the diet of coastal inhabitants around the world. Generally, green, brown, or red seaweeds can be washed and eaten raw or dried. Avoid the parts that are round and filled with gas; only eat the leafy parts. If you're not sure it's safe, you can touch the seaweed to your lips and wait a while to see if there is any ill effect. Be forewarned that seaweed tends to have a laxative effect and takes some "getting used to".

There's a lot more to survival at sea that what is mentioned here, but you get the idea. Have supplies available that you can fit into your raft, and you'll have the time you need to get rescued. It won't be easy, but you'll have a shot.

Near-Drowning

During warm weather, our nation's families will be traveling on vacation to the beach, lake, or other waterfront areas. They will be at risk for injuries, and one of the most harrowing and heartbreaking is drowning.

From 2005-2009, there were an average of close to 4000 drownings annually in the United States. Non-fatal water submersion injuries are about five times greater; some of these involve long-term brain damage.

Drowning is seen much more often in males, and the younger the person, the higher the rate of risk (ages 1-4 years highest). It's also the second leading cause of death from injuries in children 1-14 years old, surpassed only by car wrecks.

Drowning Safety Precautions

Here are some things you should know to keep your family safe from drowning:

- Take Swimming lessons: Don't go into swimming-depth water if you don't know how to swim. Swimming lessons are provided by many municipalities throughout the country, even for very young children. So are CPR classes, which are very important when it comes to aiding victims.
- Strictly supervise minors: Children in the water should always be supervised by a responsible, sober adult. For preschool children, the adult should be close enough to touch the child and not involved in any other activity.
- Utilize the "Buddy System": Everyone, even adults, should always swim with another person or persons.
- On the beach, beware of rip currents: Know the meaning of flags on supervised beaches. High waves, discolored water, debris, and channels of water moving away from shore are signs of dangerous conditions. If caught in a rip current, swim parallel to shore until free, then diagonally towards the beach.
- Be aware of the weather. Thundershowers often whip up the water with strong winds, increasing the risk of drowning.
- Be physically fit: Swimming involves exertion, so make sure you're up to the challenge.
- Don't drink alcohol: Any water activity is more dangerous, both to you and children you supervise, if you're drinking.

- Don't hyperventilate: Taking rapid deep breaths for a contest to see who can stay underwater longest may cause a blackout.
- In the wilderness, be wary of river crossings. Fast moving water may knock you off your feet, even if just a foot deep.

Reach, Throw, Row, Go

At the beach or in the wilderness, you might encounter a distressed person in the water. Your first response will be to jump in and help, but remember that the hazards that are causing the problem are probably still there. Also, the person in question will likely be panicking and flailing around. To avoid injury and reduce the risk that you'll become the next victim, consider these strategies in order: Reach, Throw, Row, Go.

- **Reach** out to the person with a stick or oar.
- **Throw** the person a lifeline, life preserver, or other floating object.
- **Row** out to the person in a canoe or other boat if available.
- **Go** into the water only when there is no other option.

In circumstances where you encounter a person face down in the water:

- Shout for help
- Remove the person from the water
- Check for pulse and breathing
- Begin CPR if not breathing, using rescue breaths. Chest compressions alone are insufficient for drowning victims
- If an automated external defibrillator is available, use it.

Needless to say, outcomes worsen significantly in an austere environment where emergency services aren't available.

VOLCANO PREPAREDNESS

A **volcano** is a rupture on the crust of the earth which allows hot lava (molten rock), ash, and gases to escape from below the surface. Volcanoes are not the disaster that most people think of as a risk to life and limb. Few think that a volcanic eruption will affect them during their lifetime. You never know where the long and wandering road will lead you, however, so a little knowledge about volcano safety just might be useful.

Most have the impression that a volcano is a conical mountain with smoke and lava spewing from the top. In actuality, volcanos have a number of forms. In Yellowstone National Park, a huge dormant super-volcano looks more like flat land than a cone. Geysers like 'Old Faithful" are evidence that there's still a great deal of pressure and molten rock below the surface.

One doomsday scenario includes the eruption of this huge land feature, which is called a "**caldera**" (meaning "cauldron" or "cooking pot"). This disaster last happened 640,000 years ago, but is thought to be an event that is likely to occur again "soon". In geologic time, "soon" means sometime in the next 40,000 years or so.

If you live in a volcanically active area, there are things that you can do to avoid becoming a victim. Vigilance is a virtue, so monitor volcanic activity reports and evacuate the area if authorities believe an eruption is imminent. Plan to get the family together and have several routes out of the area.

This isn't always easy to do. Lava flow can block your main route of exit and can mix with water to form mudslides, essentially a moving mass of wet concrete. Thick ash can damage engine parts, so drive at slow speeds.

Items for your medical storage that will be useful include masks, goggles, and flashlights for every member of your family. Ash may fall thick and heavy, and this could make breathing and seeing difficult. If you don't have masks, a damp cloth over your nose and mouth will do. Have sturdy boots, hand protection, and thick clothing that will protect as much of your head and body as possible.

If you find yourself unable to leave your home, close all windows and doors. Block chimneys to prevent ash from getting in, and be aware that layers of ash can be so heavy as to cause a roof cave-in. Have food, water, a medical kit, and other general survival items in your storage.

ALLERGIC REACTIONS AND ANAPHYLAXIS

In the face of a disaster, we may have to vacate our home and head to unfamiliar territory. During our travels, we'll expose ourselves to insect stings, strange food items, and plants like poison ivy. When a negative immune response occurs as a result, we call it an "**allergy**".

Foreign substances that cause allergies are called "**allergens**". Our response to them can be minimal or it can be life-threatening. If severe enough, we refer to a major allergic reaction as "**anaphylaxis**" or "anaphylactic shock". Anaphylaxis is the word used for serious and rapid allergic reactions, usually involving more than one part of the body.

Minor And Chronic Allergies

Mild allergic reactions usually involve local itching and the development of red patchy bumps on the skin called "**hives**". Hives, also known as "urticaria", can be caused by allergies to food, pollen, pet dander, drugs, or other substances. The most common foods that cause hives are: peanuts, chocolate, eggs, milk, nuts, shellfish, and berries. The skin effects of hives are usually transient and go away by themselves or with the help of medications such as Diphenhydramine (Benadryl) or other antihistamines.

Allergies may also manifest as "**dermatitis**", a longer lasting inflammation of the skin. Dermatitis presents as a rash that is red and itchy. The appearance of the rash depends on the amount of time it has been present:

Acute dermatitis:	Blisters
Subacute dermatitis:	Scaling or Crusting
Chronic dermatitis:	Skin thickening

The most common dermatitis is known as "**eczema**". This is a red patchy rash which is itchy and flaky. Eczema usually responds well to 1% hydrocortisone cream (non-prescription), although sometimes a stronger steroid cream such as Clobetasol (prescription) may be necessary. In the very worst cases, chronic dermatitis may require oral steroids such as Prednisone. For more information on skin conditions, refer to the chapter on the topic later in this book.

If the allergic reaction is minor, there are various natural remedies you can apply to get relief: Many of these are essential oils:

- Peppermint
- Lavender
- Chamomile (German or Roman)
- Calendula
- Myrrh
- Cypress
- Helichrysum
- Wintergreen
- Eucalyptus
- Blue Tansy

To use the above oils, you would dilute 50/50 with carrier oil (olive or coconut, for example) and apply 2 drops to the affected area.

Other natural substances that you could apply to a rash include witch hazel, oatmeal baths or compresses, Aloe Vera, Shea butter, and vitamin E oil. Use as needed.

Hay Fever

Hay Fever, also known as "allergic rhinitis" or "seasonal allergy", is a collection of symptoms, mostly affecting the eyes and nose, which occur when you breathe in something you are allergic to. Sufferers of allergic rhinitis would present with:

- Nasal congestion
- Sneezing
- Red eyes with tearing
- Itchy throat, eyes, and skin

Antihistamines such as Loratadine (Claritin) and Diphenhydramine (Benadryl) are old standbys for this type of allergy. Alternative therapies for hay fever include essential oils for use on the skin:

- German chamomile
- Roman chamomile
- Lavender
- Eucalyptus
- Ginger

Apply 2 drops to each temple, 2-4 times per day. Steam inhalation is another option: 1 drop of the oil to a bowl of steaming water and inhale slowly for 15 minutes. Covering the head with a towel concentrates the steam. A number of teas to drink that may be useful are licorice root, stinging nettle, and St. John's Wort. Drink 1 cup daily 3 times a day.

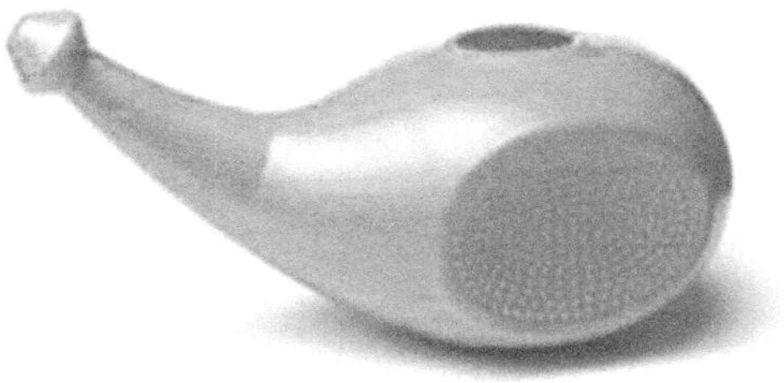

Neti Pot

A Neti Pot is a useful item to deal with allergic reactions affecting the nasal passages. It looks like a small teapot. Neti pots help wash out pollen, clear congestion and mucus, and decrease nasal inflammation. Use with *sterile* saline (salt water) solution daily in the following fashion:

- Bend over a sink.
- Tilt your head to one side.
- Keep your forehead and chin are at the same level to keep water out of your mouth.
- Breathe through your mouth during the procedure.
- Insert the spout gently into your uppermost nostril.

- Pour the solution so that it drains through the lower nostril.
- Blow your nose to clear your nostrils.
- Change head position and repeat with the other nostril.

There have been concerns voiced about neti pots from the Food and Drug Administration (FDA). They warn that, if not used properly, the patient runs the risk of developing serious (even life-threatening) infections. Neti pots are meant to be used with *sterilized* saline; in 2011, two people lost their lives after using contaminated tap water.

Allergy Or Side Effect?

A medical caregiver has many responsibilities in a disaster. Everyone knows that their duty is to deal with injuries and illness, but few are aware of their obligation as medical archivist; that is, they are responsible for knowing the medical history of the people under their care. Part of that medical history includes what medicines to which a patient is allergic.

Many people will report that they are allergic to a particular drug. The reasons for this could be:

- It causes symptoms that makes them feel unwell.
- A family member was once diagnosed as being allergic to the drug, and they assume that they might be also.
- Their parents told them about an incident in their childhood that resembled an allergy, so better safe than sorry.
- They read something negative about it online or saw it on TV, and they don't want to ever take it.
- They are philosophically opposed to a particular type of drug (antibiotics, psychiatric meds).
- They might actually be allergic to the drug.

We place an actual allergy to a drug last on this list because, according to the World Allergy Organization, less than 10% of reactions to medications really relate to allergies. Most symptoms that people get after taking medicine are what we call adverse or "side" effects.

What's the difference? A **drug allergy** is a negative response by your immune system after exposure to a medicine. An adverse reaction is a well-documented negative consequence of its use in a percentage of patients. In an allergic reaction, the immune system recognizes a substance as foreign. This starts a cascade of reactions that is normally protective, but when excessive, may be harmful. If a drug normally causes, say, intestinal spasms in a percentage of cases, then cramps would be a side-effect instead of an allergy.

We hear reports of people claiming an allergic response the "first" time they take a certain medicine. The body, however, will usually not respond immunologically the first time it's exposed to a drug. We believe, if it's a true allergy, that an unknown previous exposure was involved.

Why is it important to know whether a symptom is related to a side effect or an allergy? Here's an example: A man has chest pain and a history of heart disease. You suspect a heart attack, but he says that he is allergic to aspirin, the only medicine you have available. Do you give it?

Here's another: A woman has a severe infection that has proven resistant to many antibiotics, leaving you with one or two options, both of which are listed as allergies in her medical history. What do you do?

Give the medication in the two cases above, and you may save the patient. Unfortunately, you also might kill the patient if they are truly allergic. To claim a side effect as an allergy ties a medical provider's hands, and can cause a big difference in the final outcome. Therefore, it's important to know the usual adverse reactions to common drugs. Having a reference book that lists these, like the Physician's Desk Reference, is a good addition to your survival medicine library.

Asthma

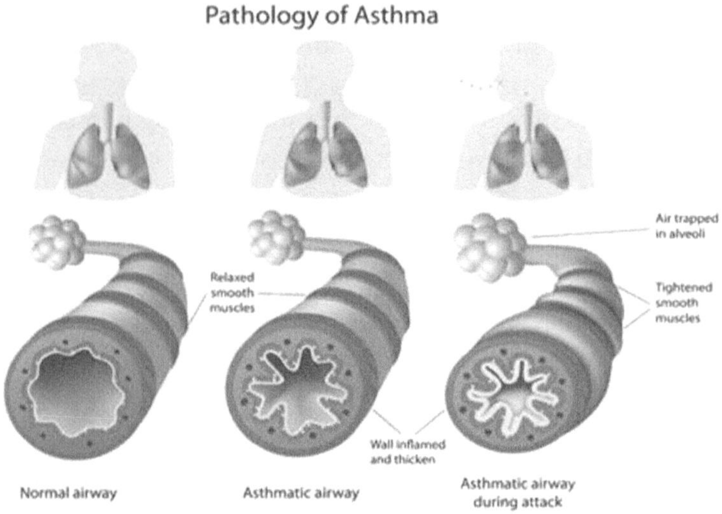

Asthma is a chronic condition that limits your ability to breathe. It affects the airways, which are the tubes that transport air to your lungs. When people with asthma are exposed to a substance to which they are allergic (an "**allergen**"), airways become swollen and filled with mucus. As a result, air can't pass through to reach the part of the lungs that absorbs oxygen (the "**alveoli**").

During an episode of asthma, you will develop shortness of breath, tightness in your chest, and start to wheeze and cough. This is referred to as an "asthma attack". In rare situations, the airways can become so constricted that a person could suffocate from lack of air.

Here are common allergens that trigger an asthmatic attack:

- Pet or wild animal dander
- Dust or the excrement of dust mites
- Mold and mildew
- Smoke
- Pollen
- Severe stress

- Pollutants in the air
- Some medicines
- Exercise

There are many myths associated with asthma; the below are just some:

- Asthma is contagious. (False)
- You will grow out of it. (False; it might become dormant for a time but you are always at risk for it returning)
- It's all in your mind. (False)
- If you move to a new area, your asthma will go away. (False; it may go away for a while, but eventually you will become sensitized to something else and it will likely return)

Here's a "true" myth: Asthma is, indeed, hereditary. If both parents have asthma, you have a 70% chance of developing it compared to only 6% if neither parent has it.

Physical Signs And Symptoms Of Asthma

Asthmatic symptoms may be different from attack to attack and from individual to individual. Some of the symptoms are also seen in heart conditions and other respiratory illnesses, so it's important to make the right diagnosis. Symptoms may include:

- Cough
- Shortness of Breath
- Wheezing (usually sudden)
- Chest tightness (sometimes confused with coronary artery spasms/heart attack)
- Rapid pulse rate and respiration rate
- Anxiety

Besides these main symptoms, there are others that are signals of a life-threatening episode. If you notice that your patient has become "cyanotic", they are in trouble. Someone with **cyanosis** will have a blue/gray color to their lips, fingertips, and face.

You might also notice that it takes longer for them to exhale than to inhale. As an asthma attack worsens, wheezing may take on a higher pitch. Once the patient has spent enough time without adequate oxygen, they will become confused, drowsy, and possibly lose consciousness.

To make the diagnosis, use your stethoscope to listen to the lungs on both sides. Make sure that you listen closely to the bottom, middle, and top lung areas as described in the section on physical exams.

In a mild asthmatic attack, you will hear relatively loud, musical noises when the patient breathes. As the asthma worsens, less air is passing through the airways and the pitch of the wheezes will be higher and perhaps not as loud. If no air is passing through, you will hear nothing, not even when you ask the patient to inhale forcibly. This person may become cyanotic.

Sometimes a person might become so anxious (a "panic attack") that they become short of breath and may think they are having an asthma attack. To resolve this question, you can measure how open the airways are with a simple diagnostic instrument known as a **peak flow meter**. A peak flow meter measures the ability of your lungs to expel air, a major problem for an asthmatic. It can help you identify if a patient's cough is part of an asthma attack or whether they are, instead, having a panic attack or other issue.

To determine what is normal for a member of your group, you should first document a peak flow measurement when they are feeling well. Have your patient purse their lips over the mouthpiece of the peak flow meter and forcefully exhale into it. Now you know their baseline measurement. If they develop shortness of breath, have them blow into it again.

In moderate asthma, peak flow will be reduced 20-40%. Greater than 50% is a sign of a severe episode. In a non-asthma related cough or upper respiratory infection, peak flow measurements will be close to normal. The same goes for a panic attack; even though you may feel short of breath, your peak flow measurement is still about normal.

Treatment Of Asthma

The cornerstones of asthma treatment are the avoidance of "trigger" allergens, as mentioned previously, and the maintenance of open airways. Medications come in one of two forms: drugs that give quick relief from an attack and drugs that control the frequency of asthmatic episodes over time. In panic attacks, however, these medicines are ineffective; treatment for anxiety is discussed later in this book.

Quick relief asthma drugs include "bronchodilators" that open airways, such as Albuterol (Ventolin, Proventil), among others. These drugs should open airways in a very short period of time and give significant relief. These drugs are sometimes useful for people going into a situation where they know they will exposed to a "trigger", such as before strenuous exercise. Don't be surprised if you notice a rapid heart rate on these medications; it's a common side effect.

If you find yourself using quick-relief asthmatic medications more than twice a week, you are a candidate for daily control therapy. These drugs work, when taken daily, to decrease the number of episodes and are usually some form of inhaled steroid. There are long-acting bronchodilators as well, such as ipratropium bromide (Atrovent). Another family of drugs known as Leukotriene modifiers prevents airway swelling before an asthma attack even begins. These are usually in pill form and may make sense for storage purposes. The most popular is Montelukast (Singulair).

Often, medications will be used in combination, and you might find multiple medications in the same inhaler. U.S. commercial product Advair, for example, contains both a steroid and an airway dilator. Remember that inhalers lose potency over time. Expired inhalers, unlike many drugs in pill or capsule form, have less effect than fresh ones.

It's important to figure out what allergens trigger your asthma attacks and work out a plan to avoid them as much as possible. Furthermore, make sure to stockpile as much of your asthma medication as possible in case of emergency. Physicians are usually sympathetic to requests for extra prescriptions from their asthmatic patients.

In mild to moderate cases, you might consider the use of natural remedies. There are actually quite a few substances that have been reported to be helpful:

Ginger: A study published in the American Journal of Respiratory Cell and Molecular Biology indicates that Ginger is instrumental in inhibiting chemicals that constrict airways. Animal tests find that extracts of Ginger helps ease asthmatic symptoms in rodents. Use as a tea or extract twice a day.

Ginger and Garlic Tea: Put four minced garlic cloves in some ginger tea while it's hot. Cool it down and drink twice a day. Some have reported a beneficial effect with just the garlic.

Other herbal teas: Ephedra, Coltsfoot, Codonopsis, Butterbur, Nettle, Chamomile, and Rosemary all have been used in the past to improve an asthmatic attack.

Coffee: Black unsweetened coffee is a stimulant that might make your lung function better when you are having an attack. Don't drink more than 12 ounces at a time, as coffee can dehydrate you. Interestingly, coffee is somewhat similar in chemical structure to the asthma drug Theophylline.

Eucalyptus: Essential oil of eucalyptus, used in a steam or direct inhalation, may be helpful to open airways. Rub a few drops of oil between your hands and breathe in deeply. Alternatively, a few drops in some steaming water will be good respiratory therapy.

Honey: Honey was used in the 19th century to treat asthmatic attacks. Breathe deeply from a jar of honey and look for improvement in a few minutes. To decrease the frequency of attacks, stir one teaspoon of honey in a twelve ounce glass of water and drink it three times daily.

Turmeric: Take one teaspoon of turmeric powder in 6-8 ounces of warm water three times a day.

Licorice and Ginger: Mix licorice and ginger (1/2 teaspoon of each) in a cup of water. Warning: Licorice can raise your blood pressure.

Black Pepper, Onion, and Honey: Drink ¼ cup of onion juice with a tablespoon of honey, after adding 1/8 tablespoon of black pepper.

Mustard Oil Rub: Mix mustard oil with camphor and rub it on your chest and back. There are claims that it gives instant relief in some cases.

Gingko Biloba leaf extract: Thought to decrease hypersensitivity in the lungs; not for people who are taking aspirin or ibuprofen daily, or anticoagulants like Coumadin.

Vitamin D: Some asthmatics have been diagnosed with Vitamin D deficiency.

Lobelia: Native Americans actually smoked this herb as a treatment for asthma. Instead of smoking, try mixing tincture of lobelia with tincture of cayenne in a 3:1 ratio. Put 1 milliliter (about 20 drops) of this mixture in water at the start of an attack and repeat every thirty minutes or so.

Further research is necessary to determine the amount of effect that the above remedies have on severe asthma, so take standard medications if your peak flow reading is 60% or less than normal.

Don't underestimate the effect of your diet on your condition. Asthmatics should:

- Replace animal proteins with plant proteins.
- Increase intake of Omega-3 fatty acids.
- Eliminate milk and other dairy products.
- Eat organically whenever possible.
- Eliminate trans-fats; use extra-virgin olive oil as your main cooking oil.
- Always stay well-hydrated; more fluids will make your lung secretions less viscous.

Finally, various breathing methods, such as taught in Yoga classes, are thought to help promote well-being and control the panic response seen in asthmatic attacks. Acupuncture is thought by some to have some promise as well in treating the condition.

Anaphylactic Reactions

In a small percentage of people, a response to an allergen may affect more than just a local area. Severe allergic reactions involve various organ systems and can be quite dangerous.

Anaphylactic reactions were first identified when researchers tried to protect dogs against a certain poison by desensitizing them with small doses. Instead of being protected, many of the dogs died suddenly the second time they got the poison. They were killed by their own immune systems going out of control.

The word used for preventative protection is "**prophylaxis**". Think of a condom, also known as a prophylactic. A condom protects you from pregnancy and prevents sexually transmitted diseases. The word "**anaphylaxis**", therefore, means the *opposite* of protection. The dog experiment allowed scientists to understand that the same "anti-protective" (harmful) effect can occur in humans. Anaphylaxis can be caused by drug exposure, insect venoms, or pollutants, but even foods like peanuts can be to blame.

Why does our immune system go awry during anaphylactic events? Anaphylaxis happens when the body makes an antibody called immunoglobulin E (IgE for short) in response to exposure to an allergen. IgE sticks to cells; these cells then release substances that affect blood vessels and air passages.

The first time you're exposed is called the "**sensitization**". Usually, nothing exciting happens with the first exposure. The second time you are exposed to that allergen, however, your immune system recognizes them as foreign and goes into overdrive. Your blood pressure can drop and generalized swelling (also called "edema") can occur. In severe cases, the airways can tighten and arteries can spasm. Respiratory difficulty and cardiac effects ensure, sometimes leading to anaphylactic shock and even death.

Anaphylaxis has become a timely issue because more and more people are experiencing the condition. Why the increase? The explanation is likely that we are simply exposed to more pollutants these days, and are using a lot of pharmaceuticals. Developing countries like China are experiencing terrible air quality issues. Widespread use of antibiotics and other medications are exposing us to more possible allergens to trigger an event.

Cases of asthma and hay fever are becoming more common all over the world. Pollutants and pesticides in our food might certainly be a factor, but the food itself is changing. More people are ingesting genetically-modified (GMO) food. A GMO salmon that grows twice as fast as natural salmon has been approved by the FDA. They can now produce pigs that glow in the dark by controlling their genes. More and more genetic modifications are likely in the future, and the effect on humans is uncertain.

Some of the above is conjecture, but proven causes of anaphylaxis include:

- Drugs: dyes injected during x-rays, antibiotics like Penicillin, anesthetics, aspirin and ibuprofen, and even some heart and blood pressure medicines.
- Foods: Nuts, fruit, seafood.
- Insects stings: Bees and Yellow Jacket Wasps, especially.
- Latex: Rubber gloves made of latex, especially in healthcare workers.
- Exercise: Often after eating (yes, you can actually be allergic to exercise).
- Idiopathic: This word means "of unknown cause"; a substantial percentage of cases.

Signs And Symptoms Of Anaphylaxis

It's important to recognize the signs and symptoms of anaphylaxis because the faster you treat it, the less likely it will become life-threatening. A person having an anaphylactic reaction will present with:

- Rashes: Often at places not associated with the actual exposure. For example, an all-over rash in someone with a bee sting on the arm.
- Swelling: Can be generalized, but sometimes isolated to the airways or throat.

- Breathing difficulty: Wheezing is common, as you would see in asthmatics.
- GI symptoms: Diarrhea, nausea and vomiting, or abdominal pain.
- Loss of consciousness: The patient may appear to have fainted.
- Paresthesia: Strange sensations on the lips or oral cavity, especially with food allergies.
- Shock: Blood pressure drops and respiratory failure leads to coma and death.

Fainting is not the same thing as anaphylactic shock. You can tell the difference in several ways. Someone who has fainted is usually pale in color, but anaphylactic shock will often present with the patient somewhat flushed. The pulse in anaphylaxis is fast, but a person who has fainted will have a slow heart rate. Most people who have just fainted will rarely have shortness of breath and rashes, but these will be very common signs and symptoms in an anaphylactic reaction.

In food allergies, victims may notice that the effects of anaphylaxis occur very rapidly; indeed, their life may be in danger within a few minutes. Sometimes, the reaction occurs later. People who have had a serious anaphylactic reaction should be observed overnight, as there is, on occasion, a second wave of symptoms. This can happen several hours after the exposure. Some reactions are mild and probably not anaphylactic, but a history of mild symptoms is not a guarantee that *every* reaction will be minor.

Treatment Of Anaphylaxis

During anaphylactic reactions, our immune system produces a substance called "histamine". **Histamine** triggers the inflammatory response that causes the symptoms of anaphylactic shock. Medications which counteract these ill effects are known, therefore, as "**antihistamines**".

Oral antihistamines may be helpful in mild to moderate allergic reactions but meds like Diphenhydramine (Benadryl) take about an hour to get into the bloodstream. In an anaphylactic reaction, this isn't fast enough to save lives. It may be all you have, however, so chew the pill to get into your system more quickly.

Other oral antihistamines like Claritin come in wafers that melt on your tongue and are faster acting. They are an alternative, but probably too weak for any severe reaction. It's important to know that the same cells to which IgE antibodies attach may release other substances which cause ill effects; oral antihistamines do not protect you against these.

As such, we look to another medicine that is more effective: Adrenaline, known in the U.S. as Epinephrine. Adrenaline (Epinephrine) is a hormone that is produced in small organs near your kidneys called the "adrenal" glands. This substance activates the well-known "flight or fight" response.

Epinephrine makes your heart pump faster, widens the air passages so you can breathe, and raises your blood pressure. It works successfully against all of the effects of anaphylaxis. Therefore, you should make it a part of your medical storage if you are going to responsible for the well-being of your family in any long-term disaster scenario.

Unfortunately, Adrenaline (Epinephrine) comes in an injectable solution. You might consider an inhaler to be more appropriate, but anaphylactic reactions can cause breathing difficulties: If you can't inhale, you won't get much benefit from an inhaler.

The "**Epi-Pen**" is the most popular of the various commercially available kits to combat anaphylaxis. It's important to learn how to use the Epi-Pen properly. Perform these simple steps:

- Remove the Epi-Pen from its case.
- Hold it firmly in your fist.
- Remove the safety cap (some have two caps).
- Have the patient sit or lie down.
- Press the end firmly against the mid-outer thigh in a perpendicular fashion; it should click.
- Hold for 10 seconds.
- Massage the injection site.
- Dispose of the needle safely.

You can cause more harm than good if you fail to follow the above instructions. Adrenaline (Epinephrine) can constrict the blood vessels if injected into a finger by mistake, and prevent adequate circulation to the digit. In rare cases, gangrene can set in. Also, remember that the Epi-Pen won't help you if you don't carry it with you or don't have it readily accessible. Any allergic members of your family or group should always have it in their possession.

Since it's a liquid, Adrenaline (Epinephrine) will not stay effective forever, like some pills or capsules might. Be sure to follow the storage instructions. Although you don't want to store it someplace that's hot, the Epi-Pen shouldn't be kept in any situation where it could freeze, which will damage its effectiveness significantly.

If the solution changes color, it may be losing potency. It can lose effectiveness without changing color also, so use with caution if expired. Adrenaline (Epinephrine) must be protected from light and usually comes in an opaque container.

You will have limited quantities of this drug available, so when do you break into those precious supplies? An easily remembered formula is the **Rule of D's**:

- Definite reaction: Your patient is obviously having a major reaction, such as a large rash or difficult breathing.
- Danger: Any worsening of a reaction after a few minutes, especially difficulty breathing.
- Deterioration: Use the Epi-Pen before the condition becomes life-threatening.
- Doubt: When in doubt, use it.

If you are ever in doubt, go ahead and give the injection. The earlier you use it, the faster a person will resolve the anaphylaxis. One injection is enough to save a life, but have more than one handy, just in case. This is especially pertinent when you are away from your retreat or base camp.

Some people may not be able to take Adrenaline (Epinephrine) due to chronic heart conditions or high blood pressure. Advise your people to consult with their healthcare providers before a disaster occurs to determine that it's safe to receive the drug.

In a collapse, you'll be exposed to a lot of strange things and you never know when you might be allergic to one of them. Stockpile the appropriate drugs, especially if you have family members with histories of reactions. If you learn the signs and symptoms of anaphylaxis and act quickly, you'll stay out of trouble.

POISON IVY, OAK, AND SUMAC

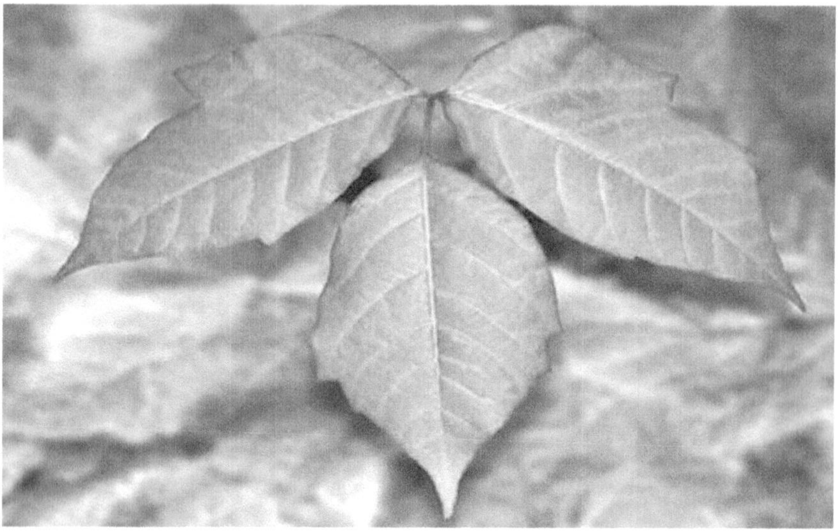

Poison Ivy

In the aftermath of a disaster, you may find yourselves outdoors a lot more often. Unless you live in Alaska, Hawaii, a mountaintop, or the middle of the desert, the outdoors will have a population of **poison ivy, poison oak, and/or poison sumac**. Once exposed to one or the other, 85% of people will develop antibodies against it that will generate an itchy rash of varying degrees of severity. Winter does not eliminate the possibility of a reaction, as you can react against even the dormant vines or shrubs.

The old saying goes: "Leaves of three, let it be". Although it is true that poison ivy comes in "leaves of three", so do many other plants. View images of poisonous plants native to your area so you can more easily avoid them.

Poison ivy and poison oak are very similar, with the same chemical compound (called "urushiol") as the main irritant. Poison ivy leaves are generally almond-shaped and pointed. Poison oak often looks more like, well, oak leaves, with scalloped or lobed edges. You'll find one or the other just about everywhere in the continental United States.

Poison Sumac is a shrub or small tree, growing up to nearly 30 feet in height in parts of the Eastern United States. Each leaf has 7–13 pointed leaflets. Although poison sumac has the same irritant present in poison ivy and poison oak, it is far more powerful. Simply inhaling smoke from burning poison sumac has been reported to be life-threatening.

All of these plants contain toxic oil that causes a reaction after the first sensitizing exposure. The oil is in just about every part of the plant, including the vines, leaves, and roots. The best strategy, of course, is not touching the plant and getting the toxin on your skin. If you can't avoid exposure, here is advice before you head out into the woods:

- Long pants, long-sleeved shirts, work gloves, and boots are imperative if you're doing work in areas known to have poison plants.
- Some recommend an over-the-counter lotion called Ivy Block as a preventative. Apply it like you would a sunblock to likely areas of exposure. Theoretically, it will prevent the oil from being absorbed by your skin.

Unfortunately, many times people don't identify the exposure before it's too late. The rash takes from several hours to several days to become apparent, and will appear as red itchy lumps that tend to be patchy. Sometimes the rash contains blisters and appears almost linear. Itching can be prolonged and severe.

The resin or oil from the plant that causes the reaction will remain active even on your clothes, so thorough laundering with special agents will be required. Routine body washing with soap will not be useful after 30 minutes of exposure, as your system will already be producing antibodies. Hot water seems to help the oil absorb into the skin, so use only cold water early on. After all the irritant has absorbed, however, hot water baths are actually recommended by some to relieve itching.

Cleansers that remove toxic resin or oil include Fels-Naptha soap or Tecnu Poison Oak and Ivy Cleanser. These products are more effective than regular detergent and can be used even several hours after exposure. Rubbing alcohol is another reasonable option and easily carried as hand sanitizers or prep pads, but dries the skin.

The good news is that, even if you choose not to treat the rash, it will go away by itself over 2-3 weeks. Even though it is temporary, it could be so itchy as to make you absolutely miserable. Diphenhydramine (Benadryl) at 25-50 mg dosages 4 times a day will be helpful in relieving the itching. It's important to know that the 50mg dosage will make you drowsy. Unfortunately, calamine lotion, an old standby, and hydrocortisone cream will probably not be very effective.

Severe rashes have been treated with the prescription Medrol dose pack, (a type of steroid known as Prednisone). Prednisone is a strong anti-inflammatory drug and will be more effective in preventing the inflammatory reaction that your antibodies will cause.

Some astringent solutions such as Domeboro have been reported to give relief from the itching. The active ingredient is aluminum acetate, which is similar to the aluminum chlorohydrate in many antiperspirants.

There are several alternative treatments for poison ivy, oak and sumac:

- Cleansing the irritated area with apple cider vinegar.
- Essential oils mixed with Aloe Vera gel, such as tea tree, lemon, lavender, peppermint, geranium, and chamomile.
- Baking soda paste
- Epsom salt baths.
- Jewelweed (mash and apply)
- Chamomile tea bag compresses

For those who prefer drinking their tea, passion flower, skullcap, and chamomile are all thought to be soothing to victims of poison ivy.

RADIATION SICKNESS

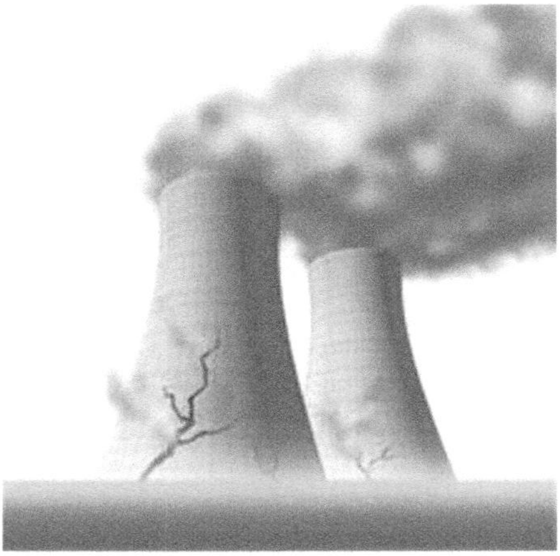

Some of the most common Doomsday scenarios involve atomic weapons and the decimation of the population from thermal blasts and radiation. Although populated areas have experienced nuclear blasts only twice, (Hiroshima and Nagasaki in 1945), nuclear reactor meltdowns and other events have occurred from time to time since then.

In an atomic explosion, radiation is just one of the possible causes of casualties; thermal blast and kinetic energy damage near the blast will cause deaths and injuries close to ground zero. Radiation, however, can have devastating effects far from an actual detonation.

Our utilization of nuclear reactors for power places us at risk for radiation exposure when they malfunction or are damaged. Examples include the "meltdowns" at Chernobyl (1986) and Fukushima (2011). A **meltdown** (technically known as a "core melt accident") happens when reactor heat increases beyond safe levels, causing a nuclear element to exceed its melting point.

Meltdowns usually occur as a result of failure of the nuclear plant coolant system. This failure can occur as a result of damage caused by natural disasters, such as earthquakes or tsunamis. They can, however, also be caused by human error or terrorist attack. Regardless of the cause, the melted radioactive elements are released into the atmosphere. This has serious implications for populations living both near and far from the event.

Radiation released into the atmosphere is known as "fallout". **Fallout** is the particulate matter (dust) that is thrown into the air by a nuclear explosion. This dust can travel hundreds (if not thousands) of miles on the prevailing winds, coating fields, livestock, and people with radioactive material.

The higher the fallout goes into the atmosphere, the farther it will travel downwind. This material contains elements that are hazardous if inhaled or ingested, like Radioiodine, Cesium, and Strontium. Even worse, fallout is absorbed by the animals and plants that make up our food supply. In large enough amounts, it is hazardous to your health.

A nuclear power plant meltdown is usually less damaging that a nuclear blast, as the radiation doesn't make it as high up in the sky as a mushroom cloud from an atomic bomb. The worst effects will be felt by those in the area of the reactors. Lighter particles, like radioactive iodine, will travel the farthest, and are the main concern for those far from the actual explosion or meltdown. The level of exposure depends on the distance that radioactive particles have to travel from the meltdown, and the time it took for the radiation to arrive.

The medical effects of exposure are collectively known as "**radiation sickness**" or "Acute Radiation Syndrome". A certain amount of radiation exposure is tolerable over time, but your goal is to shelter your group as much as possible.

To accomplish this goal, we should first clarify what the different terms for measuring the quantities of radiation mean. Scientists use terms such as RADS, REMS, SIEVERTS, BECQUERELS or CURIES to describe radiation amounts. Different terms are used when describing the amount of radiation being given off by a source, the total amount of radiation that is actually absorbed by a human or animal, or the chance that a living thing will suffer health damage from exposure:

BECQUERELS/CURIES – these terms describe the amount of radiation that, say, a hunk of uranium gives off into the environment.

Named after scientists who were the first to work with (and die from) radioactivity.

RADS – the amount of the radiation in the environment that is actually absorbed by a living thing.

REMS/SIEVERTS – the measurement of the risks of health damage from the radiation absorbed.

This is somewhat confusing, so, for our purposes, let's use RADS. A RAD (Radiation Absorbed Dose) measures the amount of radiation energy transferred to some mass of material, typically humans.

An acute radiation dose (one received over a short period of time) is most likely to cause damage. Below is a list of the effects on humans corresponding to the amount of radiation absorbed. For comparison, assume that you absorb about 0.6 RADs per year from natural or household sources. These are the effects of different degrees of acute radiation exposure on humans:

- **30-70 RADS:** Mild headache or nausea within several hours of exposure. Full recovery is expected.
- **70-150 RADS:** Mild nausea and vomiting in a third of patients. Decreased wound healing and increased susceptibility to infection. Full recovery is expected.
- **150-300 RADS:** Moderate nausea and vomiting in a majority of patients. Fatigue and weakness in half of victims. Infection and/or bleeding may occur due to a weakened immune system. Medical care will be required for many, especially those with burns or wounds. Occasional deaths at 300 RADS exposure may occur.
- **300-500 RADS:** Moderate nausea and vomiting, fatigue, and weakness in most patients. Diarrheal stools, dehydration, loss of appetite, skin breakdown, and infection will be common. Hair loss is visible in most over time. At the high end of exposure, expect a 50% death rate.
- **Over 500 RADS:** Spontaneous bleeding, fever, stomach and intestinal ulcers, bloody diarrhea, dehydration, low blood pressure, infections, and hair loss is anticipated in almost all patients. Death rates approach 100%.

The effects related to exposure may occur over time, and symptoms are often not immediate. Hair loss, for example, will appear at 10-14 days. Deaths may occur weeks after the exposure.

In the early going, your goal is to prevent exposures of over 100 RADS. A radiation dosimeter will be useful to gauge radiation levels and is widely available for purchase. This item will give you an idea of your likelihood of developing radiation sickness.

There are three basic ways of decreasing the total dose of radiation:

1) **Limit the time unprotected**. Radiation absorbed is dependent on the length of exposure. Leave areas where high levels are detected and you are without adequate shelter. The activity of radioactive particles decreases over time. After 24 hours, levels usually drop to 1/10 of their previous value or less.
2) **Increase the distance from the radiation.** Radiation disperses over distance and the effects will be decreased. To make an analogy, you have less chance of drowning the farther away you are from deep water.
3) **Shield people to decrease radiation where they are.** Shielding will decrease exposure exponentially, so it is important to know how to construct a shelter that will provide a barrier between your people and the source. A dense material will give better protection that a light material.

Barrier effectiveness is measured as "**halving thickness**". This is the thickness of a particular shield material that will reduce gamma radiation (the most dangerous kind) by one half. When you multiply the halving thickness, you multiply your protection.

For example, the halving thickness of concrete is 2.4 inches or 6 centimeters. A barrier of 2.4 inches of concrete will drop exposure to one half. Doubling the thickness of the barrier drops it to one fourth (1/2 x 1/2) and tripling it will drop it to one eighth (1/2 x 1/2 x 1/2), etc. Ten halving thicknesses will drop the total radiation exposure to 1/1024.

Here are the halving thicknesses of some common materials:

Lead:	0.4 inches or 1 centimeter
Steel:	1 inch or 2.5 centimeters
Concrete:	2.4 inches or 6 centimeters
Soil (packed):	3.6 inches or 9 centimeters
Water:	7.2 inches or 18 centimeters
Wood:	11 inches or 30 centimeters

To take an example, let's assume you are in a concrete bunker (2.4 inches halving thickness). You would need it to be 24 inches thick to drop your radiation exposure to 1/1024 of the outside environment.

Emergency treatment of radiation sickness involves dealing with the symptoms. Antibiotics may be helpful to treat infections, fluids for dehydration, and drugs like Zofran (Ondansetron) to treat nausea. In severely ill patients, stem cell transplants and multiple transfusions are indicated but will not be options in an austere setting. This underscores the importance of an adequate shelter.

There is protection available against some of the long term effects of radiation, however. Potassium Iodide (known by the chemical symbol KI) is a 130 mg tablet that prevents radioactive Iodine from damaging the specific organ that it targets, the thyroid gland. **Radioactive Iodine** is the most common component in fallout that is not in the immediate area of the nuclear event.

Taking KI 30 minutes to 24 hours prior to a radiation exposure will prevent the eventual epidemic of thyroid cancer that will result if no treatment is given. Radiation from the 1986 Chernobyl disaster has accounted for more than 4,000 cases of thyroid cancer so far, mostly in children and adolescents.

Although there is a small amount of KI in ordinary iodized salt, not enough is present to confer any protection by ingesting it. It would take 250 teaspoons of household iodized salt to equal one Potassium Iodide tablet.

If radiation exposure is expected, take the KI tablet once a day for 7-10 days, or longer if prolonged or multiple exposures are expected. Children should take 1/2 the dose (65 mg). It is also recommended to consider 1/2 tablet for large dogs, and 1/4 tablet for small dogs and cats.

Don't depend on supplies of the drug to be available after a nuclear event. Even the federal government will have little KI in reserve to give to the general population. In recent power plant meltdowns, there was little or no Potassium Iodide to be found anywhere for purchase. If you have a limited supply, it is important to know that children are the most likely to develop thyroid cancer after an exposure and should be treated first.

If you find yourself without any KI, consider this alternative: 2% tincture of Iodine solution (brand name Betadine). "Paint" 8 ml of Betadine on the abdomen or forearm 2-12 hours prior to a radiation exposure and re-apply daily. Enough should be absorbed through the skin to give protection against radioactive Iodine in fallout.

Apply 4 ml. on children 3 and older (but under 150 lbs. or 70 kg.). Use 2 ml for toddlers and 1 ml for infants. This strategy should also work on animals. If you don't have a way to measure, remember that a standard teaspoon is about 5 milliliters. Discontinue the daily treatment after 3-7 days or when Radioiodine levels have fallen to safer levels.

Be aware that those who are allergic to seafood will probably be allergic to Iodine. Adverse reactions may also occur if you take medications such as diuretics and Lithium. It is also important to note that you cannot drink Betadine; it is poisonous if ingested.

Although many in the preparedness community don't view a nuclear event as the most likely disaster scenario, it's important to learn about all the possible issues that may impact your family in uncertain times.

BIOLOGICAL WARFARE

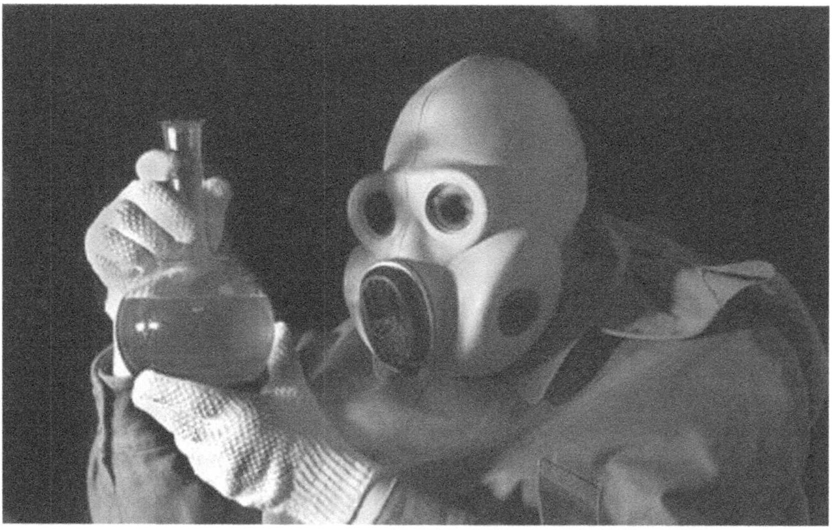

There are many calamities that can befall a population: Economic collapse, solar storms, global warming, and civil unrest are just a few. There is one scenario, however, that few consider as a possible cause of a long-term survival scenario: biological warfare.

Biological warfare is the term given to the use of infectious agents such as bacteria, viruses, fungi, or their toxins to attack a specific population. As a result, the attacker achieves control over an area or a segment of the population by weakening the ability to resist. Biological weapons don't necessarily have to kill humans: unleashing a horde of locusts to destroy crops or agents that kill livestock can be just as effective.

This type of weapon has been used since ancient times, and even appears in the bible as part of the plagues visited upon Pharaoh by a wrathful God. Medieval accounts of Bubonic plague-ridden corpses catapulted into besieged cities abound; this method was used as late at 1710, when the Russians attacked the Swedish city of Reval (present day Tallinn) in this manner.

The Western hemisphere was changed forever by an act of inadvertent biological warfare: the introduction of smallpox into the Native

American population. This had the result of killing 90% in some areas and opening vast swaths of land for European colonization. In addition, purposeful biological warfare occurred against Native Americans when the British presented a large "gift" of infected blankets as a "peace" offering during Pontiac's War in the mid-1700s.

As time progressed, new infectious agents (Anthrax) were used in certain situations during World War I. The use of biological weapons was banned by the Geneva Protocol in 1925, but research and production was still carried out by both sides during World War II. Research into the use of Anthrax by the United Kingdom left their laboratory area in Scotland contaminated for the next five decades.

In 1972, the storage, production, and transport of biological warfare agents was banned by the Biological Weapons Convention (BWC). The Treaty does allow the stockpiling of biological agents and toxins for "prophylactic, protective or other peaceful purposes". Despite this, there have been a number of violations of the treaty by the former Soviet Union, Syria, and Iraq; various others are suspected. As of 2015, 173 countries have signed the BWC pact.

The perfect biological weapon would have these characteristics:

- Be infectious and contagious in a large percentage of those exposed.
- Cause severe long-term debilitation or death of the infected organism.
- Have few available antidotes, preventives or cures.
- Be easily deliverable to the area or population targeted.
- Have low likelihood of causing damage to those using the agent.

The concerns about "accidents" affecting the aggressor have most countries reluctant to use such weapons in normal tactical situations. During the largest such accident in 1979, a Russian lab released anthrax into the surrounding area, killing 42 people, infecting sheep over 200 miles away, and causing the immediate area to be off-limits even today.

Some candidates for use as biological agents include Anthrax, Smallpox, Viral hemorrhagic Fevers such as Ebola, and Pneumonic Plague.

Anthrax can be contracted in several ways: skin contact, inhalation, and gastrointestinal infection. More common in livestock than people, **Anthrax** is not an ideal "weapon of mass destruction" in that no person-to-person contagion occurs, except in skin cases (the least lethal form). A "cloud" of Anthrax would be necessary to affect a large population, although large numbers of infected livestock could result in an epidemic of the disease in humans.

Anthrax exists as spores which, in the right environment, release toxins that cause a flu-like syndrome which eventually destroys cells in lymph nodes. It becomes highly lethal when it spreads to the lungs and blood. Although Penicillin, Doxycycline, and Ciprofloxacin (Fish-Pen, Bird-Biotic, and Fish-Flox, respectively) are effective against this bacteria as a preventative or for early treatment, full-blown inhalation Anthrax may be difficult to survive; the toxins released by the spores remain even if the spores are killed.

Inhalation Anthrax can progress to shock and death in many cases; luckily, not everyone exposed will get symptoms. Because of higher risk of exposure, certain individuals, such as livestock workers, are often offered a vaccine against the disease.

Another example of biological warfare is the **Plague**. "Pneumonic" is one of three types of Plague and, by far, the most contagious, easily spread by coughing bacteria into the air. It is caused by a bacterium known as Yersinia Pestis, usually found on rodents and other small animals in their fleas. Also starting off as a flu-like syndrome, it quickly develops into pneumonia with fever, weakness, shortness of breath, and cough (often with blood).

Pneumonic plague is different from Bubonic plague in that the patient will not have the classic swellings in the groin or armpit (called "Buboes"). Unlike inhalation Anthrax, which may take weeks to develop symptoms, patients with pneumonic plague may be dead in 2-4 days if not treated early.

Tetracycline (veterinary equivalent: Fish-Cycline), Doxycycline (Bird-Biotic) and Ciprofloxacin (Fish-Flox), and IV Gentamycin are effective treatments for victims of Plague. Oxygen is often used to support the sick individual, and protective masks, gloves, and gowns are imperative for those who are caring for them.

There are several types of viral fevers that have been considered as possible agents for biological warfare. **Hemorrhagic Fevers** like **Ebola** start off with fever, diarrhea, and weakness, but progress to more serious problems relating to internal and external hemorrhaging. Patients may bleed from eyes, ears, nose, mouth, or rectum and may have bruising on the skin from subcutaneous bleeding.

Normal antivirals don't seem to cure this disease, and death rates may be as high as 90%. The illness is spread by bodily fluids and other contact, so masks, gloves, and gowns, again, are extremely important for health care workers.

You would think that Ebola would be an excellent choice as a biological weapon. It isn't. Ebola virus is very sensitive to its environment and just doesn't last long outside a host. It doesn't tolerate sunlight and needs high temperature and humidity to survive. Most cities in developed countries don't have the climate conducive to Ebola's survival.

It's also not easy to work with. Even if a terrorist kidnapped an Ebola victim, working with the virus in anything less than an advanced microbiology lab (called a "Biosafety Level 4") would likely result in the villain's death. As well, Ebola virus is too sensitive to survive the complex process of refining, enriching, etc. that is necessary for weaponization.

Smallpox is another viral illness that is highly contagious and was responsible for the decimation of the Native American population. Related to the chickenpox virus, smallpox differs in that all the blisters develop at the same time, rather than their being at different points of developing and healing.

Contact with these blisters causes the disease to be contagious. Fever and fatigue accompany the illness. Although rare in developed countries now, it was prevalent in the past and the government still stockpiles Smallpox vaccines in enough quantity to vaccinate every U.S. citizen. No curative treatment is currently available, and complications can lead to shock and death.

By-products released by microbes and plants walk the fine line between biological weapons and chemical weapons. Toxin released by the bacteria that causes botulism causes paralysis of muscles, and is used in small quantities in the cosmetic agent Botox. Castor beans contain Ricin, a potent toxin that causes respiratory and circulatory failure. 3 mg. of ricin is potent enough to kill an average-sized adult if inhaled.

A classic example of old-time survivalism that may be useful is the "**gas mask**". A gas mask is placed over the face to protect the wearer from inhaling airborne pollutants and toxic gases. It forms a sealed cover over the nose and mouth with filters that allow safe breathing. Gas masks will often cover the eyes or the entire face. Although cumbersome, they are superior to surgical masks as a barrier. The user is still vulnerable to chemicals that can penetrate the skin, however, unless they are wearing a protective suit as well.

SECTION 6

✚ ✚ ✚

INJURIES TO SOFT TISSUES

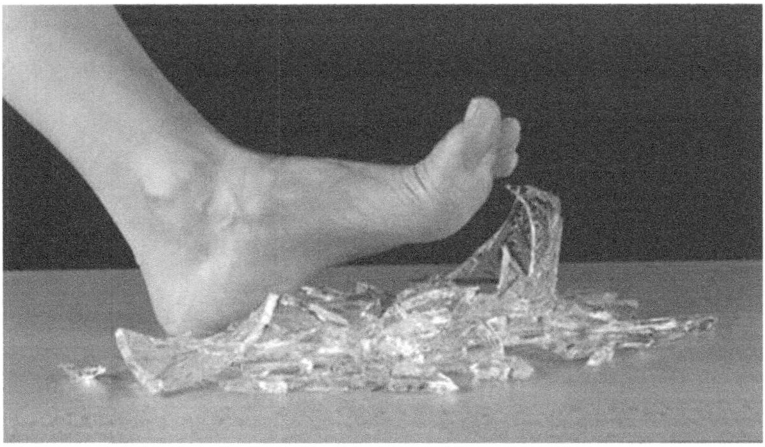

In long-term survival, the performance of tasks like chopping wood, cooking food, etc. will likely lead to a number of soft tissue injuries (those that do not involve bony structures). From a simple cut to a severe burn, any damage to skin is akin to a chink in your body's protective armor.

Your skin is a considered an organ, indeed, the largest organ in the body. It serves as a barrier against infection and loss of fluids. When this barrier is weakened by an injury, your health is in jeopardy. Rapid and effective treatment of these injuries will prevent them from becoming life-threatening.

Some rugged individualists shrug off minor injuries as inconsequential. Yet, any minor injury has the potential to cause trouble down the road. As a healthcare provider during troubled times, you must monitor the healing process of every wound.

Each wound is different and must be evaluated separately. If not present at the time the wound is incurred, the medic should begin by asking the simple question: "What happened"? A look around at the site of the accident will give you an idea of what type of debris you might find in the wound and the likelihood of infection. Always assume that a wound incurred outdoors is dirty initially. Other questions to ask are whether the victim has chronic medical problems, like diabetes, and whether they are allergic to any medications.

The physical examination of a wound requires the following assessment: Location on the body, length, depth, and the type of tissue involved. Circulation and nerve involvement must also be evaluated. If an extremity is injured, have the patient show you whether they have full range of motion during your examination. This is especially important if the injury involves a joint.

This section will deal with various injuries, their evaluation, and treatment. With close observation, you will be best able to assure a full recovery for your patient.

MINOR WOUNDS

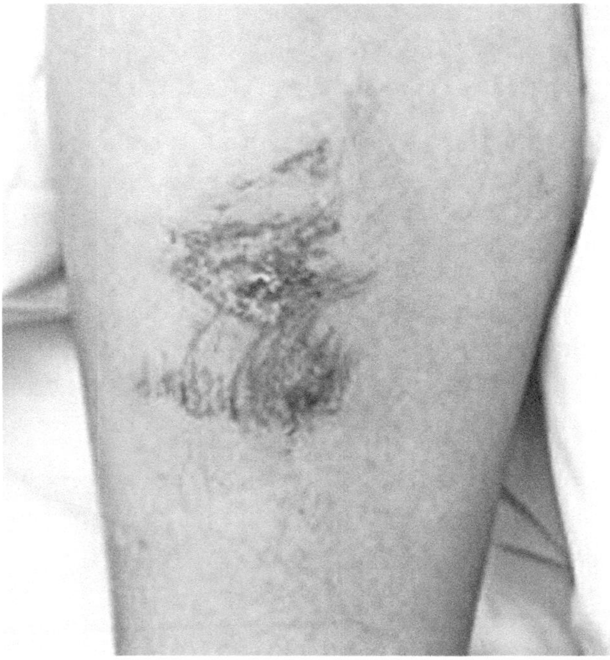

A soft tissue injury is considered minor when it fails to penetrate the deep layer of the skin, called the "**dermis**". This would include cuts, scrapes and bruises.

- **Cuts and Scratches:** These tears in the skin only penetrate the "**epidermis**" (superficial skin layer) and are rarely problematic in a healthy person.
- **Abrasions or Scrapes:** A portion of the epidermis has been scraped off. You probably have experienced plenty of these as a child.
- **Bruises or Contusions:** These result from blunt trauma and do not penetrate the skin at all. However, there is bleeding into the skin from blood vessels that have been disrupted by the impact.

All of the above minor injuries can be easily treated. Wash the wound anywhere that the epidermis has been violated. The use of an antiseptic such as Betadine (Povidone-Iodine solution), honey, or antibiotic ointment such as Neosporin or Bactroban will be helpful to prevent infection. Ibuprofen and Acetaminophen are useful over-the-counter drugs to treat minor pain. These injuries will heal over the next 7-10 days, dependent on the amount of skin area affected.

Minor bleeding can be stopped with a little pressure or a wet styptic pencil, an item normally used for shaving cuts. The wound, if it broke the skin, should be covered by a protective adhesive bandage (such as a Band-Aid).

Applying pressure and ice (if available) wherever a bruise seems to be spreading will stop it from getting bigger. Bruises will change color over time from blackish-blue to brown to yellow. Bruises may be gravity-dependent and may descend slightly and time goes on.

The Liquid Skin bandage is an excellent way to cover a minor injury with some advantages over a regular bandage. You apply it once to the cut or scrape; it dries within a minute or so and seals the wound. It also stops minor bleeding, and won't fall off during baths. There are various brands (Band-Aid Liquid Bandage, New Skin, Curad, 3M No Sting liquid bandage) and many come as a convenient spray.

You don't always have to travel the traditional road to treat many medical problems. If you have one of the minor injuries mentioned, you can choose any of a number of natural remedies. Here's an alternative process to deal with these issues:

1) Evaluate seriousness of wound; if minor, you may continue with herbal treatment.
2) Stop minor bleeding with herbal blood clotting agents such as Cayenne Pepper powder, and compress the area with gauze. Substances that clot blood are called "hemostatic" agents. These include:
    - Essential oils- Geranium, Helichrysum, Lavender, Cypress, Myrrh, or Hyssop. Apply any of these to a gauze compress.
    - Medicinal Herbs- Cayenne pepper powder or cinnamon powder with direct application or Yarrow tincture soaked in a gauze compress.

3) After minor bleeding is stopped, the wound should be cleaned with an herbal antiseptic: Mix a few drops of oil with sterile water and wash the wound thoroughly. Essential oils with this property include:
   - Lavender oil
   - Tea tree
   - Rosemary
   - Eucalyptus
   - Peppermint
4) Apply herbal antiseptic to the wound using the above essential oils. For example, use peppermint oil in a 50/50 mix with carrier oils such as olive or coconut oil. Other natural antiseptics include garlic, raw unprocessed honey, Echinacea, Witch Hazel, and St. John's Wort.
5) If needed, use natural pain relievers, such as:
   - Geranium oil
   - Helichrysum oil
   - Ginger oil
   - Rosemary oil
   - Oregano oil

   Apply 2-4 drops of a 50/50 dilution around the wound's edges.
6) Dress the wound using clean gauze. Don't wrap too tightly.
7) Change the dressing, reapply antiseptic, and observe for infection twice daily until healed.

   Infected minor wounds are discussed in the section on cellulitis in this book.

Some naturopaths advocate the use of activated charcoal to help wounds heal. To make a poultice:

- Mix 1 -2 tablespoons of activated charcoal with a small amount of water to form a moist paste.
- Add flax seed meal to help retain moisture.
- Spread the paste on gauze cut to fit the wound and fold it over.
- Apply to the injury and cover with plastic wrap.
- Tape securely in place and leave overnight.
- Evaluate the wound in the morning.

HEMORRHAGIC WOUNDS

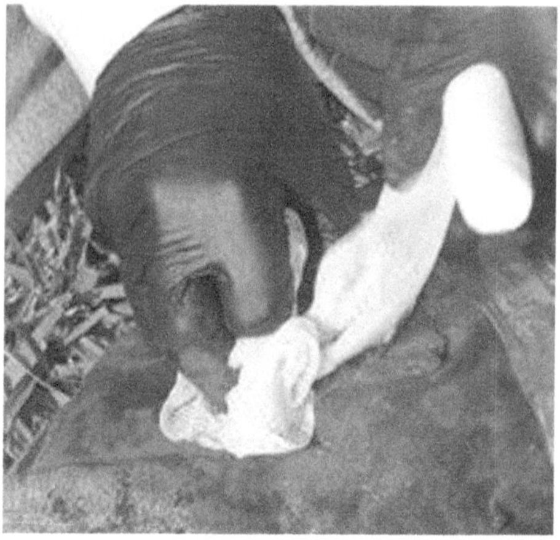

In a destabilized society, the risk of civil unrest is high. Traumatic wounds may be commonplace. Therefore, the medic for a family or group must be prepared for the worst possible injuries. Some of these, especially those that cause bleeding in the abdomen and chest, are likely to be fatal without advanced medical care. We will concentrate on those wounds that are survivable in austere settings.

Cuts in the skin can be minor or catastrophic, superficial or deep, clean or infected. Most significant cuts (also called 'lacerations') penetrate both the dermis and epidermis and are associated with bleeding, sometimes major. Knowing how to manage a hemorrhagic wound quickly and effectively will be of paramount importance.

In studies of casualties in recent wars, 50% of those killed in action died of blood loss. 25% died within the first "**golden hour**" after being wounded. A victim's chance of survival diminishes significantly after 1 hour without care, with a threefold increase in death rate for every 30 minutes without care thereafter. Indeed, it could take just a few minutes for a person to "bleed out". Perhaps we should be considering the "platinum five minutes" instead.

Venous bleeding manifests as dark red blood that drains steadily from the wound. Bleeding can also be arterial, which is bright red (due to higher oxygen content) and comes out in spurts that correspond to the pulse of the patient. As the vein and artery usually run together, a serious laceration can have both.

Once below the level of the skin, large blood vessels and nerves may be involved. Assess circulation, sensation, and the ability to move the injured area. You will notice more problems with vessel and nerve damage in deep lacerations and crush injuries.

Physical Effects Of Blood Loss

Evaluating blood loss is an important aspect of dealing with wounds. An average size human adult has about 10 pints of blood. The effect on the body caused by blood loss varies with the amount of blood loss incurred:

- 1.5 pints (0.75 liters) or less: little or no effect; you can donate a pint of whole blood, for example, as often as every 8 weeks.
- 1.5-3.5 pints (0.75-1.5 liters): The victim is usually agitated, with rapid heartbeat and respirations. The skin becomes cool and may appear pale.
- 3.5-4 pints (1.5-2 liters): Blood pressure begins to drop; the patient may appear confused. Heartbeat is usually very rapid.
- Over 4 pints (more than 2 liters): Patient is now very pale, and may be unconscious. After a period of time with continued blood loss, the blood pressure drops further, the heart rate and respirations decrease. This patient is in serious danger.

ABCDE vs. CABDE

The initial field assessment of a victim usually involves the acronym ABCDE:

- Airway: Is the airway open?
- Breathing: Is the victim breathing?
- Circulation: Is the victim bleeding?
- Disability: Can the victim feel and move extremities? Can they respond appropriately to questions?
- Exposure: Can you see the full extent of the injury? Are there other hidden injuries, such as an exit wound?

This sequence changes in the actively bleeding wound to CABDE. In these circumstances, the cause of death is more often hemorrhage which must be abated quickly. The determination of airway, breathing, and mental status can often be done simultaneously with bleeding control, as many patients will be conscious and talking.

Remember that the patient may be in shock. Keep them warm by covering them with a blanket if possible. If the wound is in an extremity, raise their legs 12 inches above the level of the heart. If the wound is in the torso, however, do not elevate the legs.

It's important to note that the bleeding may not be coming from the most visible wound. Where there is an entry wound, there is probably an exit wound, depending on the projectile. This may not be directly on the opposite side of the entrance wound. A bullet may ricochet off a bone and exit in an entirely different direction. Also, the position of the victim when wounded plays a part. If they were in a crouching position when hit in the chest, the exit wound might be in the lower back or buttocks.

Direct Pressure To Control Hemorrhage

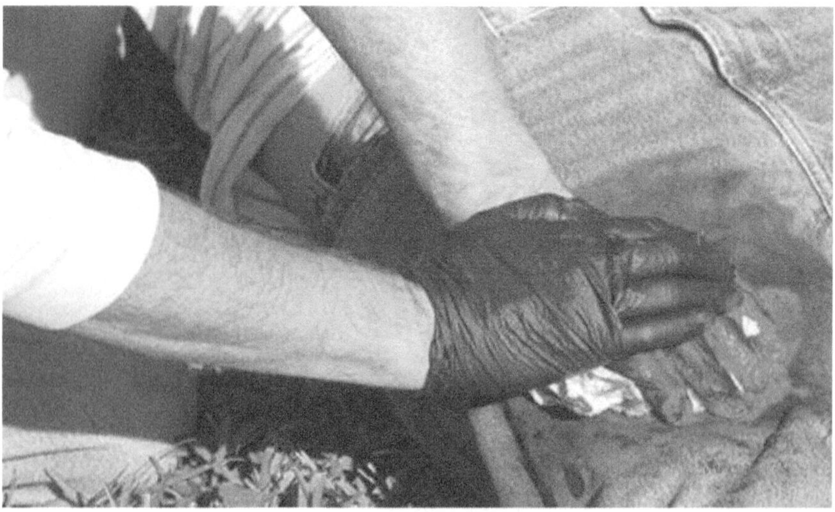

When you encounter a person with a bleeding wound, the first course of action is to stop the hemorrhage. In the grand majority of cases, direct pressure on the bleeding vessel might stop bleeding all by itself. Bleeding in an extremity may be slowed by elevating the limb above the level of the heart. This decreases the blood pressure in the extremity and, thus, the force by which blood leaves the body.

The medic should always have nitrile gloves in his or her pack; this will prevent the wound from contamination by a "dirty" hand. Try to avoid touching the palm or finger portions of the gloves as you put them on. If there are no gloves, grab a bandanna or other barrier. At the very least, use hand sanitizer. If none of the above are available, do not stop to look for supplies if the bleeding is severe.

If you have bandage dressings, use them or any clean cloth to pack the wound. Bandages are not just for sopping up blood; they are useful to apply pressure. A compact dressing that comes vacuum-packed is made by H&H Medical Corp. These compressed gauze bandages are small enough to fit several into a small kit, but each is 12 feet long.

More than one dressing may be required to keep the wound from bleeding further. If so, don't remove dressings in place: Add more on top. It's important to make sure that you put the most pressure where the blood vessel was damaged. For example, if the blood was coming from the top of a large wound, start packing there and apply firm and direct pressure.

Some advocate the use of "**pressure points**" to decrease bleeding.

Pressure points are locations where major arteries come close enough to the skin to be compressed manually. Pressing on this area will, theoretically, slow down bleeding further down the track of the blood vessel. A diagram of some major pressure points is below:

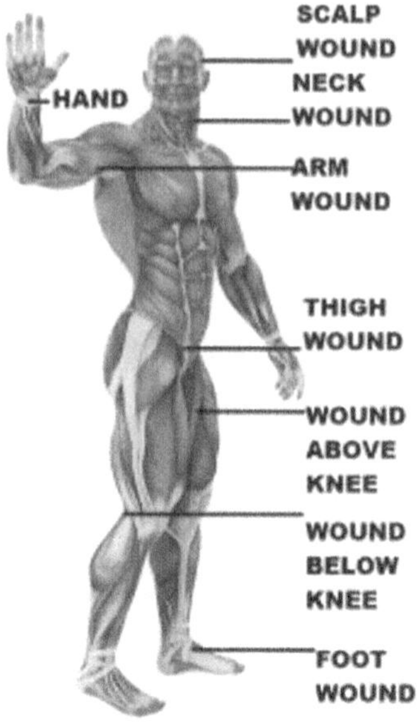

Using pressure points, we can make a "map" of specific areas to concentrate your efforts to decrease bleeding. For example, there is a large blood vessel behind each knee known as the Popliteal Artery. If you have a bleeding wound in the lower leg, say your calf, applying pressure on the back of the knee may help slow the hemorrhage.

As finding the exact location of a pressure point is not always easy for the untrained, this method should not take the place of well-aimed direct pressure on the bleeding vessel inside the wound.

For those with training, a curved instrument known as a "hemostat" can be used to clamp a damaged vessel. This should only be done if you can easily reach and clearly visualize the point of bleeding. This isn't always possible, as transected veins and arteries may retreat into the soft tissue.

Tourniquets

If all of the above fails to stop the bleeding, it may be appropriate to use a tourniquet. Although the decision to use a tourniquet should be made judiciously, current Tactical Combat Casualty Care (TC3) guidelines recommend its quick use in cases of severe hemorrhage. Situations in survival when the tourniquet will come in handy to stop bleeding:

- Injuries where transport is difficult or impossible.
- Homestead or camp accidents.
- Gunshot or stab wounds from hostile encounters.

Although your bandage dressings will be packed directly into the wound, tourniquets should be applied at least 2 inches above the bleeding area. If you use a tourniquet, be certain to tighten it until the bleeding stops. Half measures are not appropriate, even though it will be painful for the victim. Avoid placing a tourniquet on a joint.

On a bleeding wound to the forearm or lower leg, it may be advisable to place the tourniquet on the upper arm or above the knee. This is because there is only one bone in those areas as opposed to two in the forearm and lower leg, and pressure from the tourniquet will be more even. The pitfall is that more intact areas will be compressed. If one tourniquet fails to stop bleeding, adding another further up the extremity may be necessary.

Let's review some of the tourniquets available for inclusion in your survival medical storage. Note: All of the below require practice to place appropriately.

These are generally grouped in two categories: Inflatable (pneumatic) and Non-Inflatable (most commonly found in medical kits). Many of these are able to be applied with one hand on yourself if necessary. Your choices include:

The CAT (Combat Application Tourniquet): Current generation CAT tourniquets have a wide 2.4 inch Velcro band and a one-handed plastic bar called a "**windlass**". The windlass tightens the band, which should be placed 2 inches or higher above the wound. The windlass can then be secured into place to allow the caregiver use of both hands.

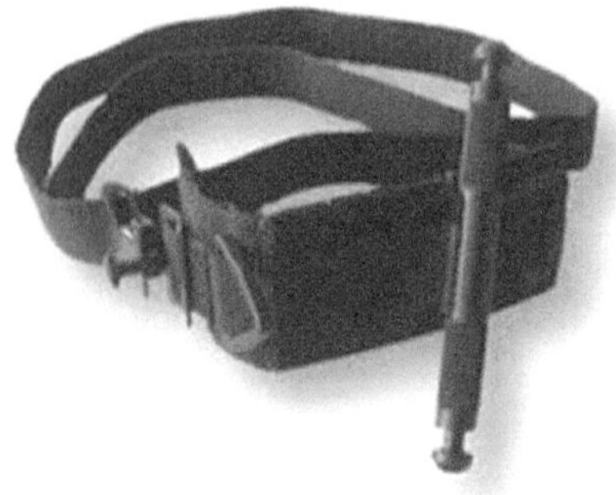

The SOF-T Tourniquet

The SOF-T (Special Operations Forces Tourniquet): Developed in response to concerns about the sturdiness of the plastic windlass in the CAT tourniquet, the SOF-T has a windlass made of fuselage-grade aluminum. A sturdy buckle eliminates the need for threading the tourniquet and secures the strap in place.

The RAT (Rapid Application Tourniquet): The RAT tourniquet is essentially a bungee cord that is wrapped around the extremity above the wound and then fitted into a metal clip to maintain pressure. Relatively inexpensive, it has been rumored to be gaining ground among the military, but must be placed appropriately to avoid ligature effects on the skin. Each successive coil of the cord must be placed next to, not on top of, the first coil around the extremity.

The MAT (Mechanical Advantage Tourniquet): This tourniquet is a cuff with a "key" that you wind like an old-fashioned wind-up toy. There is a spot on the MAT that, when pressed, releases pressure instantly. Pressure may also be released by disengaging the buckle (which must be clipped into place at the beginning of the procedure). Best used with two hands.

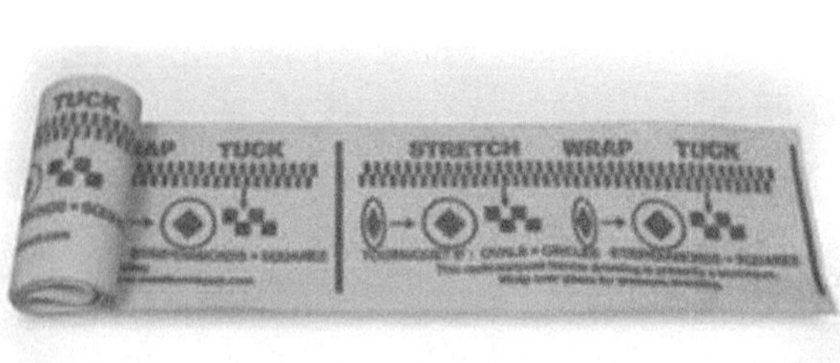

The SWAT Tourniquet

The SWAT Tourniquet: SWAT stands for "Stretch, Wrap, And Tuck". The SWAT tourniquet is a wide elastic band that can serve as a tourniquet or pressure dressing, and is very simple to use. It is compact, lightweight, and inexpensive. The SWAT is often carried as a backup to other tourniquets due to its versatility.

The Parabelt: A recent addition to the market, the Parabelt is a utility belt designed for daily wear that becomes a ratcheting tourniquet with a self-locking system. Available in 5 different sizes.

The Pneumatic Tourniquet (sometimes called the EMT or Emergency and Military Tourniquet): Commonly used in operating rooms, pneumatic tourniquets are reminiscent of a blood pressure cuff and are inflated until bleeding stops. It is important to make sure the application avoids crinkling or folding of the cuff to avoid skin damage and other issues. This item gives the ability of knowing exactly how much pressure is being applied.

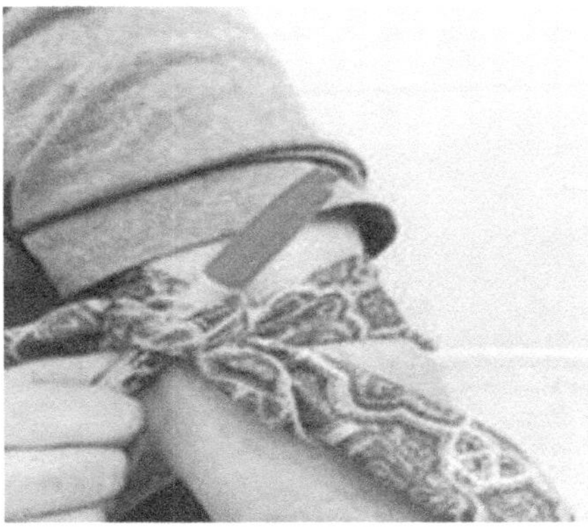

Improvised Tourniquets: Necessity is the mother of invention, and you can improvise a tourniquet with a bandanna and a stick. Wrap the bandanna or other wide strip of cloth above the wound and tie the stick in place with a knot. Twist the stick until adequate pressure is applied and then tie another knot on top to secure it. This is less effective than the commercial models, but it may be all you have.

It's important to realize that, while a tourniquet stops bleeding in a torn vessel, it also stops circulation from intact arteries and veins. As well, tourniquets are painful, and prolonged use could actually cause your patient to lose a limb. It takes less than an hour or two with a tourniquet in place to cause problems. Make sure to mark a "T" on the forehead as well as the time the tourniquet is placed.

At this point, consider placing a hemostatic agent in the wound and a pressure dressing (as discussed below). "Hemostasis" is the medical term for the control of bleeding. Once you are comfortable that major bleeding has abated, slowly release pressure from the tourniquet without removing it. This should preferably be performed within two hours.

Commercial Agents That Stop Bleeding

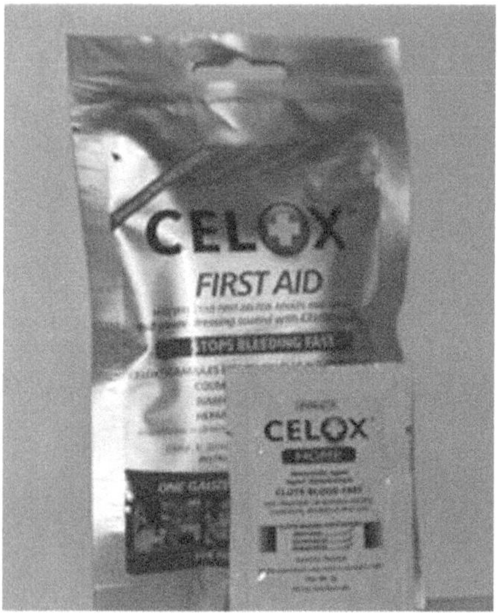

The control of major hemorrhage may be the territory of the trauma surgeon, but what if you find yourself without access to modern medical care? In the last decade or so, agents have been developed to help stop blood loss. Knowledge of their appropriate use in an emergency will increase the injured patient's chance of survival.

Although there are various types of hemostatic agents on the market for medical storage, the two most popular are Quikclot and Celox. They are two different substances that are available in powder or granule form. They also come impregnated in a dressing, which many consider easier to handle. The procedure is simple: Remove blood-soaked dressings and apply the hemostatic agent to the bleeding vessel in the wound, then apply firm direct pressure for three minutes.

Quikclot originally contained a volcanic mineral known as zeolite, which effectively clotted bleeding wounds but also caused a reaction that caused some serious burns. As a result, the main ingredient was replaced with another substance that does not burn when it comes in contact with blood. The current generation of Quikclot is made from Kaolin clay, the original ingredient in the anti-diarrheal product Kaopectate. It does not contain animal, human, or botanical components.

Contact between kaolin and blood immediately initiates the clotting process by activating Factor XII, a major player in the clotting process. The powder or impregnated gauze is applied and pressure placed for several minutes. Quikclot is FDA-approved and widely available, with a shelf life of three to five years.

One negative with Quikclot is that it does not absorb into the body and, some believe, can be difficult to remove from the wound. This was certainly true of previous generations but it is claimed to no longer be as big an issue, especially if you use the gauze dressing. If more than one dressing is required, don't remove the first one: Place the second gauze on top. Use an irrigation syringe to flush the wound after the gauze is finally removed.

Celox is another popular hemostatic agent. It is composed of chitosan, an organic material processed from shrimp shells. Despite this, the manufacturers claim that it is safe to use on those allergic to seafood.

When Celox comes in contact with blood, it bonds with it and forms a clot that appears as a gel. Like Quikclot, it also comes in impregnated gauze dressings. Unlike Quikclot, however, Celox will cause effective clotting even in those on anti-coagulants like Heparin or Coumadin without further depleting clotting factors. Chitosan, being an organic material, is gradually broken down by the body's natural enzymes and is thought to be easier to remove or absorb. Like Quikclot, Celox is FDA-approved. Both Quikclot and Celox gauze dressings have been tested by the U.S. and U.K. military in Iraq and Afghanistan.

Another product is X-STAT, a syringe full of small sponges that expand in the body. It is meant to inject into small diameter bullet wounds that are bleeding. An expensive prescription-only item with 92 pieces that must each be removed, it's an option with limited potential. Other new products we will soon see in use includes foams and gels that seal bleeding areas, even in abdominal and chest wounds.

Although they may prove to be effective, these items are not yet candidates as a first line of treatment in a bleeding patient. Pressure, elevation above the heart, gauze packing, and tourniquets should be your first steps. If these measures fail, however, hemostatic agents may save a life.

Dressing The Wound

Early in the process, don't remove bandages as you may also remove clots that are preventing further hemorrhage. Once bleeding is firmly under control, however, wound care must eventually take place. Using gloves and a 60 or 100 cc syringe, flush the wound aggressively with sterile water or a 1:10 Betadine solution. This procedure is known as "**irrigation**". You may have heard of cleaning wounds with alcohol or hydrogen peroxide; these are acceptable for a first cleaning if you have nothing else, but not for later wound care.

Once the wound has been irrigated, cover the whole area with a dry dressing for further protection. The Israeli army has developed an excellent bandage which is easy to use and is found almost everywhere survival gear is sold. The advantage of the "Israeli battle dressing" is that it not only covers a wound, but applies pressure on the bleeding area for you. It can also be used as a tourniquet if you don't have another option.

A wound that has stopped bleeding can easily start again. It may be appropriate to place a splint on an extremity to prevent movement, especially during transport.

Quick Step-By-Step Reference For Bleeding Control

1. **Put on gloves.**
2. **Expose the bleeding wound.**
3. **Using bandage or other barrier, apply firm direct pressure to wound.**

4. Use tourniquet(s) if bleeding continues.
5. Use hemostatic agents directly on bleeding vessel.
6. Wrap with tight compression dressing.
7. Cover patient with mylar blanket in shock position (legs elevated 12 inches above level of heart; not for torso wounds).
8. When transporting, immobilize an extremity wound with a splint to prevent re-bleed.

Knife And Bullet Wounds

Knife and bullet wounds are different than, say, an industrial accident in that you are, likely, in an area where there is hostile action. The first and most important goal of a medic is self-preservation. Becoming the next casualty does no one any good. Do not attempt to render aid unless you have abolished all threats to your own life. In a firefight, this may mean you should be armed and prepared to return fire.

You may have seen movies where the hero kills a villain instantly by throwing a knife at them. This is a highly improbable event. Don't be surprised if the victim is walking around with a knife in their back. In this circumstance, lie them down immediately; they can injure themselves further by fainting from loss of blood and falling onto a hard surface.

Where there is one injury, there may be more. Use a bandage scissors or EMT shears to cut through clothing and determine that you only have one wound. If the bleeding from the obvious wound is serious, however, attend to it first using the procedures previously mentioned.

In normal times, standard protocol states that you should not remove a knife or other impaled object because it can cause the hemorrhage to worsen. In these cases, keep the object in place and pack around it. This will give you time to get the patient to the hospital, but what if there are no hospitals?

In survival settings, you will have to transport your victim to your base camp and prepare to remove the knife. After all, it can't stay in there for months while you're waiting for society to re-stabilize. Getting the patient to a setting where you have control and materials is essential. Have plenty of dressings, a tourniquet, and clotting agents ready for use.

Wounds from firearms are more variable and problematic than wounds from a sharp instrument. A stabbing incident is an example of a penetrating injury, but it's unlikely to perforate through the body. A bullet wound however, may do so and it's important to look for exit wounds. These may be larger than the entry wound. Rifle rounds have a higher chance of passing through the body than those from handguns or shotguns due to their higher velocity.

Exit wounds do not always follow a straight path from the entry wound. This depends on the position the victim was in when shot, and also the structure that were impacted when the bullet entered the body. If the bullet hits a bone, for example, it can cause a fracture and then travel at an angle through the rest of the body.

Expect dirt, clothes, and other debris to have been pushed into the wound by the bullet (or even a knife). In other words, these wounds are dirty. Antibiotics will likely be necessary to prevent infection.

It's useful to have an idea of how bullets cause trauma. Ballistics is the science that deals with the launching, flight, behavior, and effects of projectiles. High-velocity projectile damage as caused by a bullet is, as you might imagine, much greater than low-velocity damage caused by, say, a knife wound. This damage depends on the amount of energy the projectile possesses due to its motion. In physics, this is referred to as **kinetic energy**. It follows the formula:

Kinetic Energy = mass of the projectile times its velocity squared, divided by 2.

The "square" of a number is the number multiplied by itself, for example, the square of 2 is 2 x 2, or 4. Because of this, you can see from the formula that the velocity, or speed, of the projectile is more important in the causing of damage than its weight, or mass.

As a missile passes through tissue, it decelerates, transferring all of this kinetic energy to the body. The result is a traumatic wound caused by several methods:

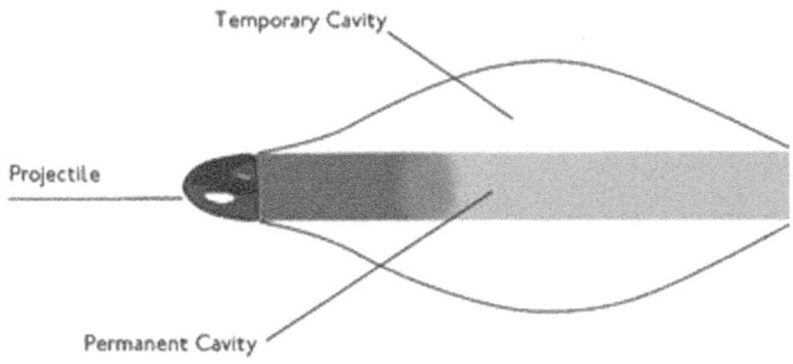

- **Permanent Cavitation:** the path permanently left by the projectile. Essentially, this is the bullet hole and the channel caused by its traverse through the body.
- **Temporary Cavitation:** A shock wave which crushes tissues beyond the actual path of the bullet. This is caused by the dissipation of kinetic energy as the missile decelerates when it meets resistance. Although various organs have differing elasticities, the shock wave may surpass the tissue's ability to absorb the energy without serious damage.
- **Deformation:** As the bullet enters the body, it may deform, increasing its diameter and, thus, the cavity it causes. This usually occurs at the expense of penetration depth. Hollow point bullets are an example of projectiles that are meant to deform ("mushroom") as they travel through the body.

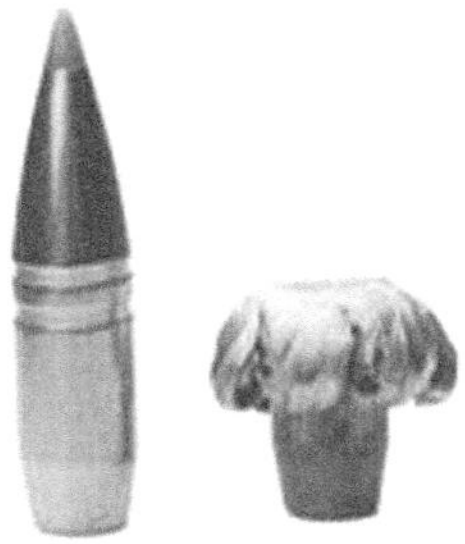

"Mushrooming" Bullet Deformation

- **Yaw:** Yaw refers to the rotation of the nose of the bullet away from the line of flight. A short, high velocity bullet begins to yaw more severely and tumble upon entering tissue. This causes a larger temporary cavitation and more tissue to be violently displaced.

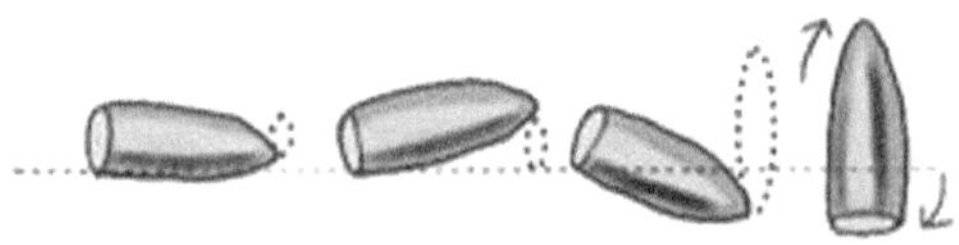

Yaw and Tumble

- **Fragmentation:** Bullets may fragment as they travel through the body. This causes multiple cavitation channels, both permanent and temporary, that can cause damage. Some bullets are specifically designed to fragment for this very purpose.

When modern medical care is available, bullets are usually removed from wounds. In austere settings, however, you will want to avoid digging into tissue for a hidden bullet. Although there are instruments for this purpose, nearby nerves and blood vessels may be damaged by your exploration. As well, contamination may lead to infection.

A historical example illustrates this well is the case of President James Garfield. In 1881, President Garfield was shot by an assassin. In their rush to remove the bullet, 12 different physicians placed their (ungloved) hands in the wound. The wound, which would not have been mortal, became infected. As a result, the president died after a month in agony. In austere settings, think twice before removing a projectile that isn't clearly visible and easily reached.

Body Armor

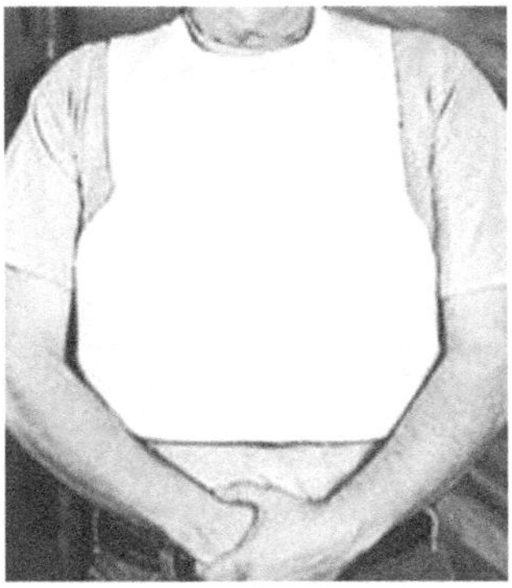

In high-risk environments, perforating trauma may be prevented by the use of body armor. The development of the protective synthetic fiber "Kevlar" by Dupont in the late 1960s led to the resurgence of body armor for use by the military and law enforcement. Lightweight and durable, more than 3000 police officers' lives and even more combat soldiers owe their lives to it over the past 30 years.

There are two types of body armor:

Soft body armor: Useful for its lightweight nature, it is protective against handgun rounds but will not stop a rifle bullet.

Hard body armor: This type is characterized by hard rigid plates which are effective even against rifle rounds. This is most commonly used by the military and police tactical units.

No body armor is entirely bulletproof; the amount of injury depends on the type you are wearing. Level I vests protect against common handgun rounds like 38 caliber. Level IV protection can protect against a round from an assault rifle.

When a bullet hits bullet proof armor, it is trapped in a web of very durable ballistic fiber. These fibers help disperse the energy from the round across the vest and prevent penetration into the body, thereby saving the wearer's life.

This doesn't mean that injuries won't happen. The bullet will cause indentation of the vest (also called "back face deformation") which can break ribs or cause large contusions, spinal injury, or internal organ damage.

The Medic Under Fire

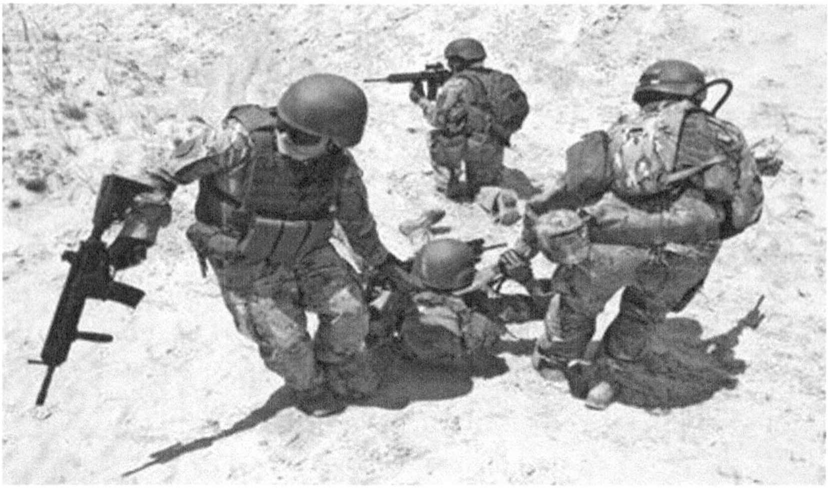

"I am dying."

This was the tweet posted by Oleysa Zhukovskaya, a 21 year old woman who volunteered to function as a medic during the Ukrainian uprising in 2013. Police snipers were targeting medics (marked with red crosses) and journalists; Zhukovskaya was struck in the neck by a bullet.

Seeing this drama unfold, we considered long term survival scenarios in which civil unrest and other events may put the group medic in harm's way. This may involve situations where the medic is with his or her group in foraging operations, or simply at "base camp" when hostile forces arrive, as in the Ukrainian example mentioned above.

Our young medic might have thought her red cross identified her as a "non-combatant" and made her immune to enemy fire. Despite the Geneva Convention, this probably could not be further from the truth: Eliminating the medics is a great way to decrease the effectiveness of the group and cause a devastating hit to morale. Therefore, a basic piece of advice is to avoid wearing a big white armband with a red cross; US military medics today wear a much less noticeable insignia.

Doing the right thing at the right time is the cornerstone of tactical combat casualty care (TCCC). This is different from what you might consider to be the practice of good medicine. In an unsafe environment, good medicine could be bad tactics, and that could get people killed.

This poses the question: Should medics be armed? An important goal in this case is to abolish all threats, and this means helping to provide suppressive fire if needed. The best medical care when under fire is eliminating the enemy, or at least keeping their heads down and weapons silent.

This tactic is hard for the medic to swallow, as they will want to attend to wounded members immediately. Without dealing with the threat, however, they are likely to become the next casualty if they run into the line of fire. History shows us that this was a common way for the medic to meet his demise, sometimes on the way to evaluate casualties that were already beyond help.

A second issue for the medic is that many of the tools used to evaluate a victim will be useless in a firefight. Forget trying to listen to a casualty's heart and lungs with a stethoscope if there is heavy gunfire. As well, it's foolhardy to use a head lamp at night to treat the wounded, as it might as well become a target bull's-eye.

When under fire, therefore, your priorities should be:

1) Abolish or suppress the threat.
2) Avoid exposure to enemy fire while attempting to reach a casualty.
3) Get the casualty and yourself to reasonable cover.
4) Use your tourniquet along with direct pressure and other hemostatic (blood-clotting) methods to stop heavy bleeding when appropriate.
5) Figure out a way to transport your victim and yourself away from hostile forces.

Notice we don't mention airway management or cervical spine immobilization, two basic steps in evaluation, care, and transport of victims of trauma in a safe environment. Stabilization of the spine is good medicine, but control of hemorrhage will be the most likely way you'll save a life in this scenario. You don't have the luxury of time to do much else.

Something that was clear to us in these settings was the importance of cross-training. Everyone in your group should know how to apply a tourniquet correctly to themselves and others, as well as other basic hemorrhage control strategies.

If the medic is the wounded party, the ability to give concise instructions to others could save a life (yours). If you are the medically responsible member in your group, think about what you would tell other group members to do if you were bleeding, broke a bone, were sick, etc. The more people that know how to deal with medical issues, the higher the chances to succeed, even if everything else fails.

By the way: Our Ukrainian medic was transported to the hospital, and survived.

SOFT TISSUE WOUND CARE

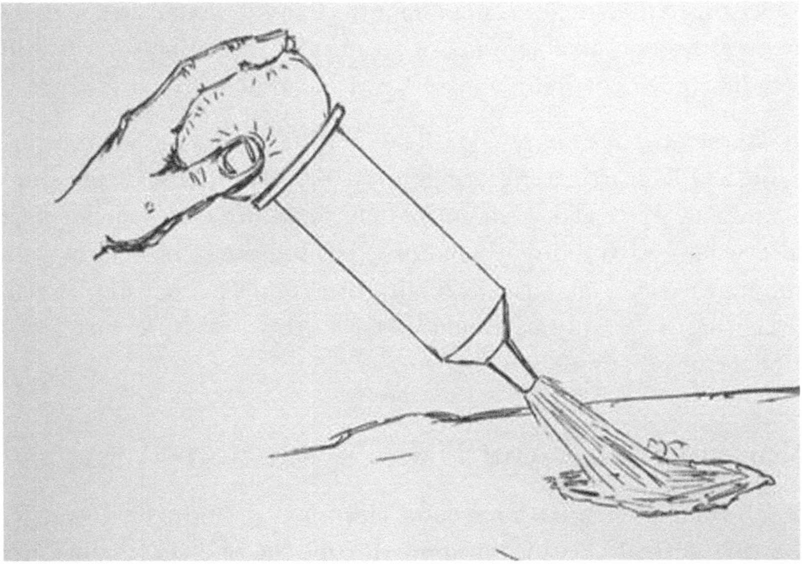

Irrigating The Wound

Once you have stopped the bleeding and applied your dressing, the emergency is over. In an austere setting, however, you must follow the status of the wound until full recovery in your role as medic. Continued diligent wound care is your responsibility.

An open wound can heal by two methods:

Primary Intention (Closure): The wound is closed in some way, such as with sutures or staples. This results in a smaller scar, but carries the risk of inadvertently sequestering bacteria deep in the wound.

Secondary Intention (Granulation): Leaving a wound open causes the formation of "**granulation tissue**". Granulation tissue is rapidly growing early scar tissue that is rich in blood vessels. It fills in spaces where the wound edges are not together. After a period of time, it turns into mature scar tissue. This scar is larger than if the wound were closed by primary intention, but proper care decreases the risk of infection.

Often, it is safest to allow a wound to heal on its own rather than suture or staple it closed. Wound dressings must be changed regularly (at least twice a day or whenever the bandage is saturated with blood, fluids, etc.) in order to give the best chance for rapid healing. When you change a dressing, it is important to clean the wound area with sterile, or at least, drinkable water or an antiseptic solution such as dilute Betadine (povidone-iodine). Use 1 part Betadine to 10 parts water.

Remember the old saying, "The solution to pollution is dilution". Using a bulb or irrigation syringe (60-100 ml) will provide pressure to the flow of water and wash out old clots and dirt. Lightly scrub any open wound with diluted Betadine, sterilized water, or normal saline. You may notice some (usually slight) bleeding. This is a sign of viable tissue that is forming new blood vessels. Apply pressure with a clean bandage until it stops.

Normal Saline And Dakin's Solution

A solution often used for wound cleaning is "normal saline". It is termed "normal" because it approximates the salt content of blood. Sterile normal saline may be purchased online, or it can be homemade. You'll need a pan with a lid, salt, water, and sterile jars with sterile lids.

Add two teaspoons of salt to a liter of water to a pan. Place a lid on the pan and bring the salt water to a roiling boil. After a short time, let the solution cool in the pan with the lid on. Then, pour into sterile jars and close with sterile lids. Sterile saline produced this way should last 30 days with the lids closed and perhaps 24-48 hours after opening.

Interestingly, most studies find that sterilized (drinkable) water is just as good as a concentrated antiseptic for wound healing (sometimes better). Although it is acceptable to perform a first cleaning with Betadine or hydrogen peroxide, later cleaning should definitely not use these concentrated products. New cells are trying to grow, and they do this best in a moist environment. Concentrated antiseptics dry out these fragile new cells and may slow down healing.

An alternative antiseptic solution that is easy to make using common storage supplies is **Dakin's Solution.** First used during WWI, Dakin's solution is used to disinfect soft tissue wounds, such as pressure sores in bedridden patients. It is inexpensive to put together and dissolves dead cells. Dakin's solution is composed of the following:

- Sodium hypochlorite solution (regular strength household bleach).
- Sodium bicarbonate (baking soda)
- Boiled tap water

To make Dakin's solution, take 4 cups of sterilized water and add ½ teaspoon of baking soda. Then, add a certain amount of bleach to reach the strength that you'll need:

- 3 teaspoons will act as a mild antiseptic effect (plenty for clean wounds that are healing)
- 3 tablespoons will give you a stronger effect for infected wounds.
- 3 fluid ounces (about 100 cc) for a full strength solution to treat the worst infections.

Do not take Dakin's solution internally and watch for allergic reactions in the form or rashes or other irritation. Store in darkness at room temperature and make a new batch every few days, as it loses potency relatively quickly. Do not freeze or heat up the solution.

The "Wet-to-Dry" Dressing

To assure rapid healing of open wounds, we use a type of dressing method known as "**wet-to-dry**". Apply a bandage that has been soaked in sterilized water and wrung out to the open wound. In this fashion, we prevent the drying out of new cells by keeping them in a moist environment. On top of the damp dressing, place a dry bandage and some type of tape to secure it in place. Thus, you have a "wet-to-dry" dressing.

It may also be a good idea to apply some antibiotic ointment around a healing wound to prevent infection from bacteria on the skin. Raw honey, lavender oil, and tea tree oil are some natural alternatives.

Black or brown material on the wound edges is non-viable and should be removed. It might easily scrub out, but you might need to take a scissors or scalpel and trim off the dead tissue. This is called "**debridement**" and removes material that is no longer part of the healing process. In some cases, certain maggots have been used to consume non-viable tissue.

WOUND CLOSURE

When a laceration occurs, our body's natural armor is breached and bacteria get a free ride to the rest of our body. Therefore, it only makes common sense that we want to close that breach to speed healing and lock out infection.

There is controversy, however, as to whether or not to close a wound. When and why would you choose to close a wound, and what method should you use? A laceration may be closed either by sutures, tapes, staples or medical "superglues" such as Derma-Bond. After rendering first aid, which includes removal of any foreign objects, hemostasis (bleeding control), irrigation, and antiseptic application, you will have to make a decision.

To Close Or Not To Close...

What am you trying to accomplish by closing a wound? Your goals are simple. You close wounds to repair the defect in your body's armor, to eliminate "dead space", and to promote healing. A well-approximated wound also has less scarring.

It sounds as if all wounds should be closed. Unfortunately, closing a wound that should be left open can do a lot more harm than good, and could possibly put your patient's life at risk. Take the case of a young woman injured some years ago in a "zipline" accident: She was taken to the local emergency room, where 22 staples were needed to close a large laceration.

Unfortunately, the wound had dangerous bacteria in it, causing a serious infection which spread throughout her body. She eventually required multiple amputations. We learn from this an important lesson: Namely, that the decision to close a wound is not automatic but involves several considerations.

The most important consideration is whether you are dealing with a clean or a dirty wound. Most wounds you will encounter in an off-grid setting will be dirty. If you try to close a dirty wound, such as a gunshot, you have sequestered bacteria and dirt into your body. Within a short period of time, the infected wound will become red, swollen, and hot. An abscess may form, and pus will accumulate inside.

The infection may spread to the bloodstream, a condition known as "**septicemia**", and become life-threatening. Leaving the wound open will allow you to clean the inside frequently and observe the healing process. It also allows inflammatory fluid to drain out of the body. The scar isn't as pretty, but it's the safest option in most cases.

Other considerations when deciding whether or not to close a wound are whether it is a simple laceration (straight thin cut on the skin) or whether it is an avulsion (areas of skin torn out or hanging flaps). If the edges of the skin are so far apart that they cannot be stitched together without undue pressure, the wound should be left open.

If the wound has been open for more than 8 hours, it should be left open. Even the air has bacteria, and there's a good chance that they have already colonized the injury.

Let's say that you're certain the wound is clean. It's less than 8 hours old. Here are some factors that would suggest that closure is appropriate:

- The laceration is long or deep. The exception would be a puncture wound from an animal bite. These bites are loaded with bacteria and should be kept open in austere settings.
- The wound is located over a joint. A moving part, such as the knee, will constantly stress a wound and prevent it from closing in by itself.
- The wound gapes open loosely, suggesting that it can be closed without undue pressure on the skin.

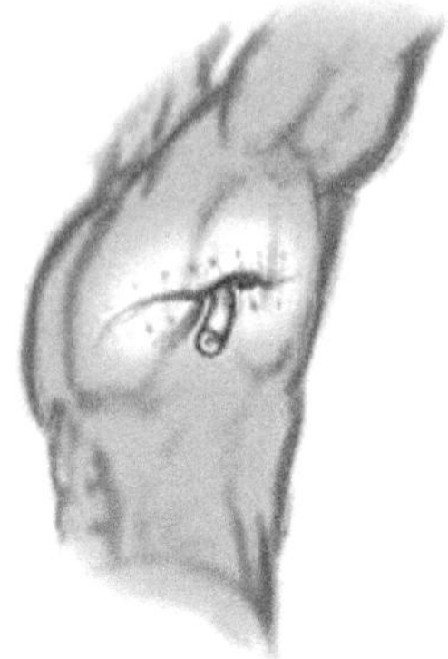

PENROSE DRAIN IN PLACE

If you are unsure, you can choose to wait 48 to 72 hours before closing a wound to make sure that no signs of infection develop. This is referred to as "delayed closure". Some wounds can be partially closed, allowing a small open space to avoid the accumulation of inflammatory fluid.

Drains, consisting of thin lengths of latex, nitrile, or even gauze, might be placed into the wound for this purpose. Penrose drains are a version of these that are still used in some operating rooms. Drains have a tendency to leak, so place a dressing over the exposed area.

Many injuries that require closure (and some that don't) also should be treated with antibiotics in oral or topical form to decrease the chance of infection. Natural substances with antibiotic properties, such as garlic or raw, unprocessed honey, may be useful in survival scenarios.

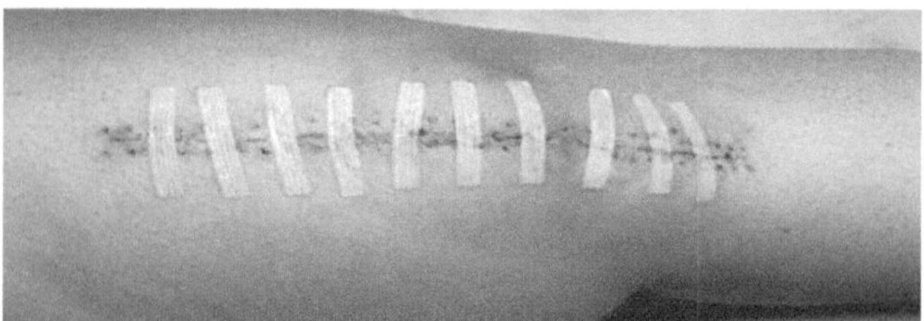

Multiple Wound Closure Methods On Same Wound

Tapes And Glues

There are several methods available to close a laceration. You should use the simplest and least invasive method that will do the job. Non-invasive methods involve the use of tapes and glues. These make sense for several reasons:

1) They are less painful for the patient.
2) Unlike sutures or staples, they don't cause additional punctures of the skin. As such, there is less risk for infection.
3) Materials are less expensive.
4) In a survival setting, more advanced closure materials like sutures and staples are no longer being manufactured, so your supply is very limited.

The easiest to use are "**Steri-Strips**" and butterfly closures. These are adhesive bandages which adhere on each side of the wound to pull it together. They don't require puncturing the skin and will fall off on their own over time. Even duct tape can be used to make a butterfly closure. For additional security, **tincture of benzoin** is applied to the skin on each side of the laceration before applying the tapes. In this way, they will usually stay on even when wet.

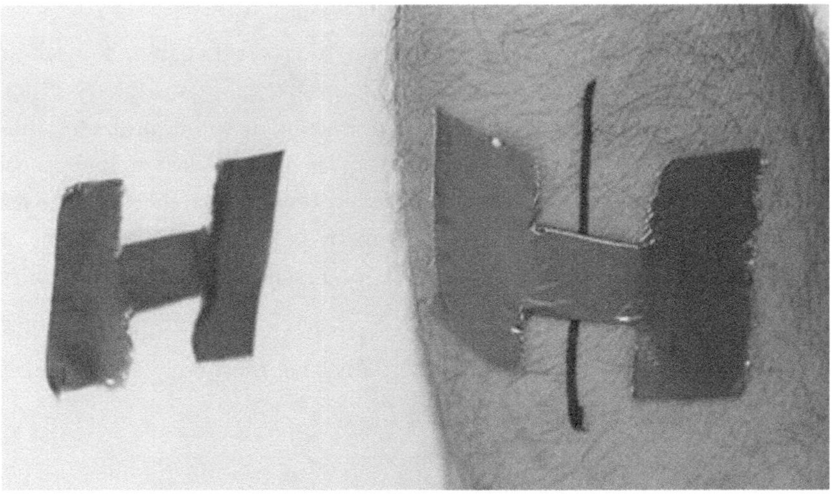

Improvised Closure With Duct Tape

Another non-invasive method is Cyanoacrylate, special "glue" sold as Derma-Bond, Surgiseal, and others, some of which are by prescription only. These are medical- grade adhesives made specifically for use on the skin. They create an environment which speeds healing and even decreases the risk of infections with bacteria like Staph. Skin glues are indicated where there is little or no tension in a dry (not bleeding) wound that is not over a joint. They are not for use inside the mouth.

To use topical skin adhesive glue:

- Approximate the wound edges carefully (best done by an assistant).
- Gently brush the glue over the laceration, taking care not to push any below the level of the skin.
- Apply about three layers of the adhesive over the wound, preferably widening the area of glue each time to increase strength of closure.
- Once completely dry, consider adding Steri-Strips to increase the strength of the closure.

Although you would use antibiotic ointment on most wound closures, avoid it in closures with skin glues; it breaks down the compound. The glue itself, however, helps protect the wound from infection.

Some have recommended (the much less expensive) household "Super-Glue" for wound closure. This preparation is slightly different chemically, and may cause skin irritation in some, and burn-like reactions have been occasionally reported. It may not last as long as the prescription version. If it's all you have, however, you may choose to use it. You can test super-glue for reactions by placing a small amount on the inside of your forearm and observe for a rash over the next 24 hours.

It should be noted that closures with butterfly closures and glues are not as strong as closure with more invasive methods like sutures or staples, especially in the first few days.

Sutures And Staples

Some wounds, especially those over joints, require a more durable closure than can be achieved with tapes or glues. Sutures and staples are closure methods that will give strong support to the healing wound. Each method has its advantages and disadvantages. They should be used only when lesser methods won't work.

Staplers were originally developed to attach loose ends of intestines together, and they are still used for that purpose in modern operating rooms. From a practical standpoint, however, you'll be using them only to close skin. Staples look and act much like office staples. They work by "pinching" the skin edges of a laceration together. Like office staples, a separate instrument called a "staple remover" is used to remove them.

Sutures are, perhaps, the most versatile closure method for serious wounds. Today, sutures are comprised of a string attached (or "swaged") onto the end of a needle. They are made of various different types of material. More knowledge, time, and training is required to place sutures than staples.

Both techniques involve putting additional punctures in the skin, which is why they are considered "invasive". When should you use one method over the other? Staples are useful in any situation where there is a straight laceration and only the skin needs to be closed. Sutures should be used for deep layers of tissue and lacerations that are irregular in appearance.

Considerations when choosing between sutures and staples:

Sutures

- Can be used on skin or deep layers
- Best for jagged lacerations
- More skill required to perform well
- Can be performed alone
- Many materials from which to choose
- More time-consuming
- Any scissors can be used to remove, or no removal at all if absorbable sutures are used.

Staples

- Should be used for skin closure only
- Best for straight-line cuts
- Less skill required to perform well
- Best performed with an assistant
- Few choices (essentially, standard or large)
- Can be accomplished very quickly
- Requires special instruments to place and remove properly

To place staples properly, an assistant is needed with two toothed tweezers called "Adson's Forceps" to hold the edges of skin together. You might find it interesting that, in stapling procedures, it's the assistants that are the skilled labor: The closure's integrity depends on whether their job was done well or not. A suture procedure, however, can be done alone.

All About Suture Material

We are asked to teach suturing more than any other first aid procedure, even though it really isn't *first* aid at all. Although stapling a wound closed is fairly straightforward for the person holding the stapler, suturing is best done by someone with experience, and you don't get that kind of experience in your typical first responder course.

Survival medical training teaches you to stabilize and transfer the patient to modern facilities as soon as possible. In survival scenarios, wound closure becomes the responsibility of the medic as the highest medical asset left. You'll need to obtain the knowledge to be able to function effectively in a long-term setting; that means learning how to close wounds. It's not just about learning how to "throw a stitch" or place a staple. It's about developing the judgement as to when a wound should be closed and when it shouldn't, plus the skill to know which closure method to use.

Let's learn more about sutures. We first starting wearing clothes about 170,000 years ago, and learned to make needles from bone and antler soon afterward. It made sense to prehistoric peoples that, if they can sew together hides to make clothing, they could sew together their own "hides" if it were necessary.

Archeological digs often turn up needles made from antler and bone. The first documentation of suturing was from the Egyptians 5,000 years ago. The Greeks and Romans, as well as various native cultures, also worked with sutures using copper needles and flax, hemp, silk, hair, animal sinew, and other natural materials. In the Roman period, the physician Galen stitched together the severed tendons and ligaments of gladiators, sometimes restoring function to a damaged extremity.

Even today, in primitive cultures, ingenious ways exist to close wounds. In some tropical rain forests, the natives would collect army ant soldiers whenever there was a wound to close. They place the jaws of the ant on the skin which causes the soldier to bite. They then twist the body off! The head stays on with the jaws shut and the skin closed. In other areas, Native Americans pull off agave cactus needles along with a strip of the plant material attached, and fashion it for use as suture.

Types Of Suture Material

Suture technology didn't really advance much until the late 19th century, when the concept of sterilization of needles and suture material came into fashion. At this time, suture material was either "catgut" (actually made from the intestinal lining of sheep and cows) or silk. Both of these materials are still available today in one form or another.

Suture "string" is either absorbable or nonabsorbable. Catgut, for example, will dissolve in the body over the course of several weeks. There are two types of catgut: Plain, which dissolves in 2 weeks and Chromic, which dissolves in 3-4 weeks. Absorbable sutures like catgut are used for deep layers or the oral cavity. They are also used to close lacerations incurred in the vagina as a result of childbirth.

More recently, synthetic absorbables have been developed such as polyglycolic acid (brand name Vicryl) and Polydioxanone (brand name PDS). These last longer than catgut, taking 2-3 months to absorb. The longer period makes them useful when suturing layers such as muscle and connective tissue.

Nonabsorbable sutures are preferably used on the skin, as they can be removed when the wound is healed. Examples of nonabsorbable sutures include silk and cotton. Synthetics developed more recently include monofilaments like Prolene and Nylon. Although meant for the skin, these sutures can be used anywhere that you can accept their permanent presence in the body.

What happens if you place permanent suture in deeper layers? The body recognizes silk, for example, as a foreign object and will wall it off as it would any invader. This forms a small nodule called a "**granuloma**" that you might feel under the skin. There is really very little, if any, ill effect other than this.

Besides different materials, sutures come in various thicknesses: 0, 2-0, 3-0, 4-0, 5-0 and 6-0 are common gauges used on humans. The higher the number, the thinner the thread will be. This is not dissimilar to buckshot: 00 is thicker than 000, just as 2-0 (pronounced two-oh) is thicker than 3-0 (three-oh). Of the above, 0 is thickest in gauge and used for large structures; 6-0, on the other hand, is used in delicate work on, for example, the face. The heavier suture has more strength, but the finer suture leaves less of a scar. For practice, consider using 2-0 or 3-0.

Needles have progressed over time, as well. Needles can be straight, curved, or a multitude of other shapes. Originally, needles were "eyed" and separate from the string. In 1920, a process called "swaging" was developed, which allowed the back end of the needle to be attached to the string. This made the two items one unit. Some swaged needles are built to "pop-off" with a quick tug after placing each stitch. This may be handy, but it is incredibly wasteful of suture material; therefore, we discourage its use unless you have unlimited supplies.

Needles are also categorized based on the point. The two most common needle points are "tapered" and "cutting", although there are various others. One is round and "tapers" smoothly to a point, like a sharpened pencil does. "Cutting" needles are triangular and have a sharp "cutting" edge on the curve of the needle. Cutting needles are best used in dense tissue, such as skin. Tapered needles are used on intestines and other delicate tissues.

HOW TO SUTURE SKIN

Here's a practice session that will give you an introduction to a brand new skill: Suturing.

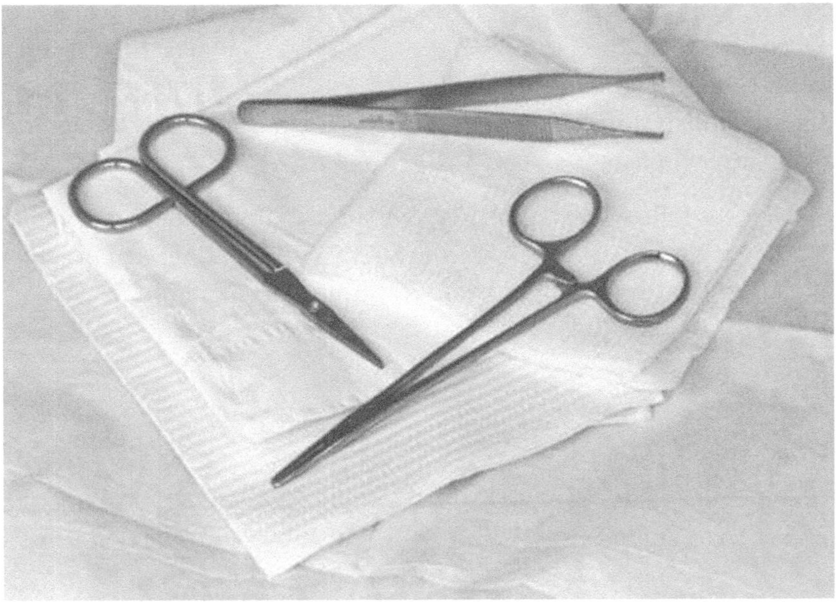

First, you'll need some supplies. Suture kits, sometimes called "laceration trays", are available commercially and are comprised of the following items:

- A needle holder to, well, hold the needle.
- An Adson forceps (looks like tweezers with teeth at the end) to steady the skin being sutured.
- Scissors to cut the string.
- Gauze pads to clean blood off the field.
- Drapes to isolate the area being repaired.

The above supplies usually arrive in a sterile package. Things you will need to add:

- Antiseptic Solution, such as Betadine (2% povidone-iodine solution) or Hibiclens (chlorhexidine).
- Gloves (Nitrile is preferable to Latex, sterile preferable to non-sterile).
- The suture you'll be using.

Of course, you'll need something to stitch together. The best material is a pig's foot. The skin of a pig's foot is probably the closest thing you'll find to human skin. Make a straight three to four inch cut through the skin with a knife or scalpel.

For the following steps below, refer to the numbered images and/or access our YouTube video: "How to Suture with Dr. Bones". This video goes through the entire process in real time with narration.

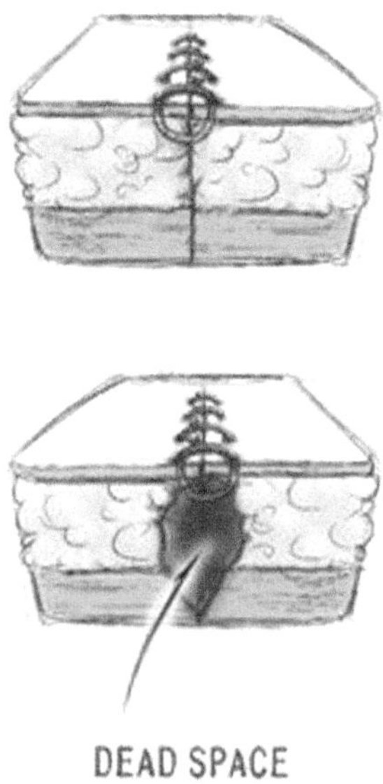

An important goal of your closure is to eliminate "dead space". Dead spaces are pockets of air or fluid in a closed wound that may lead to a major infection. Wounds that penetrate into deep layers like fat or muscle should be closed in layers, to prevent any un-approximated "dead space" from occurring. Always close the deepest layer first.

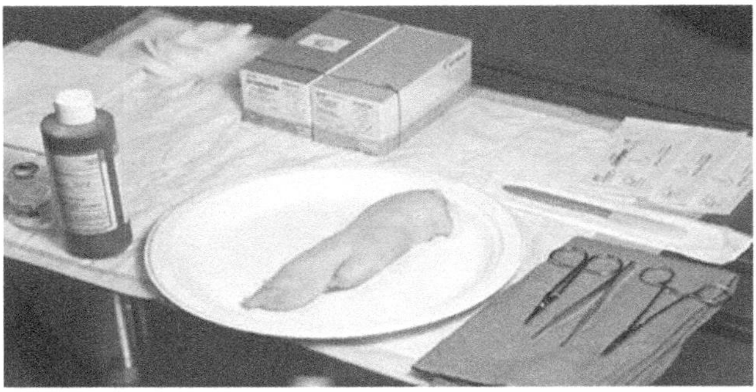

After washing and defrosting, place your pig's foot on a level surface. Put your gloves on. In a real wound, you would have irrigated the area well beforehand with an antiseptic to eliminate debris from inside the wound.

You will then perform a "skin prep". Paint the area to be sutured with a pad dipped in Betadine, Hibiclens, or other antiseptic. Alcohol may be used if nothing else is available. Start at the laceration edges and paint around them in an ever-widening oval. Don't go back over disinfected areas, as you will transport bacteria there.

Next, you will isolate the "prepped" area by placing a sterile drape. The drape will usually be "fenestrated", which means it has an opening in the middle to expose the area to be sutured. Taken together, we refer to this the "surgical" or "sterile field". Although you are suturing a (deceased, we hope) pig's foot, I'll describe the process as if you are working with living tissue.

Assuming your patient is conscious, you would want to numb the area with 1% or 2% Lidocaine solution (prescription) if you have it.

Use an alcohol wipe on the end of the bottle, then fill a small syringe with air. Inject the air into the bottle, and the local anesthetic will fill the syringe. Place an injection at a 45 degree angle to the skin, and then inject enough to form a raised area on each side of the laceration (see figure below). Within a few minutes, the area will be numb.

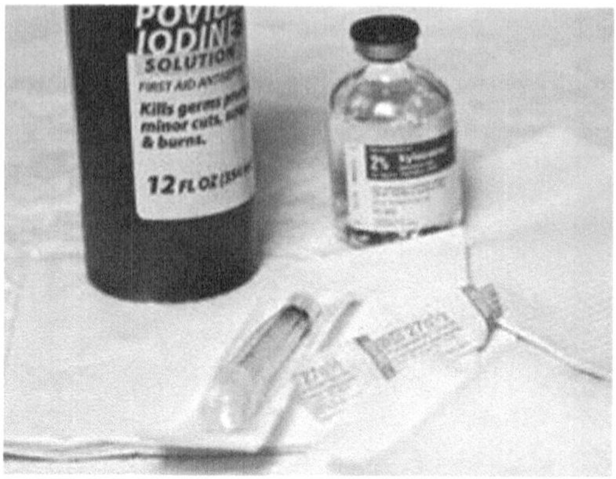

It should be noted that Lidocaine is a prescription medication and is difficult to procure. When used in subcutaneous tissue, it acts as an anesthetic; used intravenously, however, it has cardiac and other effects. An accidental injection into a blood vessel can become life-threatening, causing heart irregularities and seizures. The procedure is described more in detail in the section on local anesthesia.

To determine if you are in a blood vessel, pull the plunger back before you inject anything into the tissue. This maneuver is called "**aspiration**". Aspirating will draw blood into the syringe if it's in the wrong place. If you lack Lidocaine, you can apply an ice cube to the area to be sutured until sensation decreases.

In an austere setting, you might not even have ice. We'll just have to realize that there may not be numbing agents available if a disaster takes us off the grid. This is one reason why we recommend using the least invasive method possible of closing a wound.

Open your laceration tray and the suture packet. Take the tip of your needle holder and grasp the (usually) curved needle right in the middle. Remove it and the attached "string" from the packet. Adjust the curved needle on the needle holder so that it is perpendicular to the line of the instrument.

If you are holding the needle holder in your right hand, the sharp end of the needle should point to your left. The sharp end of the needle should point to the right for left-handers (see figure below).

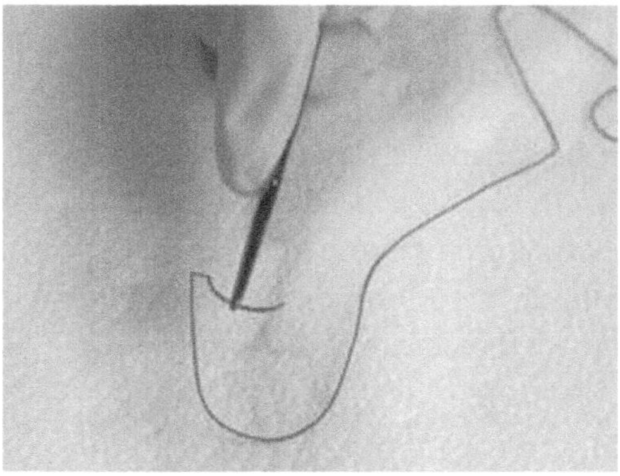

Now take your forceps (tweezers) and grasp the edge of the laceration near one end where you wish to place the first stitch (see figure below). Insert the suture needle at a 90 degree angle to the skin and drive it through that side of the laceration with a twist of the wrist The needle should enter the skin no closer than a quarter inch from the edge of the laceration, or about the width of the head of your needle driver, and exit inside the wound.

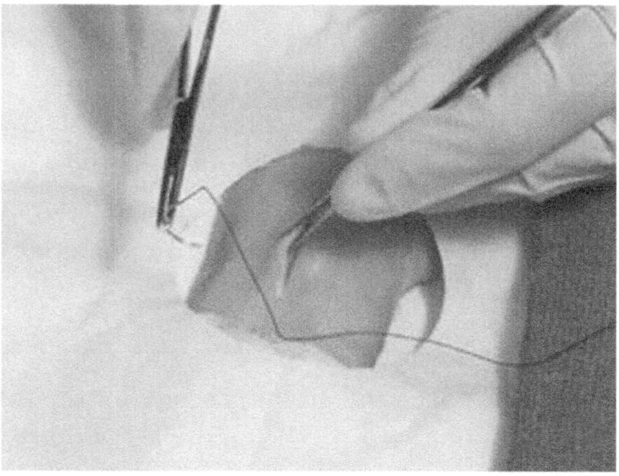

Although most suture closures begin at one end of the laceration and end at the other, an alternative is available that is especially material-conservative. Place one suture in the exact middle, then evaluate the amount of gaping in the rest of the laceration. If the skin edges close well, you can use Steri-strips or other butterfly closures to approximate the rest. If still gaping, place a suture directly in the middle of each of the two sides, then re-evaluate and place Steri-strips as needed.

Release the needle and re-clamp it on the inside of the wound and pull it through. Replace the needle on the needle holder and, going from the inside of the wound, drive the needle with a twist of the wrist through the skin on the other side of the laceration. Pull the string through, leaving a 1-2 inch length (see figure below). This should leave you with a long side (the side with the needle) and a short side.

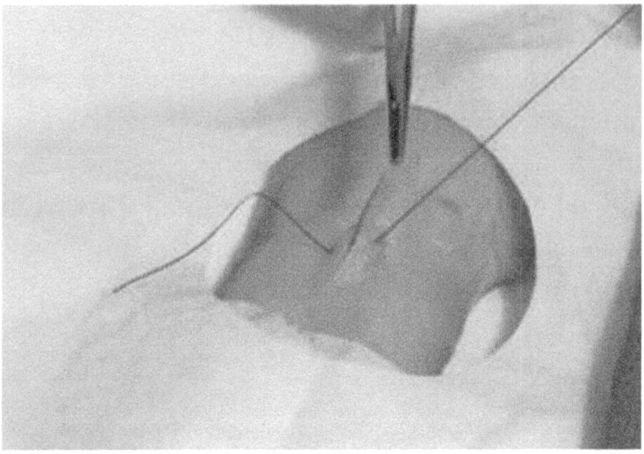

There are various ways to tie your suture, each with its own advantages and disadvantages. In our opinion, the ideal method for the survival medic 1) has multiple knots so that one faulty stitch doesn't unravel the whole closure and 2) conserves precious suture material. This method is the Instrument Tie.

Holding the needle holder loosely over the wound, wrap the long end of the string twice over and around the end of the instrument (see figure below). Then, open the needle holder end slightly and grab the very end of the short end of the suture. Pull it through the loop tightly and you will form what is called a "Surgeon's Knot. The Surgeon's Knot will stay on the skin better than most first knots. Add 4 or 5 more knots on top of the first. Although two loops are best for the first knot, only one loop around the needle holder is needed for each successive knot.

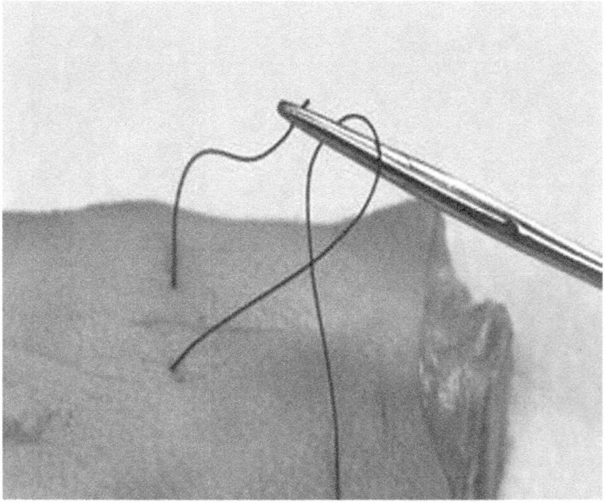

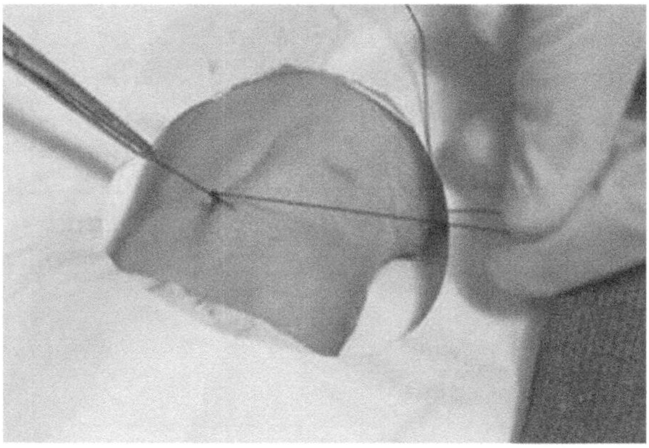

Finally, grasp the two ends and cut the remaining suture material ¼ inch from the knot with your suture scissors. If you have a good supply of suture material, place each subsequent suture about ½ inch apart from the previous one, especially if over a joint (see below). In situations where suture availability is limited, you may choose to fill in areas between sutures with tapes in areas where the laceration isn't over a joint.

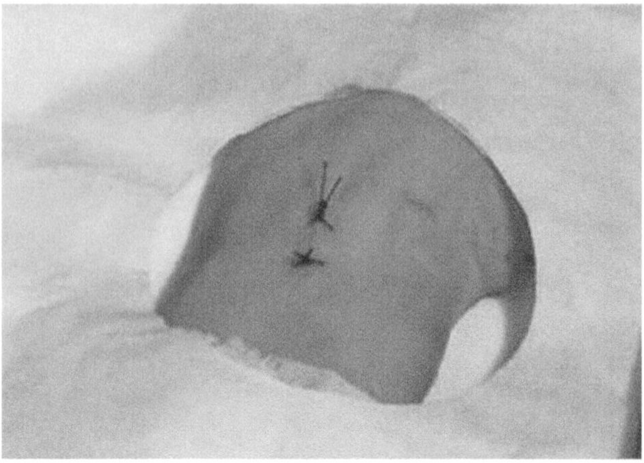

It's important to tighten your knots only enough to close the wound. Excessive pressure from a knot that is too tight will prevent healing in the area of the suture. You can easily identify sutures that are too tight: They will cause an indentation in the skin where the string is. To finish your suture job, apply some antibiotic cream or raw honey.

Cover the closure with Once the closure is done, keep the wound dry and covered for 48 hours, checking its several times a day. Sutures on the skin should be removed in 7 days (5 days if on the face); if over a joint, 14-21 days.

HOW TO STAPLE SKIN

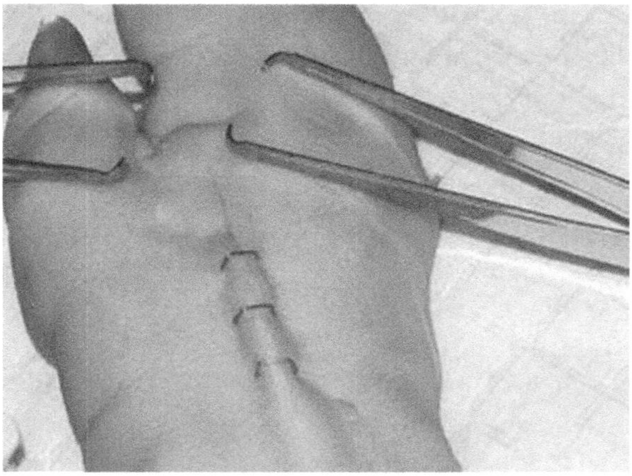

Staples vs. Sutures

For many wounds, suturing is the standard method of closure. Staples, however, are an acceptable alternative for certain lacerations. According to scientific studies, the wounds that are best served by staple closure seem to be scalp lacerations (heal faster); the worst, injuries over joints (higher incidence of infection).

Straight-line lacerations are closed faster with staples than with sutures, which make them useful in mass casualty incidents or in circumstances where quick action must be taken. Sutures are going to be difficult to place quickly, especially by the medic who was not formally trained. If adequate wound cleaning did not occur before staple placement, however, the risk of infection is high. The staples may have to be removed, thorough irrigation performed, and full evaluation to determine if closure is appropriate.

For survival purposes, staples are used only on the skin, whereas sutures may be used in deeper layers. There are staple guns for internal organs, but these procedures require special training and will have low success rates in grid-down situations.

After thoroughly irrigating the area with an antiseptic to get rid of debris, you are ready to begin. Staples are best executed if you have an assistant that can hold the skin edges together for you. As this usually requires two hands, it will be awkward for you to staple and approximate the skin in, say, a forearm wound.. The assistant, by the way, is the skilled labor on this team. Little technical skill is actually required in placing the staple.

On the other hand, suturing can be performed by one person and requires a bit of skill to achieve a cosmetic result. The trade-off is the fact that suturing is a much slower process than stapling. Also, there is the possibility that you might stick yourself with the suture needle during the procedure.

Let's say you've decided to staple the skin closed. After thoroughly cleaning a wound and applying antiseptic to "prep" the surgical field, you are ready to use your skin stapler. Your assistant will need two Adson's forceps to hold the skin for you.

Most staplers are held in the hand the same way you would hold, say, a garden hose nozzle. Stand in a position so that you have an overhead view of the laceration to be closed.

Your assistant then grasps the edges of the skin closest to you with the two forceps. Then, he/she will evert the edges (turn them inside out) slightly and hold them together.

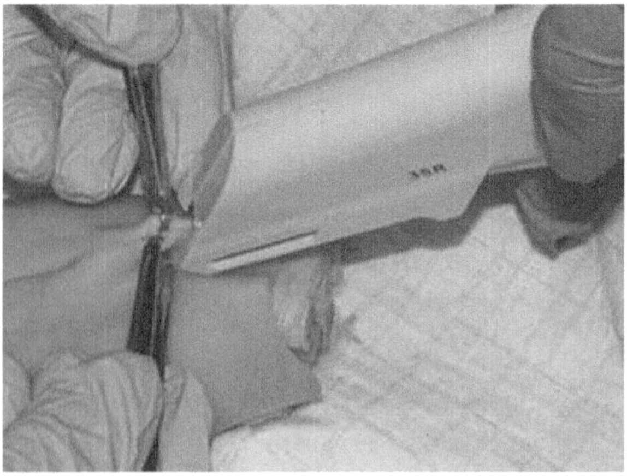

Placing a Staple

Hold your stapler at a 60-90 degree angle to the approximated edges and press firmly downward on the skin.. The line of the laceration should be right in the middle of the line of the stapler.

Press the "trigger" of your stapler to embed the staple and then release (completely) and retract. Check the staple placement and remove any that are not appropriately executed. The skin should appear slight "tented up" if the staple was placed correctly. Place subsequent staples ½ inch apart, especially in areas over a joint. In not over a joint, they can be spaced more widely apart, with steri-strips placed between in-between.

To remove staples, you will need an instrument known as a "staple remover". This instrument is similar to office staple removers of bygone days. It looks vaguely like a small scissors, but with no sharp edges.

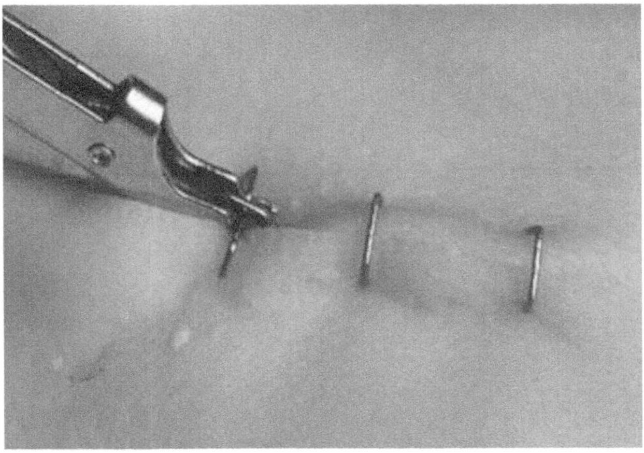

Removing a Staple

Place the "mandible" of the staple remover between the healed skin and the staple. There will be two prongs on the lower blade and one on the upper. When the two prongs are under the staple, press the handles together; the top prong will press on the staple in such a fashion that the staple is removed. Lift the staple remover and dispose of the staple safely. Repeat until all staples are removed.

Once the closure is done, keep the wound dry and covered for 48 hours, checking its several times a day. Staples on the skin should be removed in 7 days (5 days if on the face); if over a joint, 14-21 days.

LOCAL ANESTHESIA AND NERVE BLOCKS

When a person is injured and a wound must be sutured, the area will be sensitive and difficult to repair without causing significant discomfort to a person already in pain. As such, we are often asked about the use of local anesthetics like Lidocaine (brand name Xylocaine) for the purpose of preparing a laceration for closure.

There are various injectable local anesthetics on the market, such as Procaine (Novocain), Bupivacaine (Marcaine), and Mepivacaine (Carbocaine). Lidocaine is, however, the most widely used, due to the rapidity and effectiveness of its anesthetic action. Lidocaine also comes in the form of a powder, ointment, jelly, and aerosol spray. Injecting the drug in liquid form gives a much stronger effect.

It should be noted that Lidocaine is a prescription medication and is difficult to procure, although we sometimes see it for sale online. When used in subcutaneous tissue, it acts as an anesthetic; used intravenously, however, it has cardiac and other effects. An accidental injection into a blood vessel can become life-threatening, causing heart irregularities and seizures. Any unusual symptoms should abort the procedure. Those with liver or heart disease and the elderly should receive less quantities of the drug or none at all. In a survival setting, consider other alternatives due to the risks involved; our ancestors didn't use local anesthesia injections..

Although liquid Lidocaine is available by prescription in one or two per cent solution vials, it can also be purchased in powder packets that range from 25 to 2000 grams. To reconstitute Lidocaine powder into a solution, you'll need sterile saline, a pan, and a heat source.

To make a 2% lidocaine HCL solution, you'll need 300 *milli*grams (not grams) of lidocaine HCL powder, a container of sterile saline that can be measured in milliliters, and a pan of water with a heat source. You'll need a way to accurately measure out milligrams.

Take the pre-measured Lidocaine powder and mix it with 15 ml of sterile saline solution in a container that can be sealed, such as a large test tube. Seal the container and place it in a pan with water at about 180 degrees Fahrenheit (short of boiling) and leave it there for about five minutes.

The Lidocaine dissolves in the water, leaving you with a clear solution in the container. Make sure that no solid material has dropped to the bottom of the sealed container. Remove the vial from the pain and allow it to cool. If performed correctly, the procedure should give you 15 milliliters of 2% Lidocaine solution, more than necessary (or recommended) for the types of injuries you might need to treat.

To use the Lidocaine solution, proceed as follows: To load the anesthesia into a syringe, first use an alcohol pad to wipe the end of the bottle, then fill a small syringe with air. Inject the air into the bottle, and the local anesthetic will fill the syringe.

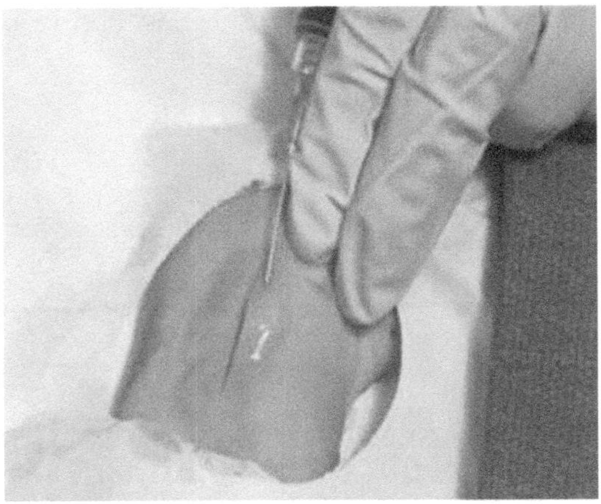

Injecting Local Anesthetic

Place an injection at a 45 degree angle to the skin, and then inject enough just under the skin to form a raised area (a "wheal") on each side of the laceration (see figure below). Within a few minutes, the area will be numb. If deeper layers must be closed, inject more Lidocaine through the wheal to reach the area. This decreases the discomfort of multiple injections by entering in an area already anesthetized by a previous injection.

To determine if you have accidentally entered a blood vessel, pull the plunger back before you inject anything into the tissue. This maneuver is called "aspiration". Aspirating will draw blood into the syringe if it's in the wrong place. If you lack Lidocaine, you can apply an ice cube to the area to be sutured until sensation decreases.

In an austere setting, you might not even have ice. We'll just have to realize that there may not be numbing agents available if a disaster takes us off the grid. This is one reason why we recommend using the least invasive method possible of closing a wound.

Once injected, you can expect full anesthetic effect in about 10 minutes after administration, and the effect should last 1-2 hours, depending on whether you use 1% or 2% Lidocaine. Epinephrine 1.200,000-1,000,000 has been used in conjunction with lidocaine to help decrease bleeding and prolong the effect further. This combination should *not* be used in areas with limited circulation, such as the fingers or earlobes. The epinephrine could constrict the blood vessels excessively and cause lack of blood flow to the tissues (also called "**ischemia**").

The Radial Nerve (Wrist) Block

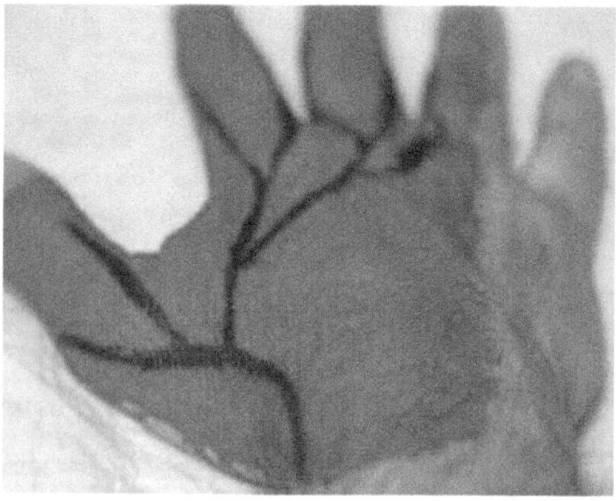

Radial Nerve Distribution

Lidocaine may be placed around the actual wound superficially or may be directed to "block" a specific nerve that serves the area to be repaired. This procedure is known as a nerve block. Each nerve block is intended to numb a portion of the course of a nerve as it travels through the body. This, in turn, numbs the area served by that nerve.

To describe every nerve block would fill an entire medical textbook, so let's take the example of a hand injury. The nerve we want to block is the radial nerve, as it supplies sensation to most of that area. You can see how helpful it can be to have a book on anatomy in your medical library. For now, see the image below to see the nerve distribution.

A nerve block here would be useful if there are multiple lacerations to the hand or fingers, imbedded foreign objects, or severe burns where extensive removal of dead tissue (called "debridement") is required.

Sterile towels and drapes will create a sterile field in which to work. In addition to Lidocaine, you'll need an antiseptic such as alcohol or Betadine, gauze 4x4s, a 6cc syringe, and a thin gauge needle (25 or 27 gauge). You can decrease the "sting" of the injection by warming the local anesthetic somewhat and/or adding 1 ml of sodium bicarbonate solution to 10 ml of Lidocaine.

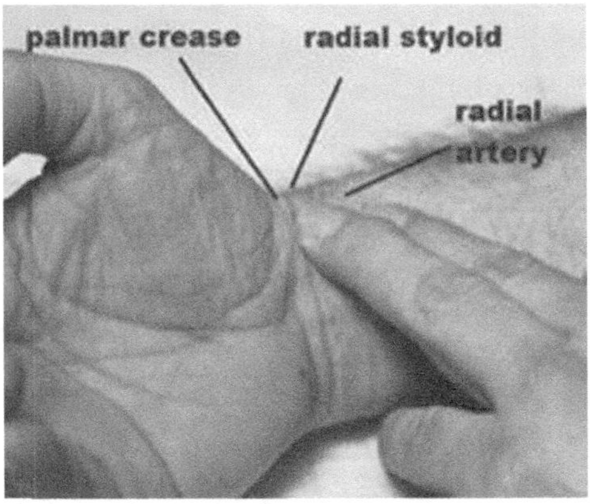

Radial Artery Pulse

You'll start with the patient's hand in the palm-up position. Clean the entire wrist and back of the hand with Betadine. Feel the radial artery pulse; this is the one that the doctor takes your pulse with when you have a physical exam. Then feel the "radial styloid"; this is the bony part of the wrist that protrudes slightly below the base of the thumb

Insert your needle between the radial artery and the styloid near the crease of the palm, and inject two or three milliliters of the anesthetic (see image below). Always pull back the plunger before you inject to make sure you haven't entered a blood vessel. Blood in the syringe should warn you to start over.

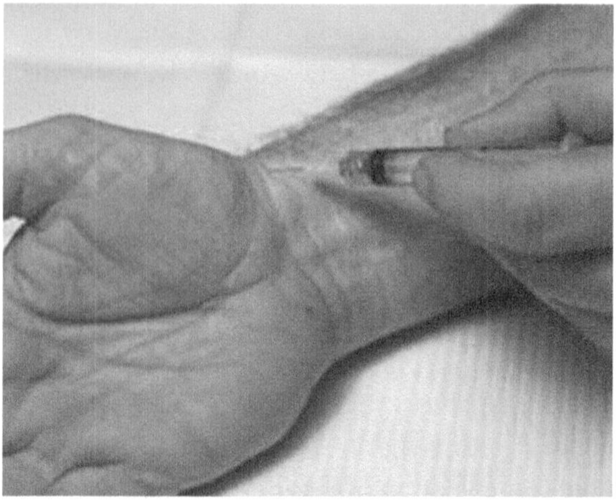

Next, you will turn the hand over. Using the same insertion site, inject another 5cc or so of Lidocaine along the back of the wrist to about the midpoint area. Use a longer needle than the one in the image below if you can; this will decrease the numbers of injections necessary.

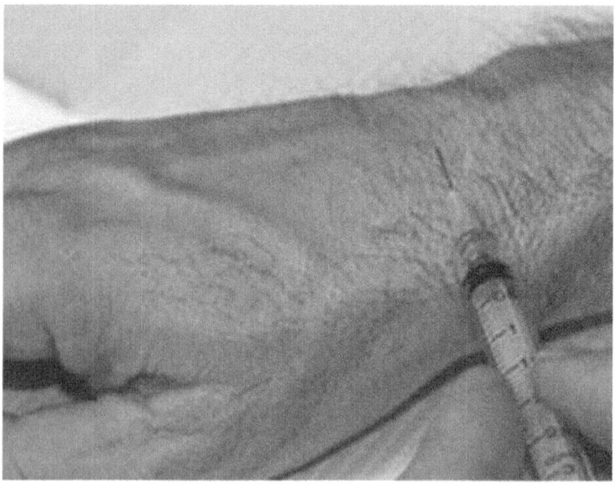

Finally, wait 10 minutes and then test the area for anesthetic effect by lightly touching the area to be sutured with a needle.

The Digital (Finger) Block

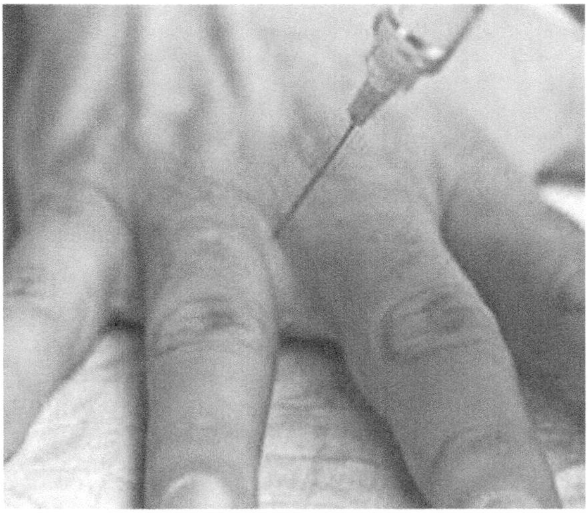

Injecting the Finger Base

The procedure to give anesthesia to a finger is relatively simple. Due to circulation issues, always use plain Lidocaine 1 or 2% *without* epinephrine.

Place the hand pronated on the sterile field (use more Betadine than we did in the photos). With your small gauge needle and a Lidocaine syringe, place a small amount of local anesthesia on either side of the base of the finger, raising a wheal (a slight swelling) just under the skin. This will make any later injections less painful.

After waiting a minute or so, insert the needle into the wheal and forward toward the base of the finger bone. Begin injecting the local anesthesia. Repeat on each side of the injured finger. One or two ml, injected as you slowly withdraw the needle, on each side should be sufficient. Too much may cause compression of blood vessels.

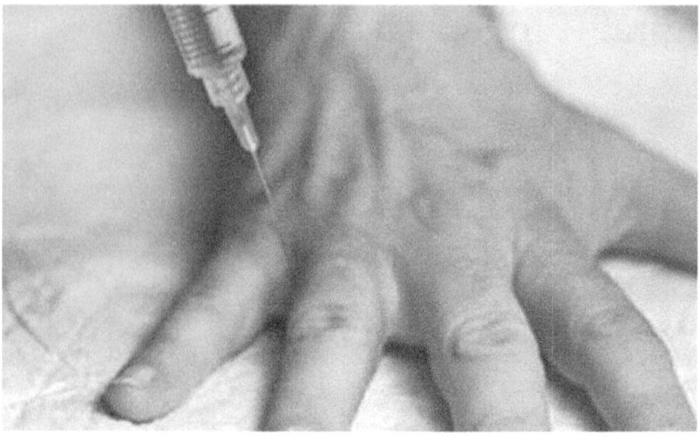

Injecting the other side

An alternative to this approach, or perhaps an addition for more complete anesthesia, is the "transthecal" finger block. The benefit is that this approach may numb the finger with a single injection, if done correctly.

To perform this type of block, turn the hand palm up, and follow the tendon of the finger down to the level of the first palmar crease line. Inserting the needle at a 45 degree angle, go down to the tendon and inject 2 ml of plain Lidocaine. If you notice resistance you are too close to the tendon and should pull back a little. Some suggest rubbing the area afterwards to distribute the medication.

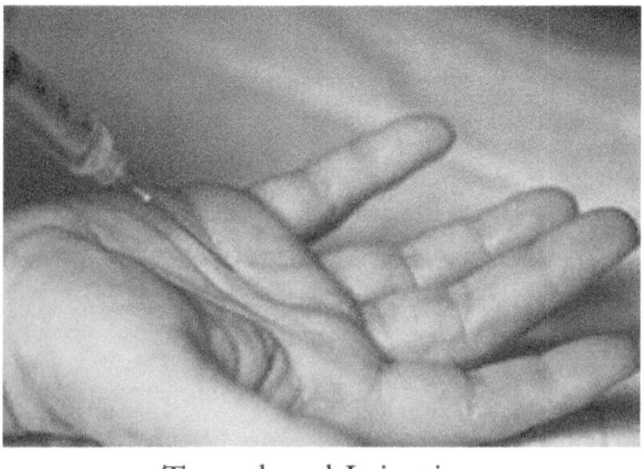

Transthecal Injection

Wait about 10 minutes or so before assessing anesthetic effect. This may be done by lightly pricking with a safety pin or applying slight pressure to the area.

After any work on the finger injury, immobilize it with a finger splint or the "buddy method" of taping the digit to an adjacent finger for support. Cover with a generous wrapping.

Some important things to review:

- Avoid clearly infected (red, swollen, warm to the touch) wounds. They should be managed as an open wound.
- Use small gauge needles to avoid hitting blood vessels and causing bleeding.
- Don't inject into any visible veins.
- Pull back on the needle before you inject anesthesia; if you see blood in the syringe, abort and try again.
- Avoid Epinephrine on fingers, toes, and earlobes.
- No more than 2 ml on each side of a finger block.
- If the injection is extremely painful, you may be hitting the nerve with the needle; abort and try again.

Finally, remember that, while we have the luxury of modern medical care, all significant injuries and wounds should be treated by qualified medical professionals. There are doctors with a lot of experience performing nerve blocks; take advantage of their expertise while they're still there for you.

BLISTERS, SPLINTERS, AND FISHHOOKS

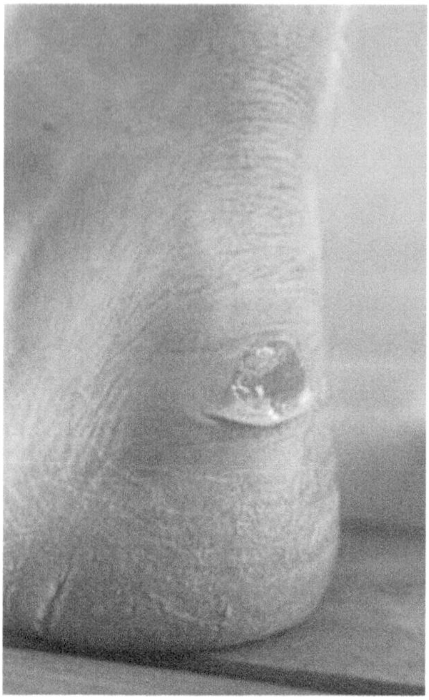

Typical broken blister

Foot Care

Anyone who has done any hiking or has bought the wrong pair of shoes has experienced a friction blister. For a relatively small soft tissue injury, a blister can certainly cause more than its share of problems. More than one hike has come to a screeching halt because the terrain was more than the footwear could handle. Never underestimate the importance of a properly-fitted pair of shoes.

Shoe size changes as you age, after a pregnancy, or even during the course of the day. You should always try new shoes on after a day of walking, when your feet are a little swollen. Most of us have one foot that's larger than the other, so make sure your boots fit both feet (especially the larger one).

Each part of your foot should be comfortable in your new boots:

- The ball of your foot should fit the widest part of the shoe without issue.
- There should be about 1/2 inch or so from the end of your toes to the end of your shoe.
- The upper part of the shoe should be flexible enough to not cause discomfort on your instep.
- Your heel should not slip up and down when you walk.

Other considerations are important: Soles should be thick Vibram or other sturdy material. High-cut boots will help prevent ankle sprains by giving more support and will protect against the occasional snake bite.

Don't buy shoes that are too tight and expect them to stretch. They might, but you'll go through a lot of discomfort to get them there. Many buy shoes online, but you really should walk in a shoe first for a while before making a purchase. Your feet are shaped differently than the next guy's, so different brands of boot might be better for different people.

Heavier boots, such as those with steel toes, are great if you're chopping wood (you get to keep all ten of your toes) but are heavy. Remember that an extra pound of weight in your boot is like 5 extra pounds of weight on your back. Getting soft, flexible uppers will help. In wet climates, waterproof materials like Gore-Tex are a good investment.

A special note: Unless you can count "shoemaker" as one of your survival skills, buy a spare pair or two before a disaster happens. Wear them a few times to break them in.

Another factor in keeping your feet healthy is your socks. Most people hike in the same pair of socks all day, even in the heat of summer.

Sweaty feet are unhappy feet; Wetness increases friction and gives you blisters.

On the trail, it's important to change wet socks; have replacement pairs in your backpack. For additional protection, consider the use of a lighter, second pair of socks (sock liners) under the thicker hiking socks you use. Use foot powders, like Gold Bond, or even corn starch to help your feet stay dry.

Blisters

If a blister is just starting, it will look like a tender red "hot spot" where the friction is worst. Cover this area with moleskin or Spenco Second Skin before it gets worse. These items are inexpensive, but if you don't have any on hand, you can make use of gauze or a Band-Aid or even duct tape. The important thing here is to add padding to prevent further friction.

Blisters will happen, however, and most people are eager to pop them right away. This shouldn't be done with small blisters as it could lead to infection. Consider that skin over a blister can serve as a dressing; a sterile one, if it's intact. Large blisters are different, as they pop easily anyway. Follow this process to deal with a blister:

- Clean the area with disinfectant. Alcohol or iodine is especially useful.
- Take a needle and sterilize with alcohol or heat it until red hot.
- Pierce the side of the blister. This allows the fluid to drain. This will ease some discomfort and allow healing to begin.
- Preserve any loose skin to protect the raw area.
- Cover the blister to offer protection and apply antibiotic cream if possible.
- Take some moleskin or Spenco Second Skin; cut a hole in the middle a little bigger than the blister.
- Place the moleskin on so that the blister is in the middle of the opening in the moleskin.
- Cover with a gauze pad or other bandage.
- Rest.

If you absolutely must keep walking, make sure that your bandage has stopped the friction to the area. Remember, bandages frequently come off, so check it from time to time to make sure it's still on. Change the bandage frequently to maintain cleanliness.

If a blister is continuously exposed to friction, there's a chance that it may turn into a foot "ulcer", A foot ulcer can be a shallow red crater that involves only surface skin or very deep, involving tendons and other deep structures. Diabetics need to be especially careful, because they're more susceptible to foot problems due to poor circulation and nerve damage.

Many home remedies for blisters exist to speed healing and prevent infection. They include:

- Cold salt water compress
- A 10 percent tannic acid solution
- A few drops of Listerine antiseptic
- Garlic oil
- Aloe Vera
- Vitamin E oil
- Zinc oxide ointment
- Witch Hazel
- Tea Tree oil
- Lavender oil

Splinters

Being out in the woods or working with wood not uncommonly leaves a person with a splinter or two to deal with. A magnifying glass will help you visualize it. Use a scalpel (#11 or #15 blade) and cut the epidermis over it. You want to cut superficially and just enough to expose the tip of the fragment. Squeezing behind or under the splinter may make it more accessible. Then, take your tweezers and grasp the end of the splinter and pull it out along the angle that it entered the skin. Don't forget to wash the area thoroughly before and after the procedure.

It's unlikely that a major infection will come from simply having a splinter, with the exception of those that have been under the skin for more than 2-3 days. Redness or swelling in the area will become apparent if an infection is brewing. You might consider antibiotics in this circumstance to avoid having problems later.

Fishhooks

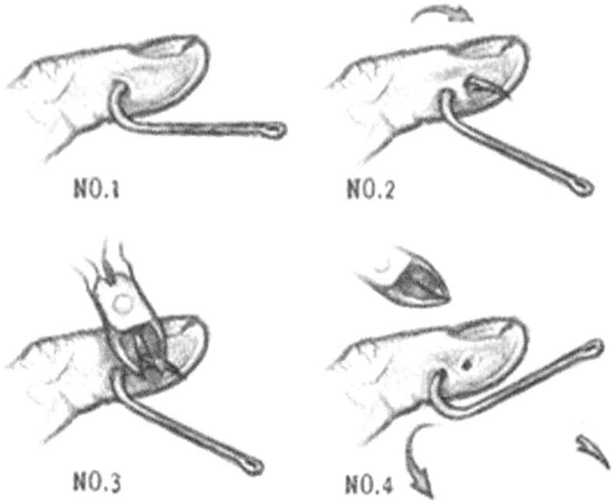

FISH HOOK REMOVAL

Even if you're an accomplished fisherman, you will eventually wind up with a fishhook embedded in you somewhere, probably your hand. Since the hook probably has worm guts on it, start off by cleaning the area thoroughly with an antiseptic.

Your hook probably has a barbed end. If you can't easily slide it out, the barb is probably the issue. Press down on the skin over where the barb is and then attempt to remove the hook along the curve of the shank.

If this doesn't work, you may have to advance the fishhook further along the skin until the barbed end comes out again. At this point, you can take a wire cutter and separate the barbed end from the shank. Then, pull the shank out from whence it came. Wash the area again and cover with a bandage. Observe carefully over time for signs of infection.

NAILBED INJURIES

Minor injuries can sometimes become a major detriment to the effective function of a member of your survival group. Although not as life-threatening as a gunshot wound or an open fracture, nail bed injuries are common; they will be more so when we are required to perform carpentry or other duties to which we're not accustomed.

Your fingernails and toenails are made up of protein and a tough substance called keratin. They are, as you might imagine, similar to the claws of animals. When we refer to issues involving nails, we refer to it as "ungual" (from the latin word for claw: unguis).

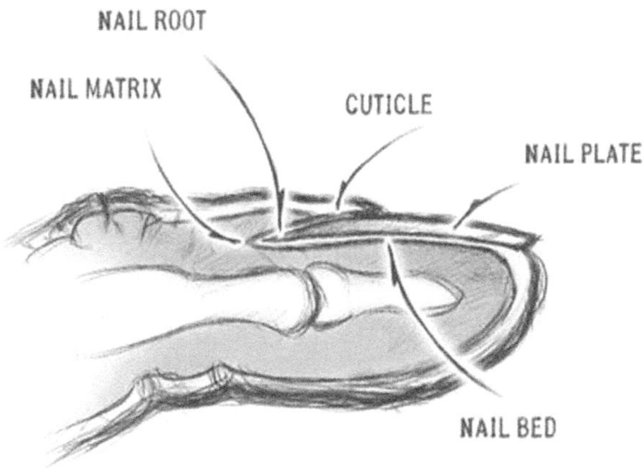

NAIL ANATOMY

The nail consists of several parts:

- **The nail plate (body):** this is the hard covering of the end of your finger or toe; what you consider to be the nail.
- **The nail bed:** the skin directly under the nail plate. Made up of dermis and epidermis just like the rest of your skin, the superficial epidermis moves along with the nail plate as it grows. Vertical grooves attach the superficial epidermis to the deep dermis. In older people, the nail plate thins out and you

can see the grooves if you look closely. Like all skin, blood vessels and nerves run through the nail bed.

- **The nail matrix:** the portion or root at the base of the nail under the cuticle that produces new cells for the nail plate. You can see a portion of the matrix in the light half-moon (the "lunula") visible at the base of the nail plate. This determines the shape and thickness of the nail; a curved matrix produces a curved nail, a flat one produces a flat nail.

In a nail "**avulsion**", the nail plate is ripped away by some form of trauma. The nail may be partially or completely gone, or may be lifted up off the nail bed. Ordinarily, depending on the type of trauma, an x-ray would be performed to rule out a fracture of the digit; you won't have this tool available without modern facilities, but you can do this:

- Numb the area by providing a digital block (discussed earlier in this book).
- Clean the nail bed thoroughly with saline solution, if available, and irrigate out any debris. Paint with Betadine (2% Povidone-Iodine solution) or other antiseptic.
- Cover the exposed (and very sensitive) nail bed with a non-adherent (Telfa) dressing. Some add petroleum jelly for additional protection. Change frequently. Avoid ordinary gauze, as it will stick tenaciously and be painful to remove.
- If the nail plate is hanging on by a thread, remove it by separating it from the skin folds using a small surgical clamp. You can consider placing the avulsed nail plate on the nail bed as a protective covering; it is dead tissue but may be the most comfortable option. Avoid scraping off loose edges, as it may affect the nail bed's ability to heal.
- If the nail bed is lacerated, suture it (once cleaned) with the thinnest gauge absorbable suture available (6-0 Vicryl is good). Be sure to remove any nail plate tissue over the laceration so the suture repair will be complete.
- Place a fingertip dressing. You might consider immobilizing the digit with a finger splint to protect it from further damage.
- Begin a course of antibiotics if the nail bed was contaminated with debris.

In some crush injuries, such as striking the nail plate with a hammer, a bruise (also called an "**ecchymosis**") or a collection of blood may form underneath (a "**hematoma**"). A bruise will be painful, but the pain should subside within an hour or two. A hematoma, however, will continue to be painful even several hours after the event. A bruise will likely appear brownish or blue, but a hematoma may appear a deep blue-black.

For a bruised nail, little needs to be done other than giving oral pain meds, such as Ibuprofen. For a significant hematoma, however, some suggest a further procedure called "**trephination**". In this instance, a very fine drill (or a hot 18 gauge needle or paper clip) is used to make a hole in the nail plate. This opening must be large enough to allow blood that has collected under the nail to escape. Once the pressure is relieved, the pain will abate.

This procedure should not be performed unless absolutely necessary, as the pain will eventually decrease over time by itself. If you go too deep through the nail, you may further injure the nail bed. The finger must be kept dry, splinted and bandaged for a minimum of 48 hours afterwards.

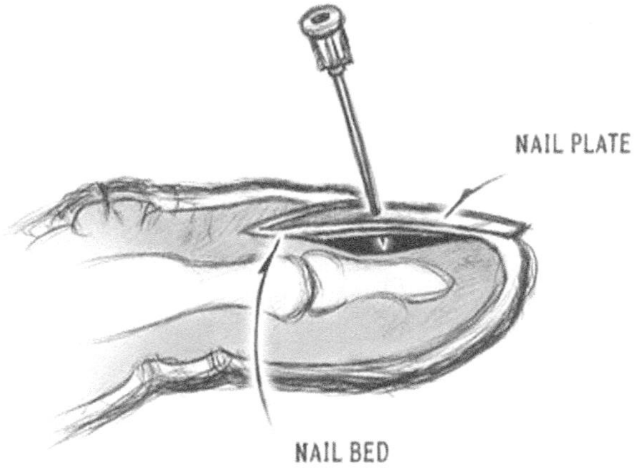

NAIL TREPHINATION

It's important to know that damage to the base of the nail (the germinal matrix) may be difficult to completely repair, and that future nail growth may be deformed in some way. In situations where modern medical care is available, a hand surgeon is often called in to give the injury the best chance to heal appropriately. Even then, a higher incidence of issues such as "ingrown" nails may occur over time. A completely torn-off nail will take 4-5 months to grow back, maybe more.

BURN INJURIES

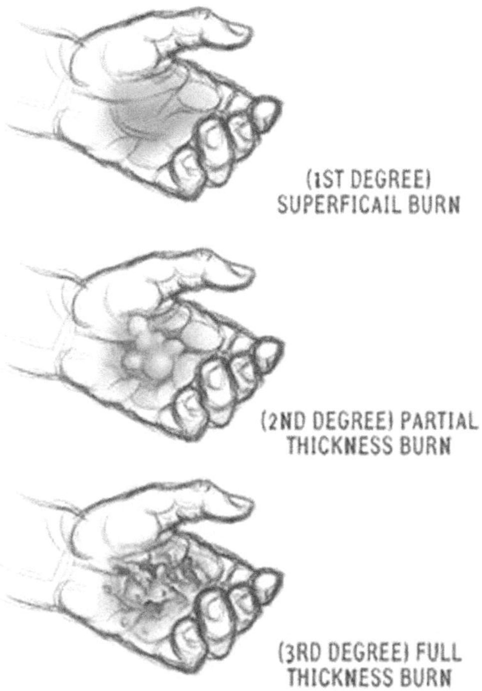

BURN CATEGORIES

Many natural and man-made disasters come with a risk of burns. Wildfires, earthquakes, terror attacks, and other events often incur burn injuries and if we find ourselves off the grid one day, we might have to cook our food over a fire.

In survival, the potential for burn injuries will rise exponentially, especially if the survival group includes small children. Kids are naturally curious and may get too close to campfires. Therefore, having the materials and knowledge to treat burns will be imperative for every group's medical provider.

The severity of a burn injury depends on the percentage of the total body surface involved, as well as the degree (depth) of penetration.

Assessing the surface percentage burned is standard practice and helpful in modern medicine. It may, however, have less practical benefit in austere settings where transport isn't an option.

First Degree Burns

Most burns you'll see will be due to excessive exposure to the sun. In most cases, these will be **first-degree burns**. In first-degree burns, only the superficial layer of the skin (the "epidermis") is injured. To avoid sunburn:

- Don't "sunbathe" (a tan is *not* healthy!).
- Avoid peak sun hours (11am-4pm).
- Wear long pants and sleeves, hats, and sunglasses.
- Spend time in the shade when possible.

If you cannot avoid extended exposure to sunlight, be certain to apply a sunblock. They should be applied prior to going outside and frequently throughout the day. Even water resistant sunscreens should be reapplied every 1-2 hours. Most people fail to put enough on their skin, so be generous in your application.

By the way, a sunblock and a sunscreen are not the same thing. Sunblocks contain tiny particles that "block" and reflect UV light. A sunscreen contains substances that absorb UV light, thus preventing it from penetrating the skin. Many commercial products contain both. Sunblocks and sunscreens should be an integral part of your medical storage.

The SPF (Sun Protection Factor) rating system was developed in 1962 to measure the capacity of a product to protect against UV radiation. It measures the length of exposure to the sun before you burn. A SPF (sun protection factor) of at least 15 is recommended. It takes about 20 minutes without sunscreen for your skin to start turning red. A product that is SPF 15 should delay burning by a factor of 15, or about 5 hours. Higher SPF ratings give more protection and are especially beneficial to those with fair skin.

Besides the sun, first-degree injuries will most likely be related to cooking or campfires. Using hand protection will prevent many of these burns, as will careful supervision of children near campfires and food preparation areas.

A first-degree burn will appear red, warm, and dry. It will be painful to the touch. In the case of sunburn, large areas of skin are frequently affected. As the injury is superficial, however, major complications are rare and treatment is focused on relieving discomfort.

Immersion in a cool bath will be helpful; at the very least, run cool water over the injury. A cool moist cloth on the burn will give some relief, as will anti-inflammatory medicines such as Ibuprofen. Aloe Vera or Zinc Oxide are effective alternatives. Expect the discomfort to improve after 24 hours. Avoid tight clothing and wear light fabrics, such as cotton.

Second-Degree Burns

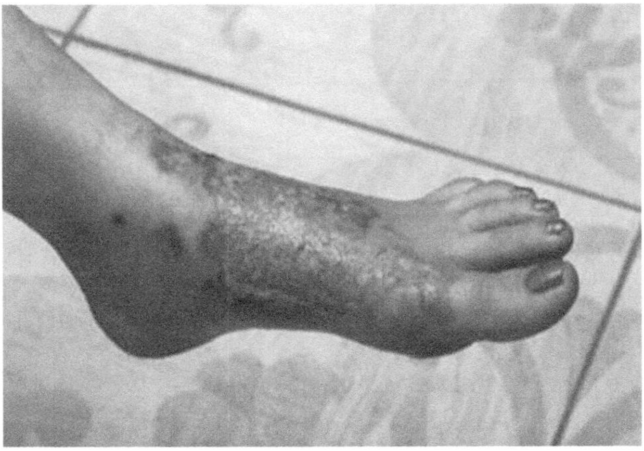

Second-degree burns are deeper injuries. They penetrate through the superficial epidermis and partially through the deeper layer of the skin (the "dermis"). Thus, they are often called "partial thickness burns".

Unlike first-degree burns, second-degree burns will be seen to be moist and have blisters with reddened bases. The area will have a tendency to weep clear or whitish fluid. Second degree burns will cause swelling, so it's important to remove rings and bracelets.

To treat second degrees burns:

- Run cool water over the injury for 10-15 minutes (avoid ice).
- Apply moist skin dressings such as Spenco Second skin or non-stick dressings (Telfa pads) with
- Give oral pain relief such as Ibuprofen.
- Apply anesthetic ointment such as Benzocaine.
- Use Silver Sulfadiazine (Silvadene) creams to help prevent infection.
- Consider antibiotic ointment if slow to heal.
- Avoid lancing blisters if possible (some very large blisters will, however, break with the slightest pressure and may benefit from a controlled way to drain them; see the section on foot blisters).
- Avoid removing burned skin.

Third-Degree Burns

Third-degree burns penetrate the full thickness of skin and enter deeper structures like fat, muscle, and bone. A third-degree burn may appear charred, or be white in color, depending on the source of heat. These burn may appear indented if significant tissue has been lost.

Third-degree burns will rapidly cause dehydration, so giving fluids is essential to keep the patient stable. The loss of fluids may be so rapid as to only be replaceable with intravenous hydration.

When a person gets burned, it's of paramount importance to remove the heat source immediately. Run cool water over any degree of burn for at least 10-15 minutes as soon as possible after the injury. Cool water is preferable to ice as it is less traumatic to the already damaged tissue. Again, be certain to remove rings or jewelry, as swelling is commonly seen in these kinds of injuries.

As the skin no longer exists in these burns, infection is very likely, especially if the wound isn't covered. Spenco Second Skin is an option as a burn wound cover. Celox combat gauze, discussed in the section on hemostatic agents, may also serve as a burn dressing. When moistened, the gauze forms a gel-like dressing that may provide a helpful barrier.

Silver Sulfadiazine (Silvadene) cream is helpful in preventing infections in third degree burns.

It should be noted that you might see fourth, fifth and sixth degree burns described in some other medical resource books. In a long-term survival scenario, they would be treated the same as a third degree burn.

Any burn this severe that is larger than, say, an inch or so in diameter, usually requires a skin graft to heal completely. A person with third-degree burns over more than 10% of the body surface could easily go into shock, and is in a life-threatening situation. Without advanced care, expect a poor outcome.

Natural Burn Remedies

If conventional medical resources aren't available, the medic must consider alternate burn treatments. Various plants and other substances have properties that can help you facilitate burn healing, even if no modern medical supplies are available. Although of limited use for severe burns, many first and second degree burns will respond to natural remedies. One of the most popular of these is **Aloe Vera**.

Studies have shown that Aloe Vera helps new skin cells form and speeds healing, making it an excellent option for first or second degree burns. Take an aloe leaf, cut it open, and either scoop out the gel or rub the open leaf directly on the burned area. Reapply 4-6 times daily. Simplicity and fast relief are the key benefits to using Aloe Vera on burns.

Many articles on natural burn remedies commonly include **vinegar** (any type) as a treatment. Vinegar works as an astringent and antiseptic and helps to prevent infections. The best way to use vinegar on smaller sized burns is to make a compress with a 50/50 vinegar/water solution and cover the burn. Re-soak the compress when it feels warm. There is no limit to how many times you can apply the vinegar soaks.

A similar method adds vinegar to a cool bath. Start with tepid water and let the water cool off while the patient is soaking. If the burn is on the torso, a cotton t-shirt soaked in vinegar will give relief and may help your patient sleep.

Another "cooling off" treatment for burns is a **Witch Hazel** compress. Use the extract of the bark, which decreases inflammation and soothes a first degree burn. Soak a cloth in full strength Witch Hazel and apply to the burned area. Reapply as frequently as desired.

Elder flower and **comfrey leaf** "decoctions" are also an excellent remedy for burns. For those unfamiliar with the term **decoction**, it is an extraction of the crushed herbs produced by boiling. Using lower water temperatures produces a "tea" instead. The decoctions of these plants can also be used for compresses or freshly crushed, hydrated, and then applied directly to the burned area with a gauze cover (a "**poultice**").

Black tea leaves have tannic acid that helps draw heat from a burn. Put two or three tea bags in cool water for a few minutes and use the water with compresses or just apply to the burned area. If your patient has to be mobile, make a stay-in-place poultice out of 2 or 3 wet tea bags. Simply place cool wet tea bags directly on the burn and wrap them with a piece of gauze and some tape to hold them in place.

Both **milk** and **yogurt** have also been found to help cool and hydrate the skin after a burn. Wrap whole-milk and full-fat yogurt inside gauze or cheesecloth and use as a compress. Replace the compress as the yogurt warms on the skin.

Yet another home remedy is the **baking soda** bath. Add ¼ cup baking soda to a warm bath and soak for at least 15 minutes or until the water cools off.

There are two essential oils that can be used on 1st or 2nd degree burns: **Lavender** and **tea tree** oils. They help with pain due to stinging and promote tissue healing. Mix tea tree oil with a small amount of water or use full-strength lavender oil as an alternative. Apply over the burned area. A loose covering of gauze over the oil may be helpful when used for second degree burns.

It is important to know that butter or lard, commonly used for burns in the past, will hold in the heat and are *not* to be used in the treatment of burns.

You can also make a poultice of marigold (**calendula**) petals pounded with small amounts of olive or wheat germ oil; this can be spread lightly over the burned area and covered by loose gauze or a sterile covering.

One of the best natural remedies for treating the burn patient is raw unprocessed honey. **Honey** is best to use in its raw unprocessed state because of its antibacterial activity and hydrating properties. This microbe-killing effect is thought to be due to an acidic pH that is inhospitable to bacteria. Raw honey helps prevent and even treat infections in many wounds. It can be used in first, second, and, if no other medical option is available, as a last resort for third-degree burns.

This is how to use honey on burns:

- Immediately after the first 15 minute cooling-down treatment, apply a generous amount of honey in a thick layer all over the burned area
- Cover the honey with plastic wrap or waterproof dressings. Use tape to hold the dressing in place. Don't use cling wrap or, at least, don't wrap all the way around an extremity; swelling may cause undue pressure.
- If the dressing begins to fill up with fluid oozing out of the wound, change the dressing. The worse the burn, the more frequently the dressing will need to be changed.
- Do not remove or wash off the honey for the first 20 days (or earlier if healing is complete). Add more honey often and fill up any deeper areas as needed. Always have a thick layer of honey extending over the edges of the wound to avoid any air getting to the burned skin. Complete coverage will help decrease the infection rate. .
- Change the dressing at least three times a day.

Treating burns without a medical system available will require aggressive care and close observation. Severe fluid losses lead to dangerous consequences for these patients, so always be certain that you do everything possible to keep them well hydrated. The damage to the skin caused by burns leaves those injured to the mercy of many pathogens, so watch for fevers or other signs of infection.

ANIMAL BITES

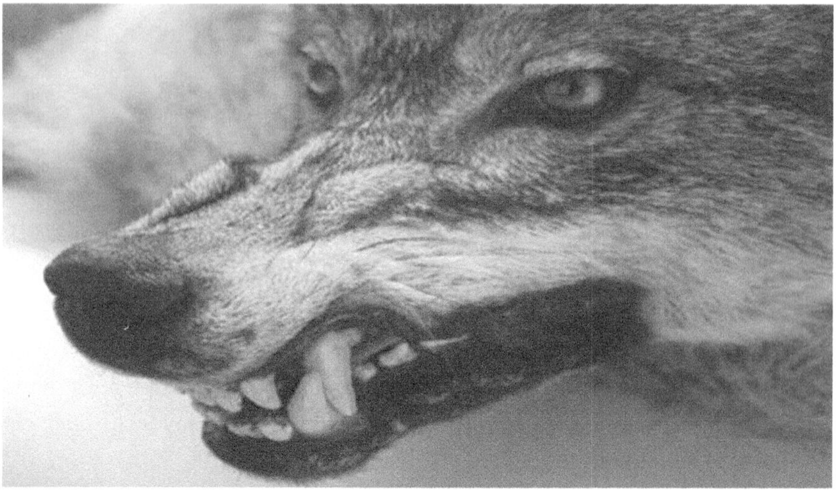

Most people have, at some time of their life, run afoul of an ornery dog or cat. There are millions of animal bites every year; they affect the hands most often in adults, but the neck, face, and head in children. Most bites caused by small animals are puncture wounds. These are likely to become infected unless treated.

Wild animals will bite when threatened, ill, or to protect their territory and offspring. Most, however, avoid humans if at all possible. Cats, dogs, small rodents, and other domestic pets are the culprits in the grand majority of cases.

Although any animal bite can lead to infection if ignored, cat bites inject bacteria into deeper tissues and seem to become contaminated more often. Dog bites are more common than cat bites but become infected less often. Despite this, their jaws are powerful and can inflict crush injuries to soft tissues.

According to a 1994 study, dog bites are:

- 6.2 times more likely to be incurred by male dogs.
- 2.6 times more likely to be incurred by dogs that haven't been neutered.

- 2.8 times more likely if the dog is chained or otherwise restrained.
- More commonly seen in children 14 years and younger than any other age group. Boys are much more likely to be the victims.

Besides the trauma associated with the actual bite, various animals carry disease which can be transmitted to humans. Here are just a few diseases, some discussed earlier in this book, and the animals involved:

- Rabies: Viral disease spread by raccoons, skunks, bats, opossums, and canines.
- Plague: Bacterial disease associated with rats and fleas.
- Tuberculosis: Bacterial disease associated with deer, elk, and bison.
- Brucella: Bacterial disease associated with bison, deer, and other animals.
- Hantavirus: Viral disease caused by mice.
- Baylisascaris (raccoon roundworm): Parasitic disease associated with raccoons.
- Histoplasma: Fungal disease associated with bat excrement.
- Tularemia: Bacterial disease usually associated with rodents, rabbits, and hares.

In addition, it is possible to develop tetanus from any animal bite. Tetanus is a potentially fatal infection of the muscles and nervous system caused by the bacteria Clostridia tetani. It is discussed elsewhere in this book.

We should take a moment to discuss rabies. Although the classic example is the rabid dog, cat bites are the most common cause of this viral infection among pets. Wildlife, however, accounts for the grand majority of cases in the United States. Raccoons, opossums, skunks, coyotes, and bats are the most common vectors. It is estimated that 40,000 persons in the United States receive rabies prevention treatment every year.

It should be noted that, in the United States, there has never been a rabies case transmitted to humans by the following animals:

- domestic cattle
- squirrels

- rabbits
- rats
- sheep
- horses

A person with rabies is usually symptom-free for a time. This varies in each case (average 30 days or so). After this "incubation period", the patient will complain of fever, headache, loss of appetite, and fatigue. The site of the bite wound may be itchy or numb. A few days after the initial symptoms, evidence of nerve damage appears in the form of irritability, disorientation, hallucination, seizures, and eventually, paralysis. The victim may go into a coma or suffer cardiac or respiratory arrest. Once a person develops the disease, it is usually fatal.

Whenever a person is bitten by an animal, several important actions should be taken:

- Control bleeding with direct pressure using gloves and a bandage or other barrier.
- Clean the wound thoroughly with soap and water. Flushing the wound aggressively with a 60-100 cc irrigation syringe filled with clean water will help remove embedded dirt and bacteria-containing saliva.
- Use an antiseptic to decrease the chance of infection. Betadine (2% povidone-iodine solution) or Benzalkonium Chloride (BZK) are good choices.
- When off-grid, don't close the wound if at all possible. Many bite wounds are stitched closed in a modern medical facility, but this may be inadvisable in a survival setting. Any animal bite should be considered a "dirty" wound; closing the wound may lock in dangerous bacteria.
- Remove any rings or bracelets in a bite wound to the hand. If swelling occurs, they may be very difficult to remove afterwards.
- Use an ice pack to decrease swelling, bruising, and pain.
- Frequently clean a recovering bite wound. Clean, drinkable water or a dilute antiseptic solution will suffice.
- Apply antibiotic ointment to the area and be sure to watch for signs of wound infection (discussed elsewhere). These may

include redness, swelling, or oozing. In many instances, the site might feel unusually warm to the touch. Warm moist compresses to the area will help an infected wound drain.

- Consider oral antibiotics as a precaution if off-grid (especially after a cat bite). Although Amoxicillin with Clavulanic acid 500mg every 8 hours for a week is a good first line therapy, a combination of Clindamycin (veterinary equivalent: Fish-Cin) 300mg orally every 6 hours and Ciprofloxacin (Fish-Flox) 500 mg every 12 hours may be considered. Azithromycin, Metronidazole (Fish-Zole), and Ampicillin-Sulbactam have also been used.

Children who suffer animal bites may become traumatized by the experience and benefit from counseling. Youngsters should be informed about the risks of animal bites and taught to avoid stray dogs, cats, and wild animals. Never leave a small child unattended around animals: Without an able-bodied person to intervene, the outcome could be tragic.

It is important to remember that humans are animals, too. In rare cases, you might see bites from this source as well. Approximately 10-15% of human bites become infected, due to the fact that there are over 100 million bacteria per milliliter in human saliva. Treat as you would any contaminated wound. A tetanus shot is indicated, if available, in those who haven't been vaccinated in the last five years.

SNAKE BITES

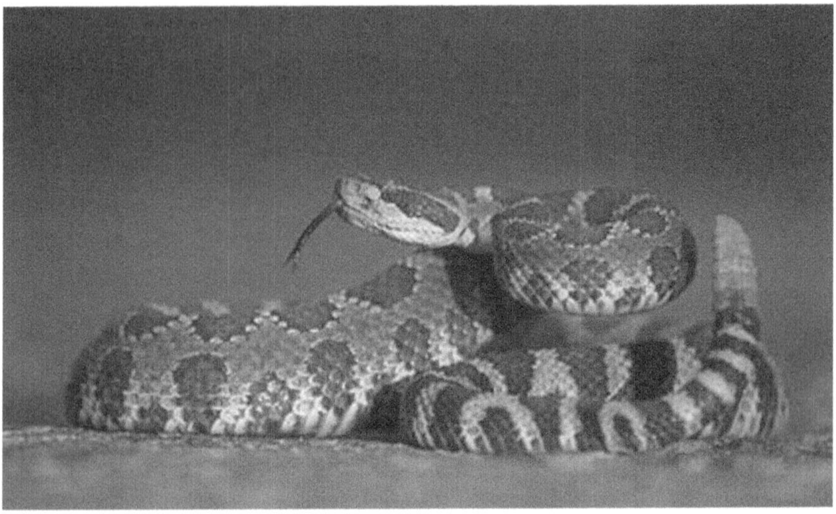

In a grid-down scenario, you will find yourself out in the woods a lot more frequently, gathering firewood, hunting, and foraging for edible wild plants. As such, you'll probably encounter a snake or two. Most snakes aren't poisonous, but even non-venomous snake bites may become infected.

Poison is, perhaps, the wrong word to use here; **venoms** and **poisons** are not the same thing. Poisons are absorbed by the skin or digestive system, but venoms must be "injected" into tissues or blood directly. Therefore, it is usually not dangerous to drink snake venom unless you have a cut or sore in your mouth (don't try it, though).

North America has two kinds of venomous snakes: The **pit vipers** (rattlesnakes, water moccasins) and **Elapids** (coral snakes). One or more of these snakes can be found almost everywhere in the continental U.S. A member of another viper family, the common adder, is the only venomous snake in Britain, but it and other adders are common throughout Europe (except for Ireland, thanks to St. Patrick).

Poisonous snakes have hollow fangs through which they deliver venom. As such, their bite appears as two puncture marks, while many other snakes' bites have a more ragged appearance.

Snakes are most active during the warmer months and, therefore, most bite injuries are seen then. Not every bite from a venomous snake transfers its poison to the victim; 25-30% of these bites will show little or no ill effects. This probably has to do with the duration of time the snake has its fangs in its victim.

An ounce of prevention, they say, is worth a pound of cure. Be sure to wear good solid high-top boots and long pants when hiking in the wilderness. Treading heavily creates ground vibrations and noise, which will often cause snakes to hit the road. Snakes have no outer ear, so they "hear" ground vibrations better than those in the air caused by, for instance, shouting.

Many snakes are active at night, especially in warm weather. Therefore, some activities, such as gathering firewood, are inadvisable without a good light source. In the wilderness, it's important to look where you're putting your hands and feet. Be especially careful around areas where snakes might like to hide, such as hollow logs, under rocks, or in old shelters. Wearing heavy gloves would be a wise precaution.

A snake doesn't always slither away after it bites you. It's likely that it still has more venom that it can inject, so move out of its territory or abolish the threat in any way you can. Killing the snake, however, may not render it harmless: it can reflexively bite for a period of time, even if its head has been severed from its body.

Snake bites that cause a burning pain immediately are likely to have venom in them. Swelling at the site may begin as soon as five minutes afterwards, and may travel up the affected area. Pit viper bites tend to cause bruising and blisters at the site of the wound. Numbness may be noted in the area bitten, or perhaps on the lips or face. Some victims describe a metallic or other strange taste in their mouths.

Pit vipers may be identified by their triangular-shaped heads and slit-like eyes. Rattlesnakes will, of course, have rattles which make noise when they're threatened. With pit viper bites, bruising is not uncommon and a serious bite might start to cause spontaneous bleeding from the nose or gums.

Coral snakes appear very similar to their look-alike, the non-venomous king snake. They both have red, yellow, and black bands and are commonly confused with each other. The old saying goes: "red touches yellow, kill a fellow; red touches black, venom it lacks". In other words, if the red band is next to the yellow band, it's a deadly coral snake. If the red band is next to the black band, it's a non-venomous king snake. This adage only applies to coral snakes in North America, however.

Coral snake bites will cause mental and nerve issues such as twitching, confusion, and slurred speech. Later, nerve damage may cause difficulty with swallowing and breathing, followed by total paralysis.

Coral snakes are not as aggressive as pit vipers and will prefer fleeing to attacking. Once they bite you, however, they tend to hold on; Pit vipers prefer to bite and let go quickly. Unlike coral snakes, pit vipers may not relinquish their territory to you, so prepare to possibly be bitten again.

The treatment for a venomous snake bite is "Anti-venin", an animal or human serum with antibodies capable of neutralizing a specific biological toxin. This product will probably be a very scarce survival commodity. The following strategy, therefore, will be useful:

- Keep the victim calm. Stress increases blood flow, thereby endangering the patient by speeding the venom into the system.
- Stop all movement of the injured extremity. Movement will move the venom into the circulation faster, so do your best to keep the limb still.
- Clean the wound thoroughly to remove any venom that isn't deep in the wound.
- Remove rings and bracelets from an affected extremity. Swelling is likely to occur.
- Position the extremity at or slightly below the level of the heart; this slows the transport of venom.
- Wrap with clean, loose bandages as you would an orthopedic injury, but continue it further up the limb than usual. Pressure bandaging is thought to be helpful for elapid bites, but may be risky for pit viper bites. Somewhat controversial as it may cause tissue damage.

- In any case, keep the wrapping less tight than when dressing a sprained ankle. If it is too tight, the patient will reflexively move the limb, and spread the venom around.
- Do not use tourniquets, which will do more harm than good.
- Draw a circle around the affected area. As time progresses, you will see the area shrink if it improves or grow if it worsens. This is a good strategy to follow for any local reaction or infection.

The limb should then be rested and, perhaps, immobilized with a splint or sling. The less movement there is, the better. Keep the patient on bed rest, with the bite site lower than the heart, for 24-48 hours. This strategy also works for bites from venomous lizards, like Gila monsters.

It is no longer recommended to make an incision and try to suck out the venom with your mouth. If done more than 3 minutes after the actual bite, it would remove perhaps 1/1000 of the venom and could cause damage or infection to the bitten area. A Sawyer Extractor (a syringe with a suction cup) is more modern, but fairly ineffective in eliminating more than a small amount of the venom unless used in the first minute after the bite is incurred. These methods fail, mostly, due to the speed at which the venom is absorbed.

Interestingly, snake bites don't cause infections as frequently as bites from cats, dogs, or humans. As such, antibiotics are used less often in these cases.

INSECT BITES AND STINGS

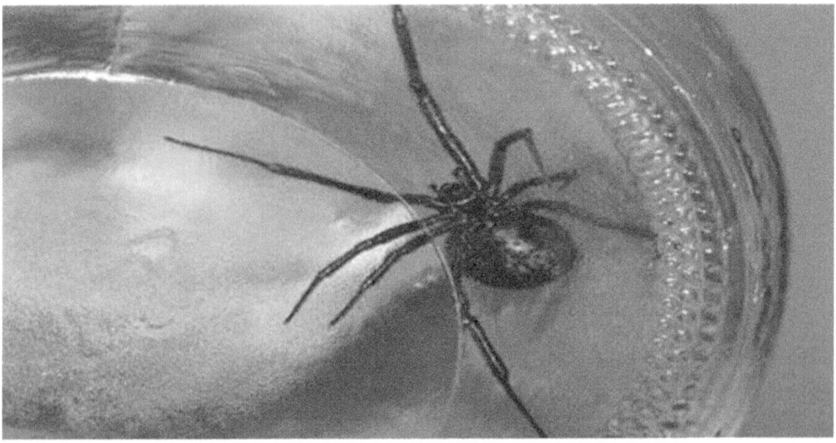

Southern Black Widow Spider

In a survival scenario, you will see a million insects for every snake; so many, indeed, that you can expect to regularly get bitten by them. Insect bites usually cause pain with local redness, itching, and swelling, but are rarely life-threatening.

The exceptions are black widow spiders, brown recluse spiders, and various caterpillars and scorpions. Many of these bites can inject toxins that could cause serious damage. Of course, we are talking about the bite itself, not diseases that may be passed on by the insect. For information on insects as vectors of disease, see the section on mosquito-borne illness.

Bee/Wasp Stings

Stinging insects can be annoyances, but for up to 3% of the population, they can be life-threatening. In the United States, 40-50 deaths a year are caused by hypersensitivity reactions.

For most victims, the offender will be a bee, wasp or hornet. A bee will leave its stinger in the victim, but wasps take their stingers with them and can sting again. Even though you won't get stung again by the same bee, they send out a scent that informs nearby bees that an attack is underway. This is especially true with "Africanized" bees, which are more aggressive than native bees. As such, you should leave the area whether the culprit was a bee, wasp, or hornet.

The best way to reduce any reaction to bee venom is to remove the bee stinger as quickly as possible. Pull it out with tweezers or, if possible, scrape it out with your fingernail. The venom sac of a bee should not be squeezed, as it will inject more irritant into the victim. The longer bee stingers are allowed to remain in the body, the higher chance for a severe reaction.

Most bee and wasp stings heal with little or no treatment. For those that experience only local reactions, the following actions will be sufficient:

- Clean the area thoroughly.
- Remove the stinger if visible.
- Place cold packs and anesthetic ointments to relieve discomfort and local swelling.
- Control itching and redness with oral antihistamines such as Benadryl or Claritin.
- Give acetaminophen or ibuprofen to reduce discomfort.
- Apply antibiotic ointments to prevent infection.

Topical essential oils may be applied (after removing the stinger) with beneficial effect. Use lavandin, helichrysum, tea tree, or peppermint oil, applying 1 or 2 drops to the affected area, 3 times a day. A baking soda paste (baking soda mixed with a small amount of water) may be useful when applied to a sting wound.

Although most of these injuries are relatively minor, there are quite a few people who are allergic to the toxins in the stings. Some are so allergic that they will have what is called an "**anaphylactic reaction**". Instead of just local symptoms like rashes and itching, they will experience dizziness, difficulty breathing, and possibly collapse. Severe swelling is seen in some, which can be life-threatening if it closes the person's airways.

Those experiencing an anaphylactic reaction will require treatment with epinephrine as well as antihistamines. People who are aware that they are highly allergic to stings should carry antihistamines and epinephrine on their person whenever they go outside.

Epinephrine is available in a pre-measured dose cartridge known as the **Epi-Pen** (there is a pediatric version, as well). The Epi-pen is a prescription medication, but few doctors would begrudge a request for one. Make sure to make them aware that you will be outside and may be exposed to possible causes of anaphylaxis. It may be wise to have several Epi-Pens in your possession. See the section on allergic reactions and anaphylaxis for a more in-depth discussion.

Spider Bites

Although large spiders, such as tarantulas, cause painful bites, most spider bites don't even break the skin. In temperate climates, two spiders are to be especially feared: The **black widow** and the **brown recluse**.

The black widow spider is about ½ inch long and is active mostly at night. They rarely invade your home, but can be found in outbuildings like barns and garages. Southern black widows have a red hourglass pattern on their abdomens, but other sub-species may not. Although its bite has very potent venom damaging to the nervous system, the effects on each individual are quite variable.

A black widow bite will appear red and raised. You may see 2 small puncture marks at the site of the wound. Severe pain at the site is usually the first symptom soon after the bite. Following this, you might see:

- Muscle cramps
- Abdominal pain
- Weakness
- Shakiness
- Nausea and vomiting
- Fainting
- Chest pain
- Difficulty breathing
- Disorientation

Each person will present with a variable combination and degree of the above symptoms. The very young and the elderly are more seriously affected than most. In you exam, you can expect rises in both heart rate and blood pressure.

The **brown recluse** spider is, well, brown, and has legs about an inch long. Unlike most spiders, it only has 6 eyes instead of 8, but they are so small it is difficult to identify them from this characteristic.

Victims of brown recluse bites report them to be painless at first, but then may experience these symptoms:

- Itching
- Pain, sometimes severe, after several hours
- Fever
- Nausea and vomiting
- Blisters

The venom of the brown recluse is thought to be more potent than a rattlesnake's, although much less is injected in its bite. Substances in the venom disrupt soft tissue, which leads to local breakdown of blood vessels, skin, and fat. This process, seen in severe cases, leads to "**necrosis**", or death of tissues immediately surrounding the bite. Areas affected may be quite extensive.

Once bitten, the human body activates its immune response as a result. Immune reactions can go haywire, destroying red blood cells and kidney tissue, and hampering the ability of blood to clot appropriately. These effects can lead to coma and, eventually, death. Almost all deaths from brown recluse bites are recorded in children.

The treatment for spider bites includes:

- Washing the area of the bite thoroughly
- Applying ice to painful and swollen areas
- Pain medications such as acetaminophen
- Enforcing bed rest
- Warm baths for those with muscle cramps (black widow bites only; stay away from applying heat to the area with brown recluse bites)
- Antibiotics to prevent secondary bacterial infection

Home remedies include making a paste out of baking soda or aspirin and applying it to the wound. The same method, using olive oil and turmeric in combination, is a time-honored tradition. Dried basil has also been suggested; crush between your fingers until it becomes a fine dust, then apply to the bite. One naturopath uses Echinacea and Vitamin C to speed the healing process. Be aware that these methods may be variable in their effect from patient to patient.

There are various devices and kits available that purport to remove venom from bite wounds. Unfortunately, these suction devices are generally ineffective in removing venom from wounds. Tourniquets are also not recommended and may be dangerous. Although antidotes known as "antivenins" (discussed in the section on snakebite) exist and may be life-saving for venomous spider and scorpion stings, these will be scarce in the aftermath of a major disaster. Luckily, most cases that are not severe will subside over the course of a few days, but the sickest patients will be nearly untreatable without the antivenin.

Scorpion Stings

Most scorpions are harmless; in the United States, only the **bark scorpion** of the Southwest desert has toxins that can cause severe symptoms. In other areas of the world, however, a scorpion sting may be lethal. In the U.S., 17,000 scorpion stings were treated in emergency rooms in 2009. Children are most at risk for major complications.

Some scorpions may reach several inches long; they have eight legs and pincers, and inject venom through their "tail". They are most commonly active at night. Interestingly, scorpion exoskeletons are fluorescent under ultraviolet light; you can find them most easily at night by using a "black light".

The nervous system is most often affected from a scorpion sting. Symptoms you may see in victims of scorpion stings may include:

- Pain, numbness, and/or tingling in the area of the sting
- Sweating
- Weakness
- Increased saliva output

- Restlessness or twitching
- Irritability
- Difficulty swallowing
- Rapid breathing and heart rate

When you have diagnosed a scorpion sting, do the following:

- Wash the area with soap and water.
- Remove jewelry from affected limb (swelling may occur).
- Apply cold compresses to decrease pain.
- Give an antihistamine, such as diphenhydramine (Benadryl). If done quickly, this may slow the venom's spread.
- Keep your patient calm to slow down the spread of venom.
- Limit food intake if the throat is swollen.
- Give pain relievers such as ibuprofen or acetaminophen, but avoid narcotics; they may suppress breathing.
- Don't cut into the wound or use suction to attempt to remove venom.

Although not likely available in an austere environment, an antivenin is now available that eliminates symptoms in children (the group most severely affected) after four hours.

Fire Ant Bites

Fire ants are about ¼ inch in length and can be red or black. If their nest is disturbed, it triggers a mass attack of, sometimes, thousands of colony members. The ants bite with their jaws and have a rear-end stinger that they can use multiple times. Hypersensitivity to fire ants causes about 80 deaths a year in the Southeastern U.S.

If you are attacked by fire ants, do the following:

- Brush them away with your hands (although it may be difficult if they have clamped their jaws into you).
- Move away from the mound.
- Remove clothes if ants have gotten inside them.
- Elevate the bitten extremity to reduce swelling.

- Place a cool compress on the area.
- Take antihistamines such as diphenhydramine (Benadryl) or apply hydrocortisone cream.
- If a blister develops, don't pop it. It will usually not get infected if it stays intact.
- If a blister pops on its own, wash with soap and water.
- Consider antibiotics, such as Amoxicillin, if the wounds appear to worsen with time.

Bedbug Bites

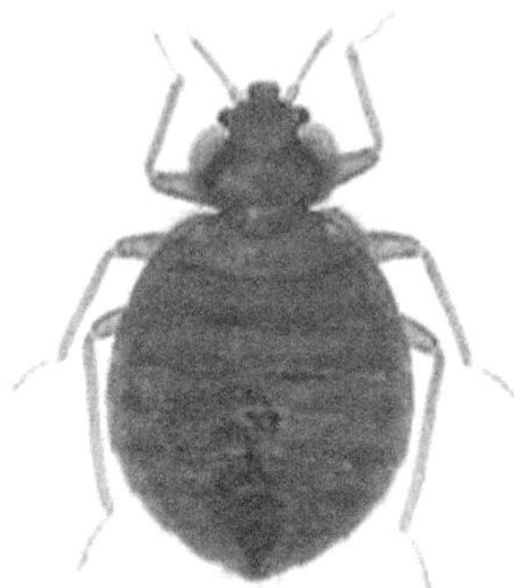

Of all the creepy-crawlies that raise an alarm in a household, few are worse than bed bugs. Although poor standards of living and unsanitary conditions have been associated with bed bug infestations, even the cleanest house in the most developed country can harbor these parasites.

Bed bugs were once so common that every house in many urban areas was thought to harbor them in the early 20th century. They declined with the advent of modern pesticides like DDT, but a resurgence of these creatures has been noted in North America, Europe, and even Australia over the last decade or so. Cities such as New York and London have seen 5 times as many cases reported over the last few years. This may have to do with the environmental restrictions on DDT-like pesticides. Another theory is that over-use of pesticides may be leading to resistance on the part of the insects.

The common bed bug (Cimex lectularius) is a small wingless insect that is thought to have originated in caves where both bats and humans made their homes. They were such a serious issue during WWII that Zyklon, a Hydrogen Cyanide gas infamously used in Nazi concentration camps, was implemented by both sides to get rid of infestations.

There are a number of species of bed bug that are found in differing climates. Unlike lice, bed bugs are not always species-specific (exclusive to humans). For example, Cimex hemipterus, a bed bug found in tropical regions, infests poultry and bats, as well as humans.

Adult bed bugs are light to medium brown and have oval, flat bodies about 4mm long (slightly more after eating). Juveniles are called "nymphs" and are lighter in color (almost translucent). There are several nymph stages; to progress to adulthood, a meal of blood (yours) is necessary.

Bed bugs are mostly active at night. They bite the exposed skin of sleeping humans to feed on their blood. They then retreat to hiding places in the seams of mattresses, linens, and furniture. Their bites are usually painless, but later on, itchy raised welts on the skin may develop. The severity of the response varies from person to person.

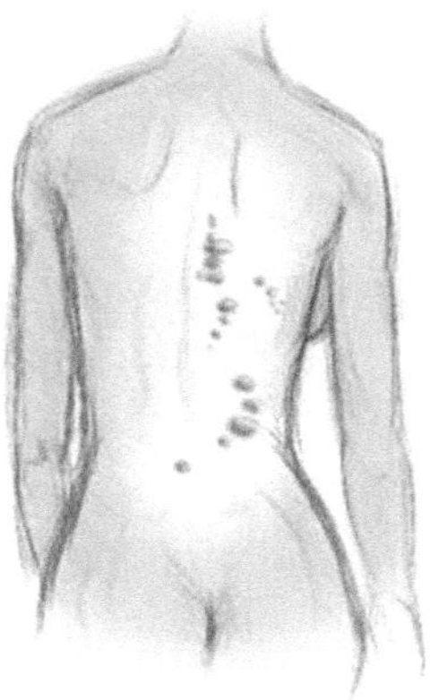

BEDBUG BITE PATTERN

Bed bugs have been known to harbor other disease-causing organisms, but there have not been, as yet, cases of illness specifically caused by them. This is in contrast to body lice or fleas, which has been associated with outbreaks of Typhus, Relapsing fever, and even Plague.

Strangely, bed bugs don't like to live in your clothes, like body lice, or on your skin or hair, like fleas. They apparently don't care much for heat, and prefer to spend more time in your backpack or luggage than your underarm.

Many confuse the bites of bed bugs with mosquitoes or fleas. Most flea bites will appear around the ankles, while bed bugs will bite any area of skin exposed during the night. Flea bites often have a characteristic central red spot. Bed bug bites may resemble mosquito bites except that bedbugs tend to bite multiple times in a straight line. This has been referred as the classic "breakfast, lunch, and dinner" pattern.

The most common treatment for bed bug bites is hydrocortisone cream to treat inflammation and the use of diphenhydramine (Benadryl) for allergic symptoms and itching. The cure, however, is to eradicate the bed bug from your shelter or camp; that's a little harder to do.

First, find their nests: Look at every seam in your mattress, linens, backpacks, and furniture. Bed bugs will also hide in joints in the wooden parts of headboards and baseboards. You will usually find bed bug "families" of various ages, along with brown fecal markings and, perhaps, even small amounts of dried blood.

Most people, once bed bugs are identified, will immediately want to treat with chemicals. Pesticides in the pyrethroid family and Malathion have been found to be effective. Propoxur, an insecticide, is highly toxic to bed bugs as well, but is not approved for indoor use in the U.S. due to health risks. One strategy that *doesn't* work: bug bombs or foggers.

If you use chemicals, be sure you cover all areas on the bed, including the frame and slats. Several treatments will probably be required to eliminate the infestation; repeat at least once every 10 days after the initial treatment.

One reasonable option is the use of bedding covers. These are impervious sheets or padding that, essentially, trap bed bugs inside your mattress until they starve. If they can't reach you to get a meal of blood, they will eventually die out. This method (known as "encasing") is the least risky, as it doesn't involve the use of chemicals.

If you have electricity, make sure to place all bedding and clothes in a hot dryer for at least an hour. Usually, washing clothes alone will not kill bed bugs although hot, soapy water over 125 degrees Fahrenheit may work. This strategy, by the way, includes your backpack when you return from a trip out of town or an extended foraging patrol. Extreme cold is also considered an effective treatment. If you live far enough north, 4 or 5 days of temperatures approaching 0 degrees Fahrenheit should kill them.

If you have access to a working vacuum, use it on flooring and upholstery. A stiff brush is helpful to scrub mattress seams before vacuuming.

Natural remedies to treat bed bugs include dusting seams with diatomaceous earth; crossing dusted areas will cut through their exoskeletons, killing them. It doesn't do much damage to their eggs, however, so regular use is necessary. Many people swear by tea tree oil and rubbing alcohol as well. Here's a time-honored herbal bedbug treatment:

- 1 Cup Water
- Lavender essential oil (10 drops)
- Rosemary essential oil (10 drops)
- Eucalyptus essential oil (10 drops)
- Clove bud essential oil (optional)
- Place in a fine mist spray bottle
- Shake well before using

As bed bugs can live for months without a meal, it's important to maintain long-term diligence in identifying these pests wherever you hang your hat during rough times. These bugs may not end your life, but they can certainly affect the quality of it.

TRAUMATIC BRAIN INJURIES

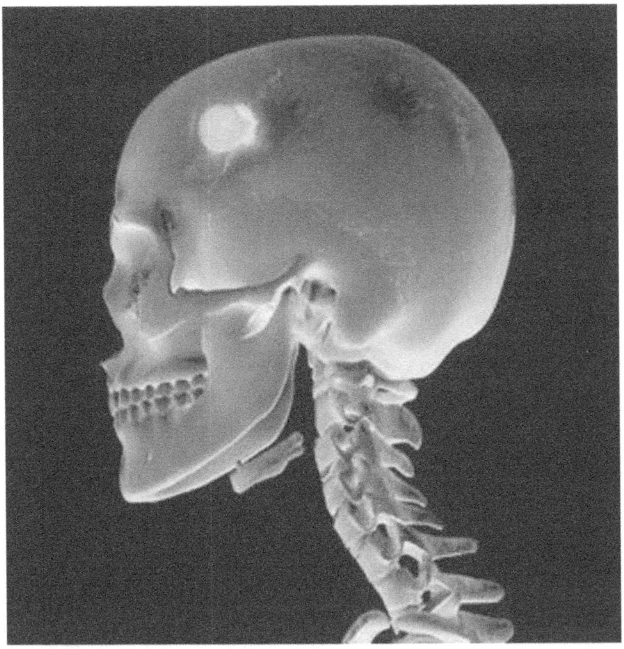

Most head injuries cause superficial damage and are not life-threatening. Indeed, most head injuries amount to only a laceration of the scalp, a black eye, or a painful bump. These wounds, however, can hide damage inside the cranium, the part of the skull that contains the brain. Injuries that affect the brain are called **traumatic brain injuries** (TBIs). It's important for the medic to recognize when trauma to the skull has caused damage that is more than superficial.

Concussions are the most common type of TBI. A concussion is associated with a variety of symptoms that are often immediately apparent. The presentation differs from one individual to the next. Although you might expect a loss of consciousness, the victim may remain completely alert. Headache is actually the most commonly seen symptom. Other symptoms include:

- Dizziness
- Confusion
- Nausea
- Loss of motor coordination
- Blurred or double vision
- Slurred speech
- Ringing in the ear (also called "**tinnitus**")
- Difficulty focusing on tasks at hand

A person with trauma to the head may be knocked unconsciousness for a period of time. In most cases, they will "wake up" in less than 2 minutes. You can expect them to be "foggy" and behave inappropriately (put me in, coach!). They may not remember the events that led to the injury. This patient will merit close observation for the next 48 hours.

You should examine for evidence of superficial injuries and determine that the patient has regained normal motor function. Make sure they can move all their extremities with normal range and strength. Even so, rest is prescribed for the remainder of the day. When your patient goes to bed, it will be appropriate to awaken them every two or three hours to make sure that they are easily aroused. In most cases, a concussion causes no permanent damage unless there are multiple episodes of head trauma over time, as in the case of boxers.

It should be noted that a physical strike to the head is not necessary to suffer a concussion. A particularly jarring football tackle or the violent shaking of an infant can cause a concussion or worse traumatic brain injury. This is because the brain "bounces" against the walls of the cranium. When injury occurs at the site of a blow to the head, it's called a "**coup**" injury. Just as often, it can occur on the opposite site of the head, known as a "**contrecoup**" injury.

In many cases, evidence of direct trauma to the skull is visible. An "open" head injury means that the skull has been penetrated with possible exposure of the brain tissue. If the skull is not fractured, it is referred to as a "closed" injury. An indentation of the skull is clear evidence of a fracture and the outlook may be grim, due to the likelihood of bleeding or swelling in the brain. A closed injury may still become life-threatening for the same reasons.

The brain requires blood and oxygen to function normally. An injury which causes bleeding or swelling inside the skull will increase the intracranial pressure. This causes the heart to work harder to get blood and oxygen into the brain. Blood accumulation (known as a "**hematoma**") could occur within the brain tissue itself, or between the layers of tissue covering the brain.

Without adequate circulation, brain function ceases. Pressure that is high enough could actually cause a portion of the brain to push downward through the base of the skull. This is known as a "**brain herniation**" and, without modern medical care, will almost invariably lead to death.

There are a number of signs and symptoms which might identify those patients that have a serious TBI. They include:

- Prolonged loss of consciousness
- Convulsions (Seizures)
- Worsening headache over time
- Nausea and vomiting
- Bruising (around eyes and ears)
- Bleeding from ears and nose
- Worsening confusion/apathy/drowsiness
- One pupil more dilated than the other
- Indentation of the skull

If the period of unconsciousness is over 10 minutes in length, you must suspect the possibility of significant injury. Vital signs such as pulse, respiration rate, and blood pressure should be monitored closely. The patient's head should be immobilized, and attention should be given to the neck and spine, in case they are also damaged. Verify that the airway is clear and breathing is regular. In a collapse, this person is in a life-threatening situation that will have few curative options if consciousness is not regained.

Other signs of a traumatic brain injury are the appearance of bruising behind the ears (**Battle's sign**) or around the eyes (**raccoon sign**) despite the impact not occurring in that area. This suggests a fracture with internal bleeding. Bleeding from the ear itself or nose without direct trauma to those areas is another indication. The fluid that drains out may be clear; this could represent spinal fluid leakage.

In addition, intracranial bleeding may cause pressure that compresses nerves that lead to the pupils. In this case, you will notice that your unconscious patient has one pupil more dilated than the other.

A severe consequence of bleeding in the brain is a **stroke**, (also known as a **cerebrovascular accident** or CVA). It represents damage to the brain caused by lack of blood supply. This could occur in a head injury due to a blockage of blood flow to a portion of the brain. This blockage could be due to a clot, a hemorrhage, or anything else that compromises the circulation in the area.

Whatever functions are associated with the part of the brain affected will be lost or impaired. These patients often present with an inability to speak, partial or complete blindness, and paralysis or weakness of one side of the body and face. The stroke is usually heralded by a sudden severe headache.

Strokes may also occur due to other reasons as well, such as uncontrolled high blood pressure. Although it may not be difficult to diagnose a major CVA in an austere setting, few options will exist for treating it. Blood thinners might help a stroke caused by a clot, but worsen a stroke caused by hemorrhage. It could be difficult to tell which is which without advanced testing.

Keep the victim on bed rest; sometimes, they may recover partial function after a period of time. If they do, most improvement will happen in the first few days.

Trauma to the head may have negligible consequences, or it could have life-threatening consequences. With certain injuries, there may be little that you, the medic, can do in a long-term survival situation.

SPRAINS AND STRAINS

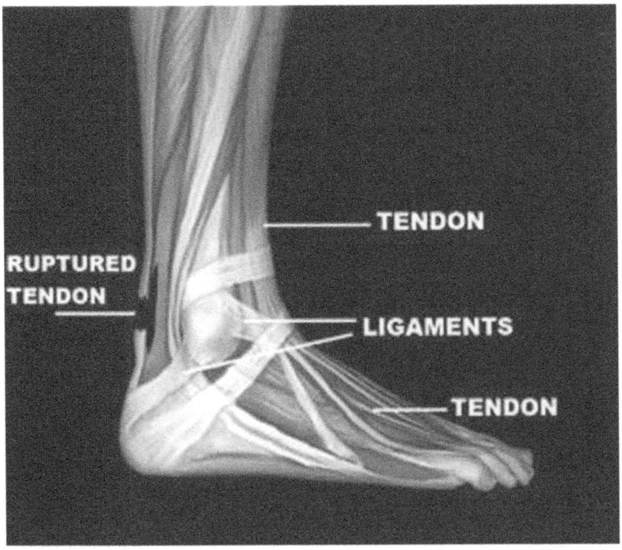

Bones, joints, muscles, ligaments, and tendons give the body support and locomotion, and there is no substitute for having all your parts in good working order. The amount of work these structures will be called upon to do after a disaster will be greatly increased. Therefore, you can expect to see sprains, strains, and fractures.

Prior to a collapse, encourage your people to use modern technology to repair whatever orthopedic issues they may have. Knees, shoulders, ankles and other joints are commonly damaged due to wear and tear, and it pays to "tune" these up while modern surgical care is still available. Many surgeries these days are done through very small incisions, and most can be done as an outpatient. You can imagine how a bum knee can impact your chances for survival.

Many people have heard of ligaments, tendons, sprains, and strains but have little idea of what they really are. Therefore, let's define some anatomical terms:

- **Joint:** the physical point of connection between two bones, usually allowing a certain range of motion. For example, the knee or elbow joint.
- **Ligament:** The fibrous tissue that connects one bone to another, oftentimes across a joint.
- **Tendon:** Tissue that extends from muscle to connect to bone.
- **Sprain:** An injury where a ligament is excessively stretched or torn by forcing a joint beyond its normal range of motion.
- **Strain:** When a muscle or its tendon is partially torn as a result of an injury.
- **Rupture:** A complete tear through a ligament or muscle.

Sprains

Our joints are truly marvels of engineering. They provide mobility and locomotion and sometimes bear an incredible amount of stress without mishap. They are moving parts, however, and moving parts wear down. In long-term survival situations, our level of physical exertion goes up a notch and the risk of joint injury increases as well.

You will find that the most common sprains involve the ankle, wrist, knee or finger. The most likely signs and symptoms are bruising, swelling, and pain. It's a rare individual who has never experienced this injury, in varying degrees of severity, over the course of their life.

Treatment for most sprains is relatively straightforward and follows the easy-to-remember **R.I.C.E.S.** protocol:

REST: It is important to avoid further injury by not testing the injured joint. You may not have a choice, but cessation of whatever actions led to the injury will give the best chance for full recovery. Continued strain will cause the weakened ligament to re-injure itself again and again.

ICE: Cold therapy decreases both swelling and pain. The earlier it is applied, the more effect it will have in speeding up the healing process. If you're in the wilderness, you might have to stick your ankle in a stream to get some cooling action, although you should always keep some "shake and break" cold packs in your medical kit.

Cold therapy should be performed several times a day for 20-30 minutes or so each time for the first 24-48 hours. This is followed each time by applying compression.

COMPRESSION: A compression bandage is useful to decrease swelling and should be placed after each cold therapy. This will also help provide support to the joint. After applying some padding to the area, wrap an elastic "ACE" bandage, starting below the joint and working your way up beyond it. The wrap should be tight, but not uncomfortably so.

Any tingling, increased pain or numbness tells you that the wrap is too tight, and should be loosened. Excessively tight wrap also may affect the circulation: You may notice the fingertips or toes becoming white or even blue.

ELEVATION: Elevate the sprain above the level of the heart. This will help prevent swelling at the site of the injury. Swelling (also called "edema") is caused by fluid that pools where the inflammation is and where gravity will allow. By elevating the leg, you allow the fluid to process itself back into your circulation and aid the healing process, or at least not impede it.

STABILIZATION: Immobilizing the injury will prevent further damage. This may be accomplished by the compression bandage alone or may best be supported with a splint or a cast. This strategy will help support the patient who is unable to place much weight on the joint.

Splints may be commercially produced, such as the versatile **SAM (Structural Aluminum Malleable) splint**, or may be improvised with sticks and cloth, or pillows and duct tape.

We are often asked how to tell the difference between a sprain and a fracture. Sometimes it's quite easy, as when a straight bone is suddenly "zig-zag" in shape. Many times, however, it's hard to determine without modern diagnostic tests (which won't be available in a long-term survival situation).

Look for one or more of these signs:

- A fracture will generally have more pronounced swelling and bruising.
- A fracture is generally so painful that no pressure may be placed on the injury at all.
- A fracture may have a deep cut in the area of the injury. This is called an "open" fracture and is particularly dangerous due to the risk of infection.
- A fracture may show motion in an area beyond the joint (if your finger suddenly has five knuckles, you probably broke it).
- A fracture may present a grating sensation when pressing upon it.
- Using a tuning fork on the bone below the level of the fracture will result in decreased sound heard with a stethoscope placed above the level of the fracture (that is, closer to the torso), compared to intact bone.

For sprains, Ibuprofen serves as an excellent anti-inflammatory and pain reliever. Natural remedies may also help. The under bark of willow, aspen and poplar trees contain Salicin, a natural pain medicine.

Most sprains, (such as wrist and ankle sprains) commonly heal well over time using the R.I.C.E.S. protocol, pain relievers, and a lot of rest. Others, however, such as severe knee sprains with torn or ruptured ligaments, may heal completely only with the aid of surgical intervention.

It's important to get joint issues dealt with while we still have modern medicine to help us. In uncertain times, you (and your joints) want to be in the best shape possible to face the challenges ahead.

Strains

By far, the most frequently seen strain will be to the back muscles. Strains, especially back strains, involve injury to the muscle and their tendons (which connects them to the bone). As the lower part of the back holds the majority of the body's weight, you can expect the most trouble here. Some of these injuries are preventable with some simple precautions:

- Every morning, you should perform some stretching exercises to increase blood flow to cold, stiff muscles and joints.
- When you lift a heavy object, such as a backpack, keep your back straight and let your legs perform the work.
- The object should be close to your body as you lift it (don't reach for it).
- For packs, keep the weight on the hips rather than the shoulders.
- If you are on rocky or unstable terrain, consider using a walking stick for balance. Remember, any weight-lifting action that you perform while off-balance is likely to result in a strained muscle.
- Cold packs will decrease swelling in the first 24 hours or so. After that, heat packs may be more effective in providing pain relief.

Ibuprofen is an excellent anti-inflammatory and pain reliever for these types of injury. For muscle injuries, prescription relaxants such as Diazepam (Valium) or Cyclobenzaprine (Flexeril) will also provide relief. If these are not available, the patient will benefit from massage.

A number of alternative remedies exist for the treatment of mild-moderate sprains and strains. Essential oils are considered helpful to clear up bruising. Apply 2-3 drops of oil of Helichrysum, cypress, clove, or geranium, mixed half and half with carrier oil such as coconut or olive, 3-5 times a day on the area of bruising.

To decrease swelling, apply Helichrysum oil, undiluted, to the affected area. Willow under bark or ginger teas have anti-inflammatory properties; drink with warm raw honey, several times a day.

Common herbal pain relievers for orthopedic injuries include direct application of Oil of wintergreen, Helichrysum, peppermint, clove, or diluted arnica to the affected area. Blends of the above may also be used in balms. Herbal teas that may give relief are valerian root, willow under bark, ginger, passion flower, feverfew, and turmeric. As always, drink warm with raw honey several times a day.

DISLOCATIONS

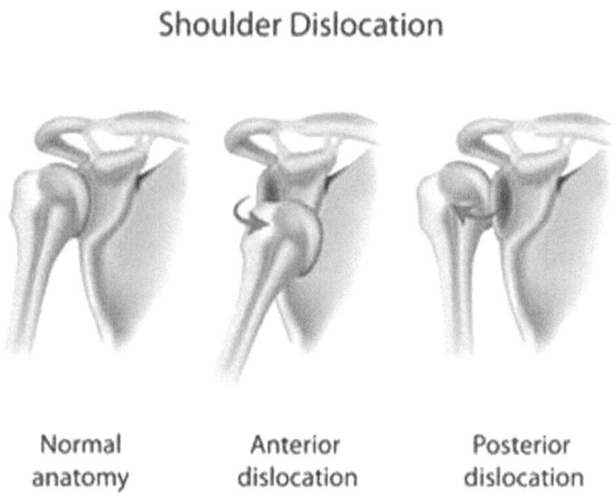

A **dislocation** is an injury in which a bone is pulled out of its joint by some type of trauma. Dislocations commonly occur in shoulders, fingers, and elbows, but knees, ankles, and hips may also be affected. The joint involved looks visibly abnormal and is unusable. Bruising and pain often accompany the injury.

If the dislocation is momentary and the bone slips back into its joint on its own, it is called a **subluxation**. Subluxations can be treated the same way that sprains are, using the R.I.C.E.S. method. It should be noted that the traditional medical definition of subluxation is somewhat different from the chiropractic one.

Of course, if there is medical care readily available, the patient should go directly to the local hospital, as general anesthesia is often needed to resolve the problem. Indeed, some dislocations may only be reduced surgically. In a collapse, however, you are on your own and will probably have to correct the dislocation yourself. This is known as performing a "**reduction**".

Reduction is easiest to perform soon after the dislocation, before muscles spasm and the inevitable swelling occurs. Not only does reducing the dislocation decrease the pain experienced by the victim, but it will lessen the damage to all the blood vessels and nerves that run along the line of the injury. The faster the reduction is performed, the less likely there will be permanent damage. Unfortunately, a dislocated joint may have a tendency to go out of place again in the future.

Expect significant pain on the part of the patient during the actual procedure. Some pain relievers like ibuprofen might be useful to decrease discomfort from the reduction. Prescription muscle relaxers such as Cyclobenzaprine (Flexeril) are also helpful.

The use of traction will greatly aid your attempt to fix the problem. Traction is the act of pulling the dislocated bone away from the joint to give room to slip back into place. Each dislocation uses a different procedure, and some have several different methods of reduction.

The patient with a shoulder dislocation will come, usually holding their forearm for support, with complaints of pain and the arm obviously out of place: The procedures for an anterior shoulder dislocation (the most common type by far) include:

Method 1: Have the patient lie face down on a surface high enough that the arm (including the shoulder joint) dangles without hitting the ground. Get the patient's arm into position slowly for the least discomfort.

Wrap a 15-20 pound weight around their forearm and wrist. Although they could hold the weight in their hand, this may tense the muscles, and you need them to relax. Once the muscles are relaxed enough (maybe 10 minutes or so), the arm should pop back into place.

Method 2: Have the patient lie on their back. With their elbow at a 90 degree angle, slowly rotate the arm outward with the palm facing the sky. This should be a slow movement; worsening pain is a sign to slow down.

Now, raise the arm so that the hand is behind their head, as if they were scratching the back of their neck. The action is similar to a baseball pitcher about to throw a ball. Once their hand is behind their head, slowly help them reach for the opposite shoulder. This motion should move the shoulder back into place.

Method 3: Place your foot against the side of the patient's chest and apply slow traction by pulling the arm while holding the wrist with the palm facing up. This, again, must be done slowly and gradually until the arm pops back into place.

If you're fortunate enough to have an assistant, wrap a towel or sheet around the upper chest of the patient and have the assistant pull in the opposite direction to provide counter-traction. This avoids having to use your foot for that purpose.

If these procedures are successful, pain and movement should be immediately improved, although it is normal to have some discomfort in the injured shoulder for some time. Your patient may benefit from the placement of a sling afterwards, although some studies suggest the effect is more psychological than anything else.

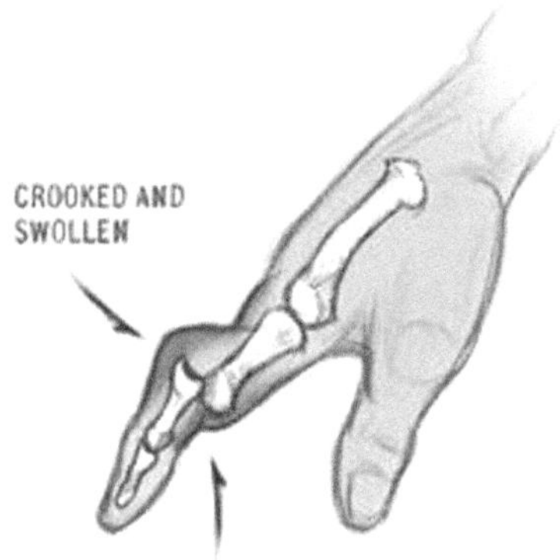

DISLOCATED FINGER

Another common dislocation is that of a finger. A portion of the digit may be displaced up or down or to the side. To reduce this deformity, use one hand to grasp and stabilize the finger above the level of the dislocation (that is, closer to the forearm). With the other, grasp the dislocated portion and pull outward and then towards the joint. A digital or wrist block, as described earlier in this section, may be performed beforehand. The reduced finger may be taped to its neighbor (the "buddy method") but may also benefit from the placement of a finger splint.

Some dislocations, such as a dislocated finger, may take as little as 2-3 weeks to regain normal function. Others, such as hip dislocations, may take many months to heal. Any dislocation may also have a fracture associated with it, and should be further evaluated.

FRACTURES

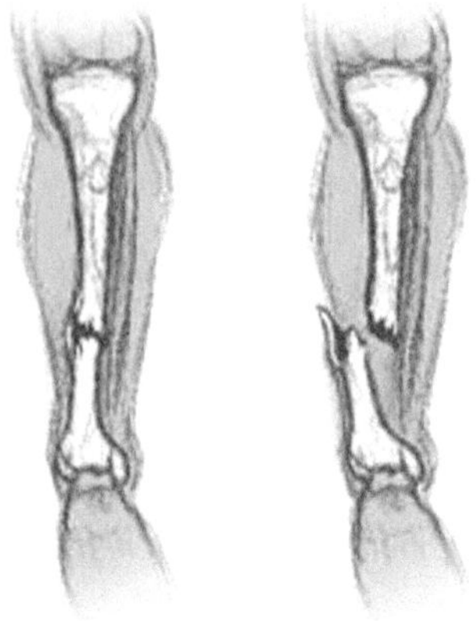

FRACTURE TYPES

If enough force is applied, an injury to soft tissues can damage the skeletal structure underneath. When a bone is broken, it is termed a fracture. There are several types of fractures:

- **Non-displaced fracture**. In the simplest fracture, the broken ends of the bone are barely out of place.
- **Displaced fracture:** The broken ends of the bone are no longer in line.
- **Open or compound fracture**. In a compound fracture, the skin is pierced by the broken bone or other penetrating trauma. The end of the bone may be exposed or may have retreated below the level of the skin..
- **Comminuted fracture:** The bone shatters into several pieces.
- **Oblique/Transverse fracture**: the line of the broken bone may be horizontal or at an oblique angle.

- **Greenstick fracture:** Sometimes called an "incomplete" fracture. One side of the bone snaps, the other remains intact. Reminiscent of the result of trying to snap live wood in two.
- **Hairline fracture:** A fracture where the line of break is so thin that the two broken ends do not separate. The break may not go through the entire bone.

For our purposes, let's assume that they are all either "open" or "closed". A closed fracture is when there is a break in the bone, but the skin is intact (all of the above except the compound fracture). In an open fracture, the skin is broken. This usually occurs as a result of the force of the fractured bone tearing through the tissue.

It stands to reason that there is usually more blood loss and infection associated with an open wound. The infection may be deep in the skin (**cellulitis**), the blood (**septicemia**), or the bone itself (**osteomyelitis**) and could be life threatening if not treated. If poorly managed, a closed fracture can become an open fracture.

Evaluating A Fracture

The diagnosis of a broken bone can be simple, as when the bone is obviously deformed, or difficult, as in a minimal, "hairline" fracture. X-rays can be helpful to differentiate a small fracture from a severe sprain, but that technology won't be available in a power-down situation. There are some ways to tell, however (also discussed under sprains):

- A fracture will manifest with severe pain and inability to use the bone (for example. The patient cannot put any weight whatsoever on a broken ankle). Someone with a sprain can probably put some weight, albeit painfully, on the area.
- More pronounced swelling and bruising is usually present on a fracture than a sprain.
- A grinding sensation may be felt when broken ends of a bone rub together.
- A deep cut in the area of the injury is a likely sign of an open fracture where the bone has retreated back into the body.

- Using a tuning fork on the bone below the level of the fracture will result in decreased sound heard with a stethoscope placed above the level of the fracture (that is, closer to the torso), compared to intact bone.
- Motion of the bone in an area where there is no joint is another dead giveaway that there is a fracture. If you notice that your finger appears to have five knuckles, you broke it.

Dealing with a fractured bone involves first evaluating the injured area for the above signs and symptoms. Use your bandage or EMT scissors to cut away the clothing over the injury. This will prevent further injury that may occur if the patient was made to remove their own clothing. First, check the site for bleeding and the presence of an open wound; if present, stop the bleeding before proceeding further.

Fractures may cause damage to the patient's circulation in the limb affected, so it is important to check the area beyond the level of the injury for changes in coloration (white or blue instead of normal skin color) and for strong and steady pulses. Usually, normal color returns to skin in the fingertips within 2 seconds of applying pressure and then releasing. This is known as the "**Capillary Refill Time**" and is further discussed in the section on mass casualty triage.

To find out what a strong pulse feels like, place two fingers on the side of your neck until you feel your neck arteries pulsing. You will do this same action on, say, the wrist, if the patient has broken their arm. Lightly prick the patient in the same area with a safety pin to make sure they have normal sensation. If not, the nerve has been injured.

If the bone has not deformed the extremity, it is called a "non-displaced" fracture. In austere settings, a simple splint held in place with elastic wraps will immobilize the fracture and promote appropriate healing. Always allow some space for swelling that may occur in the area of the injury.

Oftentimes, however, the broken ends of the bone will not be together and appear obviously deformed. These fractures must be "reduced" as we discussed with dislocations. Repositioning the fracture without surgery is referred to as a "closed" or "external reduction".

These are quite painful, but a complete recovery will not occur unless the two ends of the broken bone are realigned to their original position.

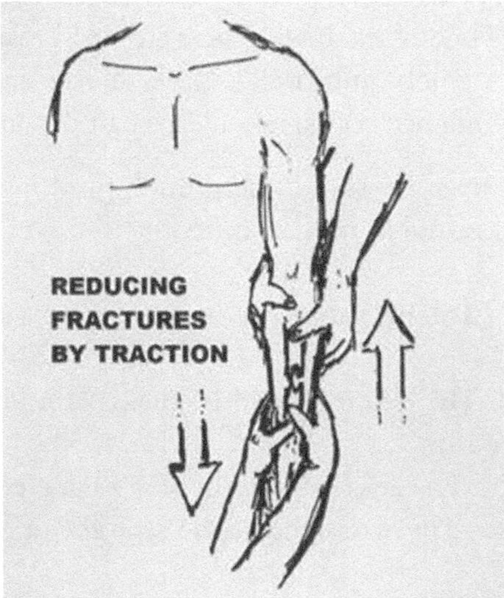

Reducing a fracture is best done under general anesthesia or significant sedation, but this won't be available to you in a disaster. It can be done, however, if necessary, by the medic and an assistant. One supports the side closest to the torso while the other exerts steady traction on the area below the fracture. In some cases, the bone may not slip back into place and you may have to move it during the procedure. Afterwards, some form of mechanical traction is often needed to keep the broken ends of the bone in place.

There are risks to this procedure: Nerves and blood vessels can be damaged, so be sure to check pulses and sensation beyond the level of the fracture before you finish.

Splint the extremity in place immediately after performing the reduction. In an open fracture, thorough washing of the wound is absolutely necessary to prevent internal infection. Infection will likely occur in a dirty wound, even if a reduction is successful. Wound care, as described previously, and antibiotics are important to prevent bacteria from contaminating the bone, marrow, or soft tissue and, as a result, entering the bloodstream. Regularly check the pulses and capillary refill time during recovery to assess the circulation beyond the level of the fracture.

Fingers and toes may be splinted by taping them to an adjoining digit. This is called the "buddy method". There are small manufactured splints that will also do the job quite well. Neck injuries may be particularly serious; immobilizing neck collars should be part of your medical storage.

To heal, an extremity should be immobilized in a position that it normally would assume in routine function:

- For legs: The leg should be straight, with a slight bend at the knee.
- For arms: The elbow should be flexed at a 90 degree angle to the upper arm.
- For ankles: The ankle should be at a 90 degree angle to the leg.
- For wrist: The wrist should be straight or slightly extended upward.
- For fingers: The fingers should be slightly flexed, as if holding a glass of water.

As previously mentioned, splints can be commercially produced (e.g., SAM splints), or may be improvised, using straight sticks or boards with bandannas or T-shirt strips to hold the splint in pace. Another option is to fold a pillow around the injury and wrap duct tape around it.

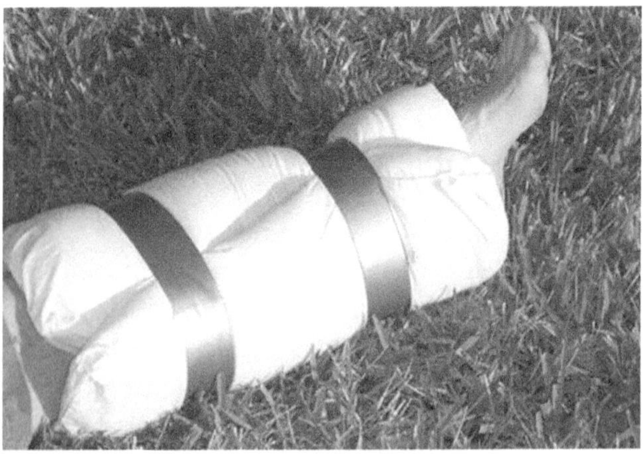

Pillow Splint

Placing A Cast

For many fractures, a splint may not be enough to ensure good healing. You will want to consider the placement of a "cast" to enforce immobilization. Casting material using plaster of Paris or fiberglass is easy to obtain and lasts a long time. Plaster is more pliable and hardens slower, giving you more time to apply the cast. Fiberglass is lighter and less messy to use. Both are useful additions to your medical supplies.

Each fracture is casted somewhat differently and with various materials, but the basic principles are the same. When placing a cast, you will first start with a liner of cotton known as a "stockinette". The stockinette should be measured and cut several inches longer than the intended cast. Place it, without wrinkling, over the area to be casted like you would put on a sock.

Then, you will need rolls of padding to form a barrier between the skin and the cast. Advance one half of the thickness of the roll each turn as you go from below the fracture towards the torso. The padding should be at least two to three layers thick and should extend and inch or two beyond the cast edge. Extra padding should be applied between digits and over bony prominences like the wrist or ankle.

At this point, rolls of plaster of Paris or fiberglass are immersed in cool water for 20 seconds or so, and then squeezed to remove excess water. Keep the end of the roll between your fingers or it will stick to the rest and be difficult to find.

Then, you will begin to slowly wrap the casting material around the area of the fracture, smoothing it out as you go along. Advance one half of the thickness of the roll each turn as you go from below the fracture towards the torso. Avoid making it too tight.

You will want perhaps three layers of casting material on the area, more in places where there is a bony prominence, such as the wrist. Roll the ends of the stockinette and padding back over the cast before the last layer is applied to form padding for the edges.

Stockinettes, padding, and casting rolls are available in different widths and lengths appropriate to the particular fracture. For comfort and cleanliness, plastic wrap is helpful to cover the cast during bathing. A wet cast is a smelly cast.

Although oscillating saws are used today to remove casts, they require the availability of electricity. There are still special heavy-duty shears available for the purpose, although some effort is needed to perform the removal.

To review: Your goal is to immobilize the fracture in a position of function. Use padding under the splint or cast as possible to keep the injured area stable and protected. Use more casting material over bony prominences.

Most fractures require 6-8 weeks to form a "**callous**"; this is newly formed tissue that will reunite the broken ends of the bone. Larger bones or more complicated injuries take longer. If a displaced fracture is not reduced, the function of the affected extremity will be permanently compromised. References to books and videos devoted to the subject are listed at the end of this volume.

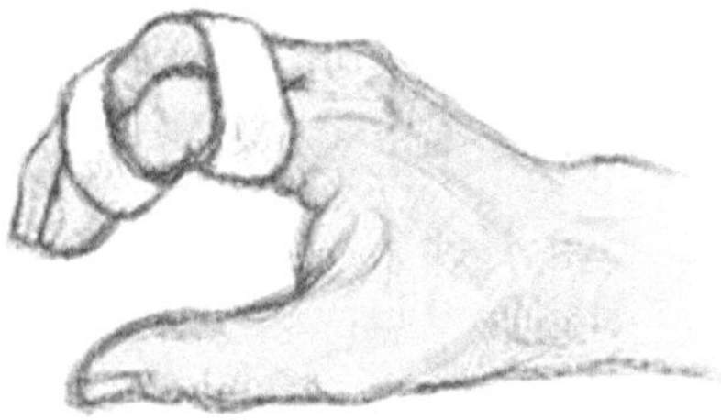

FRACTURED FINGER BUDDY

Rib Fractures and Pneumothorax

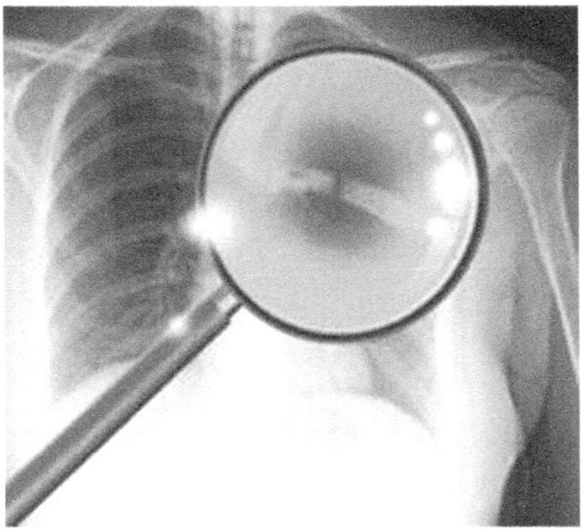

You have 12 pairs of ribs, numbered from top to bottom. These are sometimes characterized as "true ribs", "false ribs", and "floating ribs". The true ribs (ribs 1-7) connect via flexible connective tissue called "cartilage" to the breastbone. The false ribs (8-10) connect to the cartilage of the 7th rib instead. The 11th and 12th ribs "float" in front, with no connection to the breastbone at all. All ribs connect to the spine in back.

Ribs are also connected to each other by muscles (called "**intercostal**" muscles). Nerves and blood vessels travel just under each rib in the intercostal space.

Signs and symptoms of rib fractures

Rib fractures, usually caused by trauma, most often involve the middle ribs. If a rib is broken, several signs and symptoms are likely to appear. You can suspect a rib fracture if you note the following:

- A painful area, sometimes with a bump or dent, at the site of impact.
- Increased pain with breathing or movement.
- Bruising of the chest or back.
- Grating sensations or sounds when fractured bone ends rub against each other (use a stethoscope over the area to listen).
- "Splinting", the tensing of muscles in an effort to decrease pain.

In uncomplicated single fractures, there is often no change in the appearance of the chest wall itself. Previously, these injuries were treated with a binder called a "rib belt" or by tightly taping around the entire chest. Although these methods relieve some discomfort, they are now thought to cause more harm than good by preventing the ability to take deep breaths. Failure to fully inflate the lungs can lead to pneumonia.

Instead, tape could be placed from the front of the chest, over the injured rib, and back to the middle of the spine.

You can prevent pneumonia due to "under-breathing" by encouraging slow deep breathing exercises and gentle coughing every 2 hours or so. Your patient will experience less pain during this process by holding a blanket or pillow against the site of injury. Some practitioners, instead, place the arm on the affected side in a sling with padding between the arm and ribs for support during breathing exercises. Full recovery will take 6-8 weeks.

Ibuprofen and cold packs are helpful for pain. You might be surprised to find that your patient sleeps more peacefully lying with the injured side down.

More serious or multiple fractures may present with:

- Rapid, shallow breathing
- Rapid heart rate
- Bloody cough (also called "**hemoptysis**")
- Irregular appearance (bump or dent) at the site of injury
- Decreased or unusual movement of the chest wall on the affected side.

When there are multiple rib fractures they usually occur in a row. This injury is called a "Flail Chest" and can be identified by placing one hand on each side of the chest. Observe chest movement during breathing. The uninjured side will rise during inhalation as normal, but the flail injury will fall. This occurs because the "loose" rib segments are pulled into the chest cavity when inhaling. The lung is usually bruised and gets less oxygen to the body. Without modern respiratory support and, perhaps, surgical intervention, the patient is unlikely to survive.

Rib fractures are most dangerous if a jagged bone punctures organs in the chest, such as the lungs. Air enters the chest cavity through the puncture, causing a condition known as a "**pneumothorax**". As more air fills the chest, it causes pressure that prevents the lung from filling with air.

Although a person with a very small pneumothorax will complain of pain with breathing or some shortness of breath, the condition may sometimes resolve on its own or with oxygen. It may, however, progress to a "**tension pneumothorax**". Usually caused by significant trauma or penetrating wounds, the victim may have increasing signs of bluish skin coloration (called "**cyanosis**"), distended neck veins, and signs of shock. If you use a stethoscope, you will hear crackling sounds or, sometimes, no breath sounds at all on the affected side.

With a tension pneumothorax from a rib fracture, emergency needle decompression is indicated if there isn't an open wound. This procedure is *not* appropriate, however, for traumatic pneumothorax if medical facilities are readily at hand (a "chest tube", discussed below, should be placed). Decompression should only be attempted in austere settings if it's clear the patient will die without action taken on their behalf.

To perform needle decompression:

- Wearing gloves, clean the area of the chest on the affected side with Povidone-iodine solution or Chlorhexidine in the intercostal space above the third rib midway between the center of the collarbone and the nipple.
- Using a 14 gauge decompression needle catheter, enter the skin just above the rib (the blood vessels travel below) at a 90 degree angle. Go deep enough to hear a pop and a hiss as air passes through. This should allow the lung to inflate.
- Remove the metal needle and leave the plastic sleeve (the "catheter") in place.

Many are taught to place a valve of some sort over the catheter once placed. This is meant to prevent air from returning to the lung cavity. A useful item for medical storage would be a "chest seal". Asherman, Hyfin, Bolin, or other vented chest seals also have the benefit of securing the catheter in place.

When penetrating trauma like a stab or gunshot causes a tension pneumothorax (often called a "sucking chest wound"), a chest seal must be placed over the site of entrance wounds (and exit, if any). You goal is to provide a way for the air to escape from the chest cavity, but not to go back in.

Although many commercial vented seals are available, one can be improvised by taking a 4-6 inch square of plastic wrap or other airtight material and firmly taping three sides on top of the wound. The open fourth side will serve as a valve and allow air to escape and the lung to inflate, while not letting air back in. If this fails, sometimes the wound opening could be spread to allow air to exit and the seal replaced.

You must realize that, in normal times, there is much more to be done, such as placing a "chest tube", a more extensive procedure that opens a path for suction drainage of fluids and re-inflation of the lung. Inflammatory or bloody fluid is likely to accumulate in many lung wounds and must be eliminated to adequate air passage. A tube connected to a jar placed below the patient may perform this duty (very poorly) by using gravity.

No improvised system, however, will be as efficient as the suction systems and respiratory support available at your local hospital. It's important to accept that a traumatic pneumothorax will be difficult to recover from in austere settings. During the Civil War, chest wounds carried a 72% death rate. Be realistic in your expectations.

AMPUTATION

In rare circumstances, damage to a limb may be so extensive that it cannot be saved. Amputation is the surgical removal of all or part of an extremity. This procedure is performed on arms, legs, hands, feet, fingers, or toes. Amputation of a part of the leg is the most common amputation surgery.

An amputation, in a survival situation, is clearly a procedure of last resort. In many cases, your patient will not survive it. At least 25% of American civil war soldiers undergoing the procedure lost their lives due to complications. The closer to the body that the amputation was performed, the higher the death rate will be. It's unlikely there will be much improvement over Civil War statistics in future times of trouble.

There are various reasons that an amputation may be necessary. The most common is poor circulation because of damage to blood vessels. Without reasonable blood flow, tissue may not get enough oxygen to remain viable. Infection and gangrene (discussed in the section on frostbite) may set in.

Below are some reasons that an amputation may be indicated:

- Extensive injury from trauma or burns.
- Cancerous tumors
- Serious infection that fails to improve with antibiotics
- Severe frostbite
- Gangrene (tissue death due to loss of circulation)

Several methods are used to determine where to cut and how much to remove:

- Checking where an extremity loses a pulse.
- Areas when a limb loses normal temperature.
- Spreading areas of reddened skin (infection) or blackened skin (gangrene)
- Checking where the extremity is no longer sensitive to touch.
- Identifying areas where a bone has been crushed beyond repair.

Basic measures to increase the chances of a successful amputation are:

- Sedate the patient as much as possible.
- Clean the damaged area with Betadine or other antiseptics before the procedure.
- Use sterile gloves in a sterile field
- Remove debris and bits of shattered bone.
- Tie off bleeding blood vessels with suture material.
- Preserve an adequate amount of living skin and soft tissue to cover the exposed end of the bone.
- Shorten and smooth the bone enough to decrease irritation to the covering soft tissue.
- Stitch remaining muscle to the bone lining (also known as the "**periosteum**"). This is difficult without special equipment.
- Before closing completely, place a drain (discussed earlier in this book) to allow blood and inflammatory fluid to exit the surgical site.
- Adequately close the wound with sutures or staples, while allowing room for a drain to be placed).
- Change dressings regularly.
- Observe for infection and start a course of antibiotics.

Amputation is a procedure we hope you will never have to consider. In severe injuries, it may be life-saving. Realize, however, that your patient might not recover without advanced care.

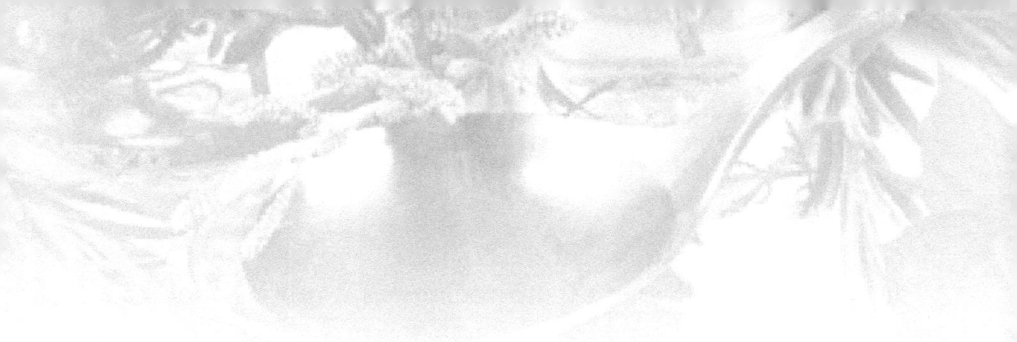

SECTION 7

CHRONIC MEDICAL PROBLEMS

As a caregiver in a long-term survival scenario, you can't expect that everyone under your care will start off in perfect health. It is likely that one or more members of your family or group will have a longstanding medical issue that cannot be ignored.

The amount and diversity of chronic medical issues may test the medic's fund of knowledge. You must formulate strategies that might be effective to control chronic medical problems in austere settings. Some of your options might not be as effective as those that modern technology can provide. Despite this, you must take action to be ready for difficult times or your patient may suffer the consequences.

You would probably be surprised at how many of your family or group members have chronic illnesses or conditions of which you're unaware. Even those you may have known for decades may not make it a habit of discussing their medical issues with you. As the person responsible for their medical well-being in a collapse, however, it is your duty to obtain full histories from everyone in your party. Without obtaining this information, you will be less effective in your role as medic.

Thyroid malfunction, diabetes, and heart disease are just some of the issues. These illnesses require medications that will not be manufactured in times of trouble. We must, therefore, think "outside the box" to formulate a medical strategy for these patients that does not include modern technology.

Its goes without saying that medical conditions that are poorly controlled now could be completely out of control in a collapse. The most important way to preserve your family's health will be to have any chronic conditions appropriately treated and monitored *prior* to a catastrophe.

While you have the benefit of modern medical care (and, perhaps, medical insurance), take full advantage of any option that will tune up chronic problems. Eliminate dental issues you might have ignored, repair that defective knee joint, or consider procedures to correct your vision. In hard times, you'll need to function at 100% efficiency. If you ignore your medical issues now, how can you expect to keep it together if things fall apart, whether it's your health or that of others?

This section will discuss some of the most common diseases that people have to deal with today. The successful caregiver will develop a plan of action in advance that will keep chronic medical problems in check. If we ever find ourselves on our own, having a plan in place will increase a medic's effectiveness and improve the health of the community.

THYROID DISEASE

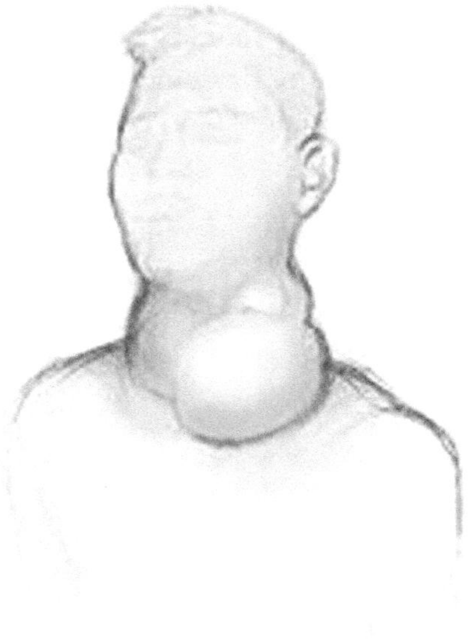

GOITER

The thyroid gland is positioned just in front of and below the Adam's apple (also known as the "laryngeal prominence") and produces hormones that help regulate your metabolism. **Hormones** are chemical messengers that glands secrete to direct the function of other parts of the body.

The thyroid gland is involved in maintaining a hormonal balance between itself and two other organs, the "pituitary gland" and the "hypothalamus". These two organs can be found near the base of the brain. When this balance is disturbed, we experience thyroid dysfunction. Thyroid conditions usually involve the production of either too little or too much of these hormones. These malfunctions may occur in anyone, but are most commonly seen in women.

A thyroid problem that might be common in an austere setting is the development of a lump (known as a "**goiter**"). This is the result of a deficiency of iodine in the body, and is one of the reasons why common table salt is "iodized". Potassium Iodide tablets (discussed in the section on radiation) may be a treatment option if no other source of iodine is available. Iodide can also be found in Kelp (a type of seaweed).

Unfortunately, the use of Iodides, while a known treatment, may actually worsen the condition in some cases. It should be noted that iodine-containing drugs should not be administered to those with allergies to seafood.

Lumps on the thyroid may develop that are not associated with iodine deficiency. They can exist without causing symptoms or even disturbed thyroid hormone levels. A lump may present as a **cyst** (a mass filled with fluid) or a **nodule** (a solid mass), and usually has no major ill effect. These are considered to be "cold" tumors. Some thyroid tumors, however, are "hot" and produce excessive amounts of hormone. Thyroid cancer is relatively uncommon and grows slowly, even in the elderly, unless there has been exposure to radiation.

Hyperthyroidism

The excessive production of thyroid hormone is known as Hyperthyroidism. Determination of thyroid malfunction depends on certain blood tests and, sometimes, a scan of the gland. These won't be an option in a collapse, so it's important to learn what a person with elevated thyroid levels looks like. Some common signs and symptoms of this condition in adults are:

- Insomnia
- Hand tremors
- Nervousness
- Feeling excessively hot in normal or cold temperatures
- Eyes that appear to be bulging out or "staring"
- Frequent bowel movements
- Losing weight despite normal or increased appetite
- Excessive sweating
- Weight loss
- Menstrual periods that are scant or cease altogether
- Growth and puberty irregularities in children
- Muscle weakness, chest pain and shortness of breath (elderly)

Poorly controlled hyperthyroidism can lead to a condition known as **thyroid "storm"**, in which very high levels of hormone cause major effects on the heart and brain. All the above symptoms may combine with elevated heart rate and blood pressure to endanger the patient's life.

Treatment of hyperthyroidism involves medications such as Propylthiouracil and Methimazole, which block thyroid function. These medications should be stockpiled if you're aware of a member of your group with hyperthyroidism, as they will be hard to find if modern medical care is no longer available.

Substances such as I-131 (also known as radioiodine) have been used to actually destroy an overactive thyroid. As you can imagine, this results in the patient producing no thyroid hormone at all. I-131 treatment is useful in severe hyperthyroidism, but is also unlikely to be available in a collapse.

Dietary restriction of nicotine, caffeine, alcohol, and other substances that alter metabolism will be important to control high thyroid conditions. Vitamins C and B12 are thought to have a beneficial effect on those with this condition, as does L-Carnitine. L-Carnitine may lower thyroid hormone levels without damaging the gland.

Foods that are thought to depress production of thyroid hormone include cabbage, cauliflower, broccoli, Brussels sprouts, and spinach. In addition, foods high in antioxidants are thought to reduce free radicals that might be involved in hyperthyroidism. These include blueberries, cherries, tomatoes, squash and bell peppers, among many others.

Hypothyroidism

More commonly seen than hyperthyroidism, hypothyroidism is the failure to produce enough thyroid hormone. Various causes of low thyroid levels exist, such as certain drugs or exposure to radiation. Also, the immune system sometimes misfires and targets the thyroid. The most commonly seen signs and symptoms of hypothyroidism in adults are:

- Fatigue
- Intolerance to cold
- Constipation
- Poor appetite
- Weight gain
- Dry skin
- Hair loss
- Hoarseness
- Depression
- Menstrual irregularity
- Poor growth (Children)

If ignored, additional symptoms might appear, such as:

- Thickened skin
- Hair loss
- Vocal changes
- Swollen appearance of hands, feet, and face

It should be noted that untreated hypothyroidism in a pregnant woman may cause birth defects in the baby.

The treatment of this condition is based on the oral replacement of the missing hormone, which is called "**thyroxine**". These drugs come in a variety of dosages, and it is important for a physician to determine the appropriate dose for your patient while modern medical care is still available. The lowest dose that will maintain normal thyroid levels is indicated; too much may cause hyperthyroidism.

Once you have determined the right dosage, you may consider, in normal times, asking a physician for additional supplies or perhaps a prescription for a higher dose. This might allow you to use, say, half of the pill in the present and stockpile the other half for the uncertain future. Only do this if you intend to follow your physician's advice as to your dose. There is no benefit (but significant risk) to taking more thyroid replacement medicine that you should. Not all physicians will take kindly to this request.

Besides standard thyroid medications such as Synthroid and Levothyroid, there are a number of other remedies that may have effect in improving hypothyroidism. A number of thyroid extracts are available which consist of desiccated and powdered pig or cow thyroid gland. The amount of thyroid hormone in these extracts may be variable; therefore, the medical establishment recommends against their use.

Having said this, in the absence of modern medications, it is better than nothing. One strategy that may help you decide what natural supplement may be right for you is to ask your physician to monitor your thyroid levels for 2-4 weeks or so while you try it out. If your thyroid levels drop precipitously, it may have little or no effect and you should research other options. If your thyroid levels remain normal on the alternative, continue monitoring long term to determine whether the product might be worthwhile to stockpile.

From a dietary standpoint, you should avoid foods that depress thyroid functions. These include cauliflower, broccoli, Brussel sprouts, spinach, and cabbage.

A number of natural supplements, such as Thyromine, are commercially available. They are combinations of various herbs that are touted as beneficial for both low and high thyroid conditions. Your experience may vary.

DIABETES

Diabetes is a common, yet devastating disease. It is characterized by high sugar (also called "glucose") levels. Uncontrolled diabetes is known to cause damage to various organs, such as the kidneys, eyes, and heart. The incidence of the disease has been increasing over time in developed countries, perhaps due to issues relating to obesity.

Diabetes is especially problematic for the survival medic in that the medications used to treat the worst cases are unlikely to be produced in a grid-down scenario. Diabetic medications in liquid form, such as insulin, lose potency over time. Therefore, an alternative strategy to keep diabetics from losing complete control of their blood sugar will have to be formulated.

Type 1 Diabetes (known in the past as "juvenile diabetes" or "insulin-dependent diabetes") results from the failure of certain cells in an abdominal organ called the "pancreas". These cells function to produce insulin. **Insulin** is a hormone that controls the level of sugar in your system. It is required to move sugar (glucose) into cells; there, glucose is stored and later used to produce energy for the body. When these pancreatic cells fail, insulin production decreases greatly or stops. The leads to elevated levels of glucose in the blood, also called "**hyperglycemia**".

The destruction of the cells in the pancreas that produce Insulin is thought to be caused by an autoimmune response. This means that the body's own immune system attacks parts of itself. Type 1 diabetes is often first diagnosed in childhood, but 60% of new cases are now found in those over the age of 40.

Type 2 Diabetes (known in the past as "adult-onset" or "non-insulin dependent diabetes") is the result of resistance to the insulin produced by the pancreas. Although Insulin is produced, the cells in the body fail to respond to it. This is called "insulin resistance". Glucose fails to enter these cells and accumulates in the blood instead.

Obesity is thought to be a major factor in Type 2 diabetes. Most people are, indeed, overweight when the diagnosis is made. More and more children are being found with the condition due to the epidemic of obesity in modern societies.

Diabetes (mild or severe) may also develop in some pregnancies, even in non-diabetic women. In serious cases, insulin injections are required. Some believe that those that get diabetes during their pregnancies may be prone to diabetic issues later in life.

The three classic symptoms of diabetes are:

1) Excessive thirst
2) Excessive hunger
3) Frequent urination.

A number of physical effects ensue due to high glucose levels. Uncontrolled diabetes causes eye and kidney problems, leading to blindness and renal failure. It worsens coronary artery disease, increasing the risk for heart attacks and other cardiac issues. Weight loss may occur despite excessive hunger and the consumption of more food. This is because the body can't access the glucose in the blood for energy to produce mass.

Cuts and scrapes, especially in the extremities, are slow to heal. Over time, nerve damage occurs which causes numbness, pins and needles sensations and, in the worst cases, gangrene. Many uncontrolled diabetics require amputation later in life.

As type 2 Diabetes is most often seen in older, heavier, and less active individuals, weight control and close attention to controlling the amounts of carbohydrates (which the body turns into sugars) in the diet is important. In some cases, decreasing excess weight and frequent small meals may reverse Type 2 diabetes in its entirety. Regular exercise will also decrease blood sugar levels, and improve glucose control. The most popular oral medication used for treatment is called Metformin, which works in various ways, including increasing the cells' sensitivity to insulin. In tablet form, it is a good candidate for medical storage.

Type 1 Diabetes is more problematic, as many with this medical problem have large swings in their sugar (glucose) levels. Insulin has been used since its formulation in the 1920s to control severe diabetes. Regular monitoring of blood glucose levels and appropriate treatment with the right amount of Insulin is necessary to remain good control.

There are two common diabetic emergencies. These are related either to very low or very high glucose levels. If a diabetic, especially Type 1, fails to eat regularly or in accordance with his Insulin therapy, he or she may develop "**hypoglycemia**". Hypoglycemia can occur very rapidly; symptoms commonly seen are sweating, loss of coordination, confusion, and loss of consciousness.

In this case, a drink containing sugar will rapidly resolve the condition. Never give liquids to someone who is unconscious, however; the fluids could go down the respiratory passages and suffocation could occur. If the patient is not mentally alert, place some sugar granules under the tongue. This will absorb rapidly without causing the tendency to choke.

On the other hand, very high glucose levels lead to a condition called "**Diabetic Ketoacidosis**". This occurs as a result of missed Insulin doses and/or chronically under-dosed Insulin. Patients will have a characteristic "fruity" odor to their breath. In addition to the usual symptoms, they will note nausea, vomiting, and abdominal pain. This is a major emergency which could lead to coma and even death. Small amounts of clear liquids are acceptable in someone with this condition, but without Insulin, the prognosis is grave.

Some forms of Insulin can be purchased without a prescription in the United States. Unfortunately, like most liquid medications, it will lose potency relatively soon after its expiration date. Due to the complexity of the manufacturing process, it is unlikely to be available in a collapse situation. What, then, can be done to maximize glucose control?

Prevention is the best way to avoid hypoglycemia and/or Diabetic Ketoacidosis. In hard times, the goal will be to prevent ketoacidosis. Diabetics will be unlikely to have perfect control, especially Type 1 diabetics, but it may be possible to keep their sugars low enough to prevent a major complication. Even a few months of less than optimal control may be survivable and might give some time for society to re-stabilize.

One therapeutic option is to stockpile the highest dose of Metformin (oral diabetes medicine) in the hope that it will have some benefit to the Insulin-deprived Diabetic. It will certainly be helpful for type 2 diabetics, but will only deal with the issue of insulin resistance. Unfortunately, it will not make the pancreas produce insulin. Metformin is not Insulin, and it's uncertain what benefit it may give a pure Type 1 case. Even if it just prevents the diabetes from going completely out of control for a time, however, it's worth a shot.

A recent study suggests that Metformin may be used along with insulin. In some diabetics, the addition of Metformin resulted in lower amounts of insulin required for control. This is of interest to the survival medic who may have expiring insulin medications that may be made more effective by adding Metformin. More study is needed regarding the use of Metformin in these cases.

Another option is to regulate diet severely and subsist on a diet almost entirely comprised of protein and fats. The key is to restrict caloric intake significantly. This will be harmful in the long run, but frequent, small, high-protein meals may give your patient some time.

Type 2 diabetics (especially obese ones) may actually improve from the increased physical exertion and dietary restrictions that will be part and parcel of a long-term survival situation. An emphasis on limiting food intake to frequent small meals will be helpful here.

HIGH BLOOD PRESSURE

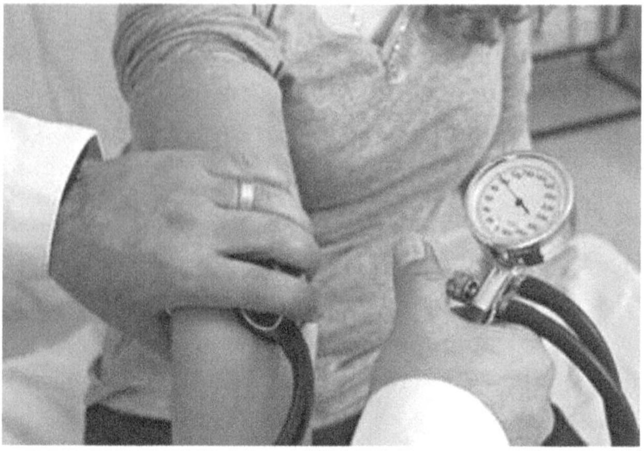

One of the most common chronic medical conditions that we will see in a collapse situation is high blood pressure (also known as "**hypertension**"). Stress associated with activities of daily survival can raise blood pressure in the short term and may worsen chronic conditions. Lack of blood pressure medications may cause complications in people who were previously under good control.

The "**blood pressure**" is the measure of the blood flow pushing against the walls of the arteries in your body. If this pressure is elevated over time, it can cause long-term damage. Many millions of adults in the U.S. have this condition, which is often **asymptomatic** (no signs or symptoms). Because of this, it has been referred to as a "silent killer". Blood pressure tends to rise with increasing age and weight.

The group medic should have, as part of his equipment, a stethoscope for listening and a pressure monitor called a "sphygmomanometer" (blood pressure cuff). This is relatively inexpensive and will allow evaluation of the blood pressures of the members of the community.

Taking A Blood Pressure

To use a sphygmomanometer, place the cuff around the upper arm and, using the attached bulb, fill it up with air until the gauge registers around 180-200. Place your stethoscope over an area with a pulse (usually the inside of the crook of the arm) and listen while looking at the gauge on the cuff. Some new compact blood pressure units are one piece and shaped like wristbands. With these, it is important to have your wrist at the level of your heart when taking a reading. The reading will appear on the screen.

When you take a blood pressure manually, you are listening for the pulse on your stethoscope. A blood pressure is measured as systolic and diastolic pressures. "**Systolic**" refers to the blood pressure when the heart beats and "**Diastolic**" refers to the blood pressure when the heart is at rest. Blood pressure readings are written as systolic over diastolic: for example: (systolic pressure) 120 over 80 (diastolic pressure). You will see it written in this manner: 120/80.

Wherever the gauge is when you *first* hear the pulse is the "systolic" pressure. As the air deflates from the sphygmomanometer, the pulse will fade away. When it fades is the "diastolic" pressure. You should be concerned with numbers that are above 140/90 while lying down or sitting.

As blood pressures tend to vary at different times of the day and under different circumstances, you would be looking for at least 3 elevated pressures in a row before making the diagnosis of hypertension. Readings above 160/100 are associated with higher frequency of complications. Persistent hypertension can lead to stroke, heart attack, heart failure, and kidney failure. Commonly seen symptoms may include:

- Headaches
- Blurred vision
- Nausea and vomiting

Sometimes, elevated pressures can cause a blood vessel in the brain to have an "accident". **Strokes** (also known as "cerebrovascular accidents" or CVAs) are bleeding episodes or clots in the brain that can occur as a high pressure event and cause damage to the nervous system. The most common initial symptom is the sudden onset of a severe headache. Suspect this condition if your patient has suddenly found themselves unable to speak, control the extremities on one side of their body, or move one side of their face.

In austere settings, you will have few options other than placing the stroke victim on bed rest and observation. Aspirin might help a stroke caused by a blood clot but could worsen a stroke caused by a hemorrhage (you'd need a CAT scan to tell the difference). Despite the damage caused by a CVA, there is often some improvement over the first 48 hours or so. Beyond this point, further recovery may be limited.

Pregnancy-induced hypertension (also called "Pre-Eclampsia") is a serious late pregnancy condition that may lead to seizures ("Eclampsia") and blood clotting abnormalities. See the section on pregnancy for more information.

The first step to controlling elevated blood pressures is to return to a normal weight for your height and age. Most people who are overweight find that their pressures decrease (often back to normal) when they lose weight. Even a loss of 10 pounds may have a beneficial effect.

Physical exercise and dietary control are the best ways to get there. Dietary restriction of sodium is paramount in importance when it comes to decreasing pressures. Excessive salt intake appears to decrease the natural elasticity of arteries. Sodium is in just about everything you eat, so stop adding salt to food. Alcohol, nicotine, and perhaps, caffeine are also known to raise blood pressures; avoiding these substances is an additional strategy. In a long-term survival situation, forced abstention may actually have a beneficial effect on overweight patients with hypertension.

The National Institute of Health recommends the **DASH** (Dietary Approaches to Stop Hypertension) diet. A major feature of the plan is limiting intake of sodium. It generally encourages the consumption of nuts, whole grains, fish, poultry, fruits and vegetables while lowering the consumption of red meats, sweets, and sugar. It's also a reasonable diet for healthy people, rich in protein, potassium, calcium, and magnesium. Studies have found that the DASH diet can reduce high blood pressure within two weeks in certain cases. These are the daily guidelines of the DASH diet:

- 7 to 8 servings of grains
- 4 to 5 servings of vegetables

- 4 to 5 servings of fruit
- 2 to 3 servings of low-fat or non-fat dairy
- 2r less servings of meat, fish, or poultry
- 2 to 3 servings of fats and oils
- 4 to 5 servings per week of nuts, seeds, and dry beans
- Less than 5 servings a week of sweets

Typical serving Sizes

-1/2 cup cooked rice or pasta
-1 slice bread
-1 cup raw vegetables or fruit
-1/2 cup cooked vegetables or fruit
-8 oz. of milk
-1 teaspoon olive oil

Optimize your results on this diet by implementing the following tips:

- Choose foods that are low in saturated and total fat, such as lean meat, poultry, and fish.
- Eat plenty of fruits and vegetables; aim for eight to ten servings each day.
- Include two to three servings of low-fat or fat-free dairy foods each day.
- Choose whole-grain foods, such as 100 percent whole-wheat or whole-grain bread, cereal, and pasta.
- Eat nuts, seeds, and dried beans -- four to five servings per week (one serving equals 1/3 cup or 1.5 ounces nuts, 2 tablespoons or 1⁄2 ounce seeds, or 1⁄2 cup cooked dried beans or peas).
- Go easy on added fats. Choose soft margarine, low-fat mayonnaise, light salad dressing, and unsaturated vegetable oils (such as olive, corn, canola, or safflower).
- Cut back on sweets and sugary beverages.

The above is good advice about nutrition in almost every circumstance, whether you are dealing with high blood pressure or not.

A number of medications with impressive names are available for the control of high blood pressure: ACE inhibitors, alpha blockers, angiotensin II receptor antagonists, beta blockers, calcium channel blockers, diuretics, and others. Those with hypertension will be placed on one or more of these medications until their readings are back to normal.

All of these drugs will be scarce in times of trouble, so consider asking for higher doses of your specific medication than what you need, so that you can break them in half and store some of it. Again, always take your medication in the dosage prescribed by your physician and realize that they might not feel comfortable with your request.

Natural supplements have been used to help lower blood pressure, as well. Any herb that has a sedative effect may also lower pressures. Valerian, Passion Flower, and Lemon Balm are some examples. Garlic and Cayenne Pepper are also well-known to have a modest lowering effect. Antioxidants like Vitamin C and fish oil may prevent free radicals from damaging artery walls. Coenzyme Q10 and Vitamin D have shown promise in some studies as well.

Don't forget natural relaxation techniques. Meditation, Yoga, and mild massage therapy will relax your patient. Take their blood pressure after a session and see what effect it has. You might be surprised at the results.

Any avenue you can find that will keep blood pressures within normal range will keep the people under your care healthier. Diet, mild natural sedatives, relaxation techniques, and conventional medications are all tools in the medical woodshed. Consider all of them with an open mind.

HEART DISEASE AND CHEST PAIN

Unlike most medical books, we will not be spending a great deal of time discussing coronary artery disease, even though it is one of the leading causes of death in today's society. Why? It will be difficult in a collapse situation to do very much about heart attacks, due to the loss of all the advances that have been made to deal with coronary disease.

The loss of the power grid would throw us back into an earlier era from a medical standpoint. There will not be a cardiac intensive care unit or a cardiac bypass surgeon at your disposal. This is a shame, as the stress associated with the aftermath of a major disaster is known to have a damaging effect on the heart. We will have to accept that some folks with heart problems will do better than others in hard times.

Heart attacks, also called "**myocardial infarctions**", involve the blockage of an artery that gives oxygen to a part of the heart muscle. That portion of the heart subsequently dies, either killing the patient or leaving them so incapacitated as to be unable to function in a post-collapse scenario. This decrease in function is most likely permanent.

Does that mean that you can't or shouldn't do anything if you suspect that your patient is having a heart attack? No, there are low tech approaches; they just won't do much if there has been a lot of damage to oxygen-starved heart muscle.

Cardio-pulmonary resuscitation (CPR) may be limited in its usefulness. It is most helpful if you have modern medical facilities at your disposal. Despite this hard reality, CPR is still compulsory for any effective medic and is described later in this book. Encourage all your group members to eat well, exercise regularly, avoid smoking, and drink alcohol only in moderation *before* a disaster occurs. It might decrease the chance that you might have to perform CPR in a survival scenario.

You would suspect a heart event if your patient experiences the following:

- "Crushing" sensation in the chest area
- Pain down the left arm
- Pain in the jaw area

- Weakness
- Fatigue
- Sweating
- Pale coloring

The main approach is to immediately give your patient a chewable adult aspirin (325 mg). This will act as a blood thinner that aids in preventing further damage to the coronary artery and preserve oxygen flow. Aspirin works within 15 minutes to prevent the formation of blood clots in people with known coronary artery disease. Studies suggest that 325 milligrams of chewable aspirin would be preferred in the setting of a heart attack or sudden onset of "**angina**" (cardiac-related chest pain). Angina occurs when not enough oxygen reaches the heart due to clogged coronary arteries.

A natural substance (Capsaicin) found in cayenne pepper may also be helpful during a myocardial infarction. The strength of peppers are based on a measurement system called Scoville heat units (H.U.). For use during a heart attack, the H.U. should be at least 90,000. Give the conscious patient a glass of warm water mixed with 1 teaspoon of cayenne pepper. An alternative is to give 2 full droppers of cayenne pepper tincture or extract underneath their tongue. Studies at the University of Cincinnati show an 85% decrease in cardiac cell death if cayenne pepper is given.

A person suffering a heart attack will feel most comfortable lying down at a 45 degree angle. Complete rest will cause the least oxygen demand on the damaged heart. Don't forget to loosen constrictive clothing; tight clothes make a cardiac patient feel anxious and cause their heart to beat faster. This would cause more strain on an already damaged organ.

Coughing forcefully and repeatedly forces blood from the chest up to the brain and may, for a short time, prevent loss of consciousness. It is, however, unlikely to make a difference in the final outcome without the availability of advanced care.

Aspirin, in small doses, is also reasonable as a *preventative* strategy. One baby aspirin (81 mg) daily is thought to help prevent the deposition of plaque inside the blood vessels. You might consider having all of your adults 40 and over on this treatment. Men are most likely to have coronary artery disease, as female hormones seem to protect women, at least until menopause. If your patient takes heart medications, administer them immediately.

Those in your survival community with coronary artery issues should stockpile whatever medications they take to deal with their symptoms. Angina (cardiac-related chest pain) can be treated with nitroglycerine tablets. Placed under the tongue, they will give rapid relief in most cases.

Cholesterol Issues

In developed countries, high cholesterol is a major cause of coronary artery disease. In an austere setting, the tests performed to follow a person's cholesterol levels will be unavailable, but you can still devise a strategy to decrease the risk of heart attack due to this problem.

Cholesterol is a fat-like substance made in the liver and other cells. It can be found in foods such as dairy products, meat, and eggs. You need some cholesterol in order to function properly, but your body makes all it needs. The presence of too much negatively impacts the heart.

There is good cholesterol (HDL) and bad cholesterol (LDL). High levels of bad cholesterol cause plaque. Plaque is a deposit that forms on the inside of arterial linings, eventually forming a blockage that can lead to a heart attack. These are the different types of cholesterol which comprise "good" and "bad":

- **Low density lipoproteins (LDL) or Very low density lipoproteins (VLDL):** LDL and VLDL can cause buildup of plaque on the walls of arteries. The more you have of these, the greater the risk of heart disease.
- **High density lipoproteins (HDL):** HDL helps the body counteract bad cholesterol in the blood. The more HDL cholesterol you have, the better. If levels of HDL are low, the chance of coronary artery disease increases.
- **Triglycerides**: Triglycerides are another type of fat that is carried in the blood by very low density lipoproteins. Sugar,

Alcohol and overly high caloric intake increase the amount of triglycerides, making your blood "fatty".

Many factors are involved in increasing "bad" cholesterol levels:

- Poor diet - Saturated fat and cholesterol in the food you eat increase cholesterol levels.
- Weight. Obesity can also increase cholesterol. Losing weight can help lower your LDL and total cholesterol levels, as well as increase HDL ("good") cholesterol.
- Inactivity: Regular exercise can lower LDL cholesterol and raise HDL cholesterol.
- Age: As we get older, cholesterol levels rise.
- Gender: Young women tend to have lower total cholesterol levels than men of similar age. After menopause, however, women's levels rise at the same rate as men's.
- Diabetes. Poorly controlled diabetes increases cholesterol. Heredity. Families may have multiple members with high cholesterol due to genetic factors.

Despite this, you can take action to improve the situation:

- Change your diet. If you have heart disease, limit daily intake of fatty foods to less than 200 milligrams. Staying away from saturated fats can make major changes in the amount of "bad" cholesterol in your system.
- Avoid Smoking. Smoking lowers HDL ("good") cholesterol levels. This trend is reversed when you quit.
- Be active. Exercise increases HDL cholesterol in some people. Daily exercise benefits weight, diabetes, and high blood pressure.
- Stockpile Medications. Make sure that your group or family members on medications for high cholesterol (called "statins" accumulate medications if at all possible.

Even if you stockpile medications, they will eventually run out in a long term survival situation. Don't despair, as various alternatives are available: Some of the herbal and nutritional supplements that may help include:

- Garlic: Garlic is an herb that has multiple beneficial effects on the body. It has been reported to decrease cholesterol levels in some people. Be aware that it may have health risks in those on blood thinners.
- Sugar Cane: Sugar cane contains policanisol, a substance that has been shown to lower cholesterol levels in several studies.
- Red Yeast Rice: Red yeast rice contains lovastatin, a substance founds in some prescription cholesterol medications. Its effect is still under study.
- Myrrh: The mukul myrrh tree contains a resin known as guggulipid. Indian studies seem to indicate that total and LDL cholesterol is lowered with regular use, although U.S. studies have failed to achieve the same results.
- Fenugreek, artichoke extract, yarrow, holy basil, ginger, turmeric, and rosemary all have been proposed as possible options to lower cholesterol.

In addition, dietary changes may be helpful. Increasing fiber, soy, omega-3 fatty acids and plant sterols may be options to help decrease "bad" cholesterol levels. Again, some of these may adversely affect those people who take blood thinners.

Other Causes Of Chest Pain

There are various other causes of chest pain. Injury to muscles and joints in the torso may mimic cardiac pain. In this type of pain, you will notice that the pain gets worse with movement of the affected area, or that you can elicit pain by pressing on it. Rest the patient and give them Ibuprofen or Acetaminophen for pain.

Acid reflux may also cause pain (usually burning in nature) in the chest area. This type of pain is usually improved with antacids in tablet form such as calcium carbonate (Tums, Rolaids, etc.) or liquid versions with magnesium hydroxide/aluminum hydroxide Maalox, Mylanta).

Relaxation techniques such as massage in a sitting position may also help. For a further discussion about acid reflux and other gastro-intestinal issues, see the next chapter.

Chest pain is also seen in some patients with anxiety issues. This is usually accompanied by tremors, a rapid heart rate, and hyperventilation.

Sedative herbs like Valerian Root, Passion Flower, and Chamomile may be helpful in this situation, as are some prescription medications such as diazepam (Valium) or alprazolam (Xanax). See the discussion of anxiety later in this book.

ULCER AND ACID REFLUX DISEASE

Ulcers

Chronic stress in survival settings can manifest itself in ways that are both emotional and physical. One of the physical effects is increased stomach acid levels. Excessive acid can cause an inflammation of the esophagus (the tube that goes from the throat to the stomach), the stomach itself and/or the next part of the bowel, called the duodenum. The irritated lining becomes weak and an erosion forms. This erosion is called an "**ulcer**" and can cause bleeding or even perforate the entire thickness of the lining.

The major symptom of an ulcer is a burning or gnawing discomfort in the stomach area and chest. This pain is often described as "**heartburn**". It usually occurs in the left or mid-upper abdomen or travels up to the breastbone. Sometimes it is described as hunger pangs or indigestion. The discomfort that goes along with this problem is hard to ignore and will decrease work efficiency. Therefore, diagnosis and treatment are important to get your group member back to normal.

There are many causes of pain in the chest and stomach areas. Chest pain caused by coronary artery disease ("**angina**") is just one of the possibilities and was discussed earlier.

To make the diagnosis of ulcer or acid reflux disease, the timing of the discomfort is important. Ulcer and acid reflux discomfort occurs soon after eating but is sometimes seen several hours after a meal. It can be differentiated from other causes of chest pain in another way: it gets better by drinking milk or taking antacids. As you can imagine, this wouldn't do much for angina.

Many ulcers are caused by a bacterium known as Helicobacter pylori. H. pylori may be transmitted from person to person through contaminated food and water, so proper water filtration and sterilization will decrease the likelihood of this infection. A commercial test exists to diagnose it. Antibiotics such as Amoxicillin and Metronidazole in combination are the most effective treatment for Helicobacter pylori ulcers you'll have off the grid.

Other causes include the use of ibuprofen or aspirin, which can be an irritant to the stomach in some people. Avoidance of these drugs may prevent these ulcers and the pain associated with them. Smoking and alcohol abuse are also known causes.

Acid Reflux Disease

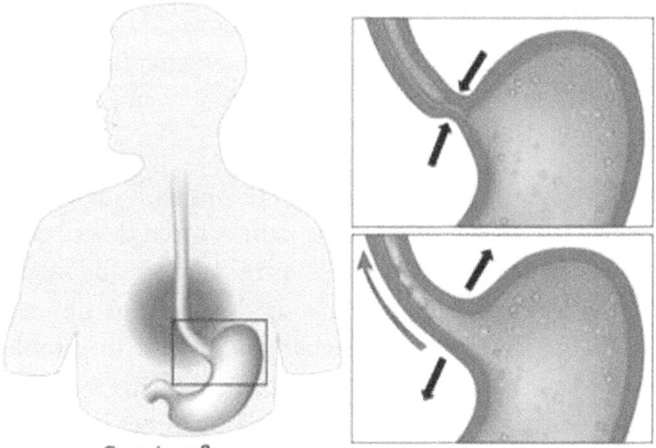

Gastric reflux

Acid reflux disease (sometimes called Gastro-Esophageal Reflux Disease or GERD) is caused by acid traveling up the esophagus. This is often related to a relaxation at the stomach-esophagus border, or by an out-pouching of the area (called a "**hiatal hernia**"). The primary symptom is heartburn, but severe disease can cause chest pain. It is usually relieved by antacids and/or by sleeping with the upper body raised.

Your patient may benefit from avoiding certain foods. These commonly include:

- Acidic fruit (for example, oranges or tomatoes)
- Fatty foods
- Coffee
- Certain teas
- Onions

- Peppermint
- Chocolate

Eating smaller meals and avoiding acidic foods is a good strategy to prevent reflux. Avoiding meals altogether for several hours before bedtime may be effective, as is sleeping with the head elevated. Obese individuals seem to suffer more from this problem, so weight loss might be helpful.

Medications that commonly relieve acid reflux include calcium, magnesium, aluminum, and bismuth antacids such as Tums, Maalox, Mylanta or Pepto-Bismol, as well as other drugs such as Ranitidine (Zantac), Cimetidine (Tagamet), and Omeprazole (Prilosec). These medications are available in non-prescription strength and are easy to accumulate in quantity.

Home remedies abound for acid reflux:

- Organic apple cider vinegar: Mix one tablespoon in four ounces of water, drink before each meal.
- Aloe Vera Juice: Mix one ounce in two ounces of water before a meal.
- Baking soda: Mix one tablespoon in a glass of water and drink right away when you begin to feel heartburn
- Glutamine: An amino acid found in milk and eggs that has an anti-inflammatory effect and reduces acid reflux.

It's important to remember to communicate with your patients. Many in the preparedness and homesteading community are rugged individualists. They may be unlikely to tell the medic about something they consider trivial, like heartburn. Anyone that is clearly in pain, losing efficiency, or unable to sleep should always be questioned about their symptoms. Offer treatment and support wherever possible.

SEIZURE DISORDERS

Seizures occur when the brain's electrical system misfires. Instead of sending out signals in a controlled manner, a surge of haphazard energy goes through the brain. These abnormal signals can cause involuntary muscle contractions, loss of bladder control, and changes in mental status. A person who has convulsions is sometimes said to have "**epilepsy**" and may be called an "epileptic". There are several types of seizures:

Seizures may involve the entire brain or just a portion. There are several types that have been identified:

- **Grand Mal seizures:** This type of seizure is what most people associate with epilepsy. Loss of consciousness, bladder control, and sometimes violent shaking and jerking. Strange sensations known as "**auras**" (smells, colors, etc.) may herald an upcoming convulsion.
- **Petit Mal seizures:** No involuntary spasms, but a temporary loss of concentration or even consciousness. Blank staring may be noticed. Auras may be noted.
- **Myoclonic seizures:** Involuntary movement of the muscles without loss of consciousness (usually).
- **Partial seizures:** Also known as "Jacksonian" seizures, these are caused by abnormal signals from one part of the brain. They may involve involuntary shaking of just one limb or specific twitching behavior. Occasionally preceded by auras. Although vision may be temporarily impaired, there may or may not be changes in mental status.

There are various causes of convulsive disorders, such as:

- High fever (in children, mostly)
- Head injury
- Meningitis (Infection of the central nervous system)
- Stroke
- Brain tumors
- Genetic predisposition

50% of seizures have no known cause. When a condition's cause is a mystery, it is referred to as "**idiopathic**".

In an austere setting, there won't be sophisticated equipment such as EEGs (electroencephalograms) and brain scans, so you will have to watch for symptoms to identify the problem. It is important to know that one seizure does not make someone an epileptic. Multiple episodes are required to be certain. In some cases (especially childhood seizures associated with fevers), a person might even "outgrow" the condition.

In addition to auras that give some warning that an attack may be imminent, there are triggers that sometimes cause a convulsion. A good example is a bright flashing light. Avoidance of these triggers will decrease the number of episodes.

The most important aspect of treatment if intravenous medication is not available will be to prevent the patient from injuring themselves during an attack. A tongue depressor with gauze taped around it and placed in the mouth was once a standard recommendation, but caused injuries to both the patient and the rescuer. Keep everything away from the patient's mouth (especially your fingers).

You shouldn't restrain the person physically, but remove nearby objects that could cause injury. An exception is if the patient is standing when the seizure starts. In this case, grab the patient and gently lower them to the floor. Placing them in the CPR "recovery" position (discussed in the CPR section of this book) will help keep their airway open and avoid aspirating vomit or other fluids down the windpipe.

Do not give oral fluids or medications to an epileptic after a seizure until they are fully awake and alert. If the convulsion is caused by a fever, as in children, cool them down with wet compresses. Anyone in your survival group with a convulsive disorder should work towards stockpiling their medicine. Popular drugs are phenytoin (Dilantin), carbamazepine (Tegretol), Valproic Acid, and Diazepam (Valium). Emphasize the importance of extra medications in cases of natural disaster or other emergencies to your family or group members.

Natural alternatives have long been claimed to decrease the frequency and severity of convulsions. Many vitamins and herbal supplements have a sedative effect, which calms the brain's electrical energy. They may be taken as a tea (1 teaspoon of the herb in a cup of water) or as a tincture (an extract with grain alcohol). Here are some that have been reported as beneficial for prevention or to decrease the frequency of episodes:

- Bacopa (*Bacopa monnieri*
- Chamomile *(Matricaria recutita)*
- Kava (*Piper methysticum*) – (too much may damage your liver)
- Valerian (*Valeriana officinalis,*
- Lemon balm (*Melissa officinalis*),
- Passionflower (*Passiflora incarnata*)
- Vitamin B12 supplements
- Vitamin E supplements

Vegetable juices may help eliminate toxins that could induce seizures. Drink a combination of carrot juice, cucumber and beet juice. Coconut oil, 3 tablespoons a day, has also been reported to decrease seizure frequency. Your experience may vary.

When a Person Collapses

Sometimes, a patient may collapse, not from a convulsion, but from simple fainting. This must be differentiated from the person who has "seized". In this circumstance, your patient won't have jerky movements as in a Grand Mal seizure or stare into space as in a petit mal seizure. A person who has had a seizure will tend to be difficult to rouse for a period of time. This is called a "**post-ictal**" **state** and will resolve on its own over time. If there has been a head injury, however, a concussion cannot be ruled out (discussed in the section on traumatic brain injury). Most people who have fainted will regain alertness relatively soon after the episode.

Dehydration, low blood sugar and various other medical conditions can cause fainting. Good hydration and appropriate dietary intake will prevent most episodes. If someone feels as if they are about to collapse, they should sit down and put their head down between their knees to increase blood flow to the brain. If you see someone who is fainting from a standing position, hold and gently lower them to the ground in a supine position. In normal times, of course, you would have someone call emergency medical services.

Evaluate the victim quickly. If someone has only fainted, they will be breathing normally and have a pulse. Raise their legs about 12 inches off the ground and above the level of their heart and head. This will help increase blood flow to the brain. Assess the patient for evidence of trauma, bleeding, or seizures. If bleeding, apply direct pressure to the wound. If the person is having a convulsion, treat as previously discussed. If no pulse or breathing, begin CPR as described later in this book.

Once you have determined that the victim is breathing, has a pulse, and is not bleeding, tap on their shoulder and ask in a clear voice "Can you hear me?" or "Are you OK?". Loosen any obviously constricting clothing and make sure that they are getting lots of fresh air by keeping the area around them clear of crowds. If you are in an area that is hot, fan the patient or carefully carry them to a cooler area.

If you are successful in arousing the patient, ask them if they have any pre-existing medical conditions such as diabetes, heart disease or epilepsy. Stay calm and speak in a reassuring manner. Don't let them get up for a period of time, even if they say that they are fine. People oftentimes are embarrassed and want to brush off the incident, but they are still at risk for another fall.

Once the victim is awake and alert (Do they know their name? Do they know where they are? What year it is?), you may slowly have the patient sit up if they are not otherwise injured. If you are not in an austere setting, emergency medical personnel are on the way; wait until they arrive before having the patient stand up. In a survival situation, however, you will have to make a judgment as to whether and when the victim is capable to return to normal activities.

Common causes of fainting include dehydration and low blood sugar, so some oral intake may be helpful. This is appropriate only if it is clear that they are completely conscious, alert, and able to function. Test their strength by having them raise their knees against the pressure of your hands. If they are weak, they should continue to rest. Close monitoring of the patient will be very important, as some internal injuries may not manifest for hours.

JOINT DISEASE

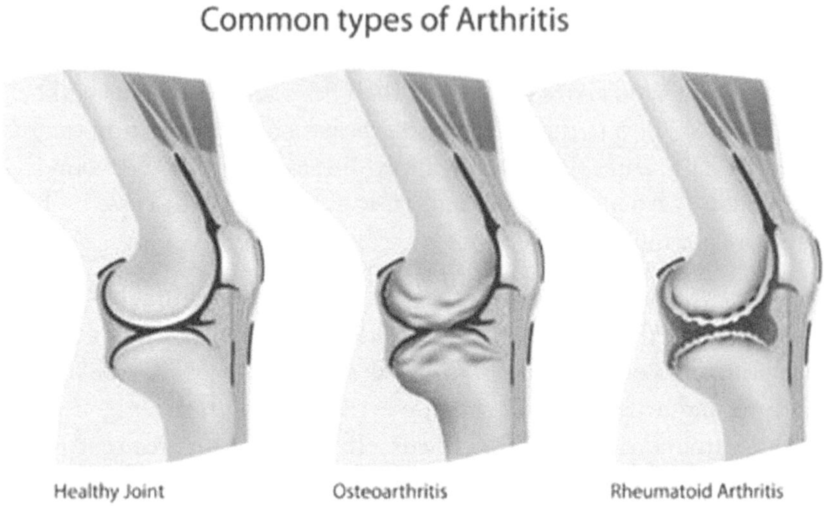

Over the course of time, the moving parts of humans suffer wear and tear just like the moving parts of any machine. Damage to ankles, knees, hips, and even the spine occurs chronically over the course of years. We can expect an acceleration of this process when demands on our body increase in times of trouble.

Degenerative damage to joints is called "**osteoarthritis**". Many advances in degenerative disease, such as hip replacements, won't be options off the grid. We will not have curative remedies, but we can still improve the quality of life of the patient.

Besides degenerative changes, inflammation of the joints (also known as "**arthritis**") can also be caused by **auto-immune** conditions. Antibodies are formed by the body that attack its own joints and sometimes cause striking deformities. Certain bacterial infections, some of which are sexually transmitted, also can significantly damage joint tissue. The cause must be identified and treated quickly.

Regardless of why the arthritis in the joint occurred, the signs and symptoms are frequently similar. You will see:

- Pain
- Swelling
- Joint stiffness and decreased range of motion
- Reluctance to use the affected joint
- Fluid accumulation in the joint space
- Muscle weakness (with chronic arthritis)
- Fever (if caused by an infection)

Types Of Arthritis

Osteoarthritis

Osteoarthritis is the most common form of arthritis, especially in older individuals. It can affect just about any joint in the body. Hands, feet, back, hip, and knees are most commonly affected, but osteoarthritis can occur even in the spinal column.

The disease is acquired by daily wear and tear on the joints, although it can also be a long term effect of a previous injury. Many athletes, for example, may develop arthritis in this manner at a relatively young age. Obesity causes increased stress on joints as well and leads to osteoarthritis.

Warm compresses are useful to treat discomfort and stiffness. Non-steroidal anti-inflammatory drugs (NSAIDs) like ibuprofen or aspirin are helpful, as is Capsaicin cream or ointment. The worst cases may require oral or injectable steroids. These, however, are unlikely to be available in austere settings. Sometimes, a needle is placed to drain excess fluid from an affected joint to give relief. This is call "**arthrocentesis**". This procedure may decrease pain, but could introduce infection into the joint if not performed with care.

Rheumatoid Arthritis

Rheumatoid arthritis is the most common auto-immune disease in the world today. It is a disorder in which the body's immune system attacks its own tissues. The attack is not only directed at the joint but to other parts of the body. Unlike some joint diseases, rheumatoid arthritis tends to affect the same joint on both sides of the body. Women are more susceptible than men.

Rheumatoid arthritis especially affects joints in the fingers and wrists, but is also common in knees and elbows. Over time, it can lead to severe deformities if not treated. Rheumatoid arthritis occurs in younger populations than osteoarthritis, even striking children on occasion.

Other symptoms associated with rheumatoid arthritis that you might not see with degenerative osteoarthritis:

- Dry mouth
- Dryness, itching, or burning in the eyes
- Insomnia
- Strange sensations in the hands or feet
- Nodules under the skin
- Chest pain when taking a breath

There is no cure for rheumatoid arthritis. Treatments concentrate on easing the symptoms. Medical therapy includes strong anti-inflammatory medications such as oral steroids (example: Prednisone).

Another auto-immune disorder that can cause joint disease is known as Systemic Lupus Erythematosus (SLE). Although usually diagnosed by blood testing, Lupus can be differentiated from rheumatoid arthritis due to its one-sided nature. You will also see patients with SLE experience hair loss and body rashes. Lupus is often treated with long-term oral steroids.

Even though rheumatoid arthritis cannot be cured, you can prevent the condition from worsening. Weight loss is one way to improve symptoms and prevent progression. Physical therapy to strengthen muscles that support joints is thought to be helpful.

Bacterial Arthritis

Bacterial arthritis (sometimes called "septic" arthritis) is often the result of some penetrating injury that allows organisms to invade the joint space. It can also occur from within, as when a blood infection (**septicemia**) or bone infection (**osteomyelitis**) has spread to a joint. Common skin bacteria, such as Streptococcus and Staphylococcus, are the usual suspects but gonorrhea, a sexually transmitted disease, can also be the cause.

Typical symptoms of a bacterial arthritis are the same as osteoarthritis, except that the patient may have a fever and may exhibit redness or warmth over the affected joint. In addition to standard treatment, antibiotics will be helpful.

Gout

Gout is another condition that destroys joints over time. Inflammation is caused by deposits of uric acid crystals in the joint. Some people simply produce too much uric acid or don't eliminate it well. Obesity is a major risk factor, as is diabetes. This illness occurs primarily in men; a history of certain types of kidney stones may be associated with gout.

The presentation of gout will appear as:

- Inflammation in one or two joints. The big toe is the classic example, but knees and ankles may also be affected.
- Warm, red, painful joints. The pain is throbbing and often severe. Even laying a sheet over it may cause pain.
- Fever.
- Episodic repeat attacks (50% of cases).

After multiple episodes, permanent damage occurs and the joint loses its range of motion. Chronic sufferers may also develop lumps composed of uric acid crystals called "**tophi**" below the skin. These occur around joints and may drain chalky material from time to time.

Specialized prescription drugs are available for gout, such as Colchicine and Allopurinol. If you have a family member with gout, encourage them to stockpile extra medications; they won't be found in your standard medic's storage.

Lifestyle and dietary changes may be helpful:

- Avoid alcohol.
- Reduce how many uric acid elevating foods you eat. These include: Liver, red meat, herring, sardines, anchovies, kidney, beans, peas, mushrooms, asparagus, and cauliflower. .
- Avoid fatty foods.
- Eat enough carbohydrates.

Natural Therapy For Joint Disease

From an alternative standpoint, there are several treatments for joint pain caused by arthritis. Various glucosamine supplements are popular; glucosamine sulfate preparations have more evidence for their effectiveness than glucosamine hydrochloride. Take 1,500 milligrams once a day on a regular basis.

Glucosamine is often paired with chondroitin sulfate. 800-1,200 milligrams a day has been shown to possibly slow progression of some arthritic conditions.

Two teaspoons of lemon juice or apple cider vinegar mixed with a teaspoon of honey twice a day is a time-honored treatment. Other oral supplements reported to be effective against joint pain are:

- Turmeric powder
- Soybean Oil
- Avocado Oil
- Rose hips
- Fish Oil
- Bathua leaf juice
- Alfalfa tea

For external use:

- Use Arnica essential oil on affected areas (good for muscle aches as well).
- Apply warm vinegar to aching joints.
- Mix powdered sandalwood into a paste; it has a cooling effect when rubbed on a joint.
- Make an ointment from 2 parts olive oil and 1 part turpentine.

Acupuncture, massage therapy, and physical therapy may alleviate muscle spasms associated with arthritis. Electricity delivered by a device known as a TENS (Transcutaneous Electrical Nerve Stimulation) unit may be helpful.

KIDNEY AND GALL BLADDER STONES

The kidney and gall bladder are two organs that have the propensity in some people to develop an accumulation of crystals. These crystals form masses known as "stones". Some are large and some are as small as grains of sand, but any size can cause pain (sometimes excruciating). These issues can put group members out of commission at a time when they are most needed.

Kidney Stones

MALE

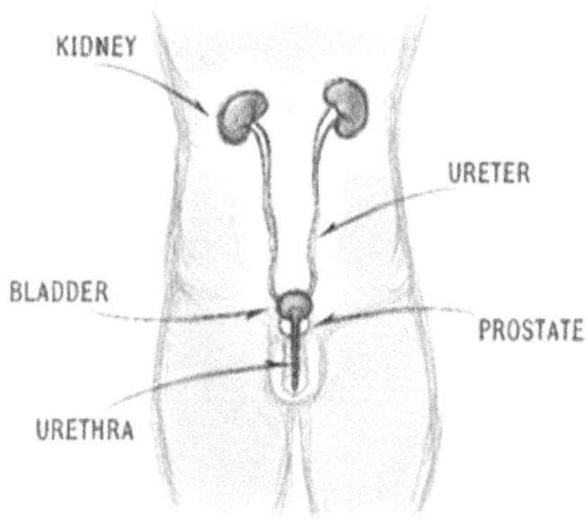

URINARY SYSTEM

Kidney stones are most commonly seen in those persons who fail to keep themselves well hydrated. Even small stones can lead to significant pain (known as "**renal colic**"), and the larger ones can cause blockages that can disrupt the function of the organ. Once you have had a kidney stone, it is likely you will get them again at one point or another. Most kidney stones are not associated with infections.

Once formed in the kidney, stones usually do not cause symptoms until they begin to move down the tubes which connect the kidneys to the bladder (the "**ureters**"). When this happens, the stones can block the flow of urine. This causes swelling of the kidney affected as well as significant pain. Kidney stones as small as grains of sand may reach the bladder without incident and then cause pain as they attempt to pass through the tube that goes from the bladder to the outside (the "**urethra**").

There are several different types of kidney stones:

- **Calcium stones:** Calcium combines with other substances, such as oxalate, phosphate, or carbonate to form a stone. The most common, they occur more often in men than in women, usually in those 20 to 40 years old.
- **Cysteine stones:** These form in people who have "cysteinuria", a condition that tends to run in families.
- **Struvite stones:** This variety is mostly found in women and can grow quite large; they can cause blockages at any point in the urinary tract. Frequent and chronic infections are a risk factor.
- **Uric acid stones:** More common in men than in women, these stones are associated with conditions such as gout (previously discussed

To diagnose a kidney stone, look for pain that starts suddenly and comes and goes. Pain is commonly felt on the side of the back (the "flank"). Lightly pounding on the right and left flank at the level of the lowest rib will cause significant pain in patients with kidney stones or kidney infections. As the stone moves, so will the pain; it will travel down the abdomen and could settle in the groin or even the urethral area.

Other symptoms of renal stones can include:

- Bloody urine
- Fever and chills
- Nausea and vomiting

Some dietary changes may prevent the formation of kidney stones, especially if they are made of calcium. Avoid foods such as:

- Spinach
- Rhubarb

- Beets,
- Parsley
- Sorrel
- Chocolate

Also, decreasing dairy intake will restrict the amount of calcium available for stone formation. This will keep them as small as possible and, therefore, easier to pass.

Your treatment goal is to assist the stone to pass through the system quickly. Have your patient drink at least 8 glasses of water per day to produce a large amount of urine. The flow will help move the stone along.

Some have used diuretic medications or cranberry juice for the same purpose. Pain relievers can help control the pain of passing the stones (renal colic). Ibuprofen will be the most available treatment of choice for pain relief. Stronger pain medications, if you can get them, may be necessary for severe cases.

Some of the larger stones will be chronic issues, as the high technology and surgical options used to remove these will not be available in a survival scenario. Medications specific to the type of stone may be helpful:

- Allopurinol (prescription medicine for uric acid stones and gout).
- Antibiotics (for struvite stones).
- Sodium bicarbonate or sodium citrate (which increases the alkalinity of the urine). These drugs decrease the likelihood of formation of uric acid stones.

A good home remedy to relieve discomfort and aid passage of the stone is lemon juice, olive oil, and apple cider vinegar. With the first twinge of pain, drink a mixture of 2 ounces of lemon juice and 2 ounces of olive oil. Then, drink a large glass of water. After 1 hour, drink a mixture of 1 tablespoon of raw apple cider vinegar with 2 ounces of lemon juice in a large glass of water. Repeat this process every 1 to 2 hours until improved.

Other natural substances that may help are:

- Horsetail tea (a natural diuretic)
- Pomegranate juice
- Dandelion root tea
- Celery tea
- Basil tea

Gall Bladder Stones

GALLSTONES

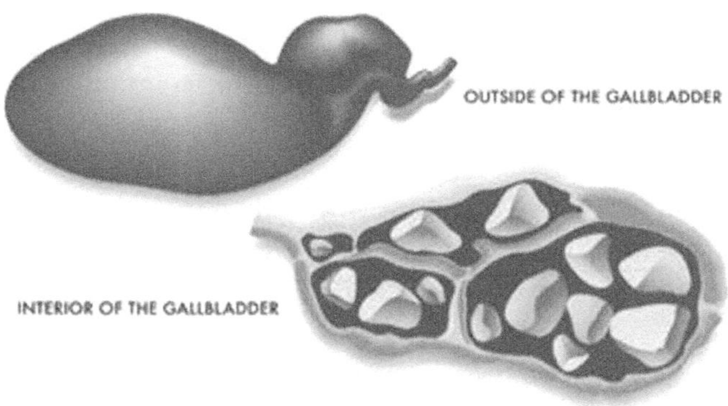

The gall bladder is a sac-like organ that is attached to the liver; it stores the bile that the liver secretes. **Gallstones** are firm deposits that form inside the gallbladder and could block the passage of bile. This blockage can cause a great deal of pain and inflammation (known as "**cholecystitis**").

There are two main types of gallstones:

1) **Cholesterol stones:** The grand majority, these are not related to the actual cholesterol levels in the bloodstream.
2) **Bilirubin stones:** These occur in those people who have illnesses that destroy their red blood cells. The by-products of this destruction releases a substance called "bilirubin" into the bile and forms a stone.

Risk factors for this condition can be described as the 4 "F's":

- **Fat:** The majority of those with gallstones are overweight.
- **Female:** The majority of sufferers are women.
- **Forty:** Most sufferers are over 40 years old.
- **Fertile:** Most women with gallstones have had children.

Additional risk factors include diabetes, liver cirrhosis (discussed in the section on hepatitis), and low blood counts ("**anemia**").

Luckily, most people with this problem don't have any symptoms. If a large stone causes a blockage, however, you may experience what is called "**biliary colic**". Symptoms of biliary colic include:

- Cramping right upper abdomen pain (constant, spreading to the back).
- Fever.
- Jaundice (yellowing of the skin and whites of the eyes).
- Discolored bowel movements (gray or grayish-white).
- Nausea and vomiting.

The classical finding on physical examination is "**Murphy's Sign**". Press with one hand just below the midline of the lowest rib on the front right. Then, ask your patient to breathe deeply. If the gallbladder is tender, the patient should complain of significant pain at the site.

Unfortunately, the main treatment for gallstones is to surgically remove the gall bladder (you can live without it and stay healthy). As surgical suites are unlikely to be available in a collapse, you might consider some alternative remedies. These are mostly preventative measures:

- Apple cider vinegar (mixed with apple juice)
- Chanca Piedra, (Phyllanthus niruri), a plant that is native to the Amazon; translated, the name means "Break Stones".
- Peppermint
- Turmeric
- Alfalfa

- Ginger root
- Dandelion root
- Artichoke leaves
- Beet, Carrot, Grape, Lemon juices

Sadly, it is very difficult to eliminate most of the risk factors for gall bladder disease. If you're forty, female, and have children, there is not much you can do about it. You may be able to do something about being fat, however. Dietary changes to decrease intake of fatty foods may help you decrease weight and the risk of gallstones.

DERMATITIS (SKIN RASHES)

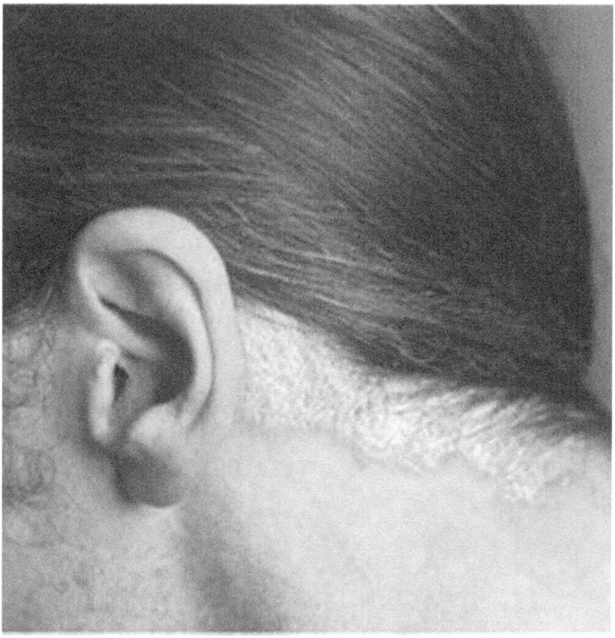

Seborrheic Dermatitis

In austere circumstances, a caregiver may consider a skin rash to be of no consequence. Symptoms associated with it, however, may cause sleep loss or irritation that make affect a group member's work efficiency. Therefore, it makes common sense to treat any condition that decreases the quality of life of a family or group member.

Dermatitis simply means inflammation of the skin. This condition has many causes and may vary in appearance from case to case. Most types of dermatitis present with swollen, flaky, reddened, and/or itchy skin. Continuous scratching traumatizes the irritated area and may lead to infections such as cellulitis once the skin is broken.

Some of the more common types of skin inflammation are:

- **Contact dermatitis:** Caused by allergens and chemical irritants. A good example would be poison ivy.

- **Seborrheic dermatitis**: A commonly seen condition that affects the face and scalp (for example, dandruff).
- **Atopic Dermatitis or Eczema:** A chronic itchy rash that can be found in various areas at once and tends to be intermittent in nature. This may be accompanied by hay fever or asthma.
- **Neuro-dermatitis:** A chronic itchy skin condition localized to certain areas of the skin (as seen in a herpes virus infection known as "Shingles").
- **Stasis dermatitis:** An inflamed area caused by fluid under the skin; commonly seen on the lower legs of older individuals. Poor circulation is a major factor.

Many of the above conditions may appear similar to the non-medical person. Indeed, some cannot be conclusively diagnosed without sending a sample of skin to a laboratory. Whatever the cause, effective treatment of symptoms will be important in a grid-down situation. Limiting trauma from repeated scratching will prevent infections at the site.

Moisturizing dry skin with lotions may be one way to help decrease frequency of outbreaks of dermatitis. Bathing is a healthy habit; it may, however, dry out your skin. You can prevent this by:

- Using mild soaps: Deodorant soaps are to be avoided in patient with significant dermatitis.
- Moisturizing: Apply any of a myriad of oils or creams to the skin while wet. This will seal in the moisture.
- Dry gently: Pat rather than rub dry with a towel.
- Bathe less: Sure enough, limiting the frequency and duration of baths may decrease symptoms.

Of all the types of skin conditions, you will most likely see contact dermatitis in a survival situation, as your people will be exposed to various substances while scavenging that may cause reactions. In good times or bad, some of these include:

- Soaps and detergents.
- Cleaning products.

- Rubber or latex.
- Metals, such as nickel.
- Plants such as poison ivy, oak or sumac.

Once you're sensitized to an allergen, future exposures may cause skin reactions. Your patient will probably experience these reactions for the rest of his or her life. Stress, sweating, temperature changes, and rough bedding or clothing may worsen the condition.

Avoidance of irritants is the cornerstone of prevention. Corticosteroid creams and cool moist compresses are a good start for treatment purposes. Use these only until the rash is improved. Antihistamines such as diphenhydramine (Benadryl) will help relieve itching. Of course, if the dermatitis was caused by contact with a specific irritant, avoid it if at all possible.

Scalp irritations caused by Seborrhea may be treated by shampoos that contain tar, pyrithione zinc, or ketoconazole. Scaly areas may be treated with mineral or olive oil if nothing else is available.

Stasis dermatitis may be improved by wearing support hose or, perhaps, elastic wraps. Pay careful attention to infections that may be developing underneath. Wet dressings may help to soften rough areas.

Neurodermatitis caused by Shingles may be treated with prescription anti-viral agents, such as Acyclovir, Famciclovir or Valacyclovir (Zovirax, Valtrex, or Famvir, respectively).

In addition to hydrocortisone cream and wet compresses, some creams that suppress local immune response such as Pimecrolimus (Elidel) may improve atopic dermatitis.

Some favor the use of light therapy. This involves exposing affected skin to controlled amounts of natural or artificial light. It may be effective in preventing recurrences of atopic dermatitis.

Other natural supplements that improve dermatitis often involve Omega-3 fatty acids, which have an anti-inflammatory effect. Used with evening primrose oil, they are thought to be especially effective. Chamomile cream is considered by some to be as potent as a mild hydrocortisone. Calendula has skin-soothing properties and may protect against contact dermatitis. Be aware, however, that it may trigger an allergic reaction on broken skin.

VARICOSE VEINS

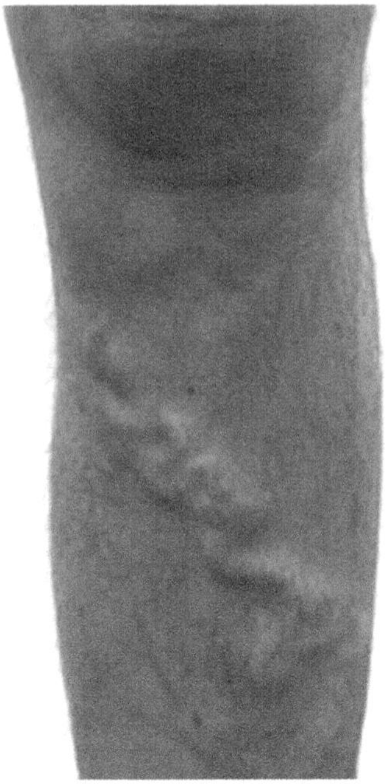

Varicose veins are enlarged blood vessels, usually in the legs, which have lost tone in the valves that control blood flow. This swelling of the vascular structures occurs in about 15% of the population, and becomes more common with age (50% over age 50). Women are several times more likely to have this problem than men.

Varicosities are gravity dependent; they may be more common in people whose occupation requires constant standing. In a power-down setting, we will be spending more time on our feet by necessity. Therefore, we must plan to prevent, if possible, and treat varicose veins before they become serious.

Varicose veins are similar to but not the same as "**spider veins**". Spider veins are formed from tiny vessels called "capillaries" that exist everywhere in your body. When they become varicose, they appear like little red or blue spider webs; you may find them on your legs, face, or just about anywhere. People with fair complexions seem to get more of them, especially if they spend a lot of time in the sun.

Classically, varicose veins are larger, blue, swollen, and stick out from the skin. They tend to look twisted or contorted. Varicosities cause the circulation to become less efficient. This causes pain and fatigue in the legs, and could lead to an inflammation known as "**phlebitis**".

You're more likely to get varicose veins if you:

- Are 50 years of age or older. The valves in your veins weaken as you age.
- Have a family history. If your mother had varicose veins, you are likely to get them as well.
- Are a woman. High levels of estrogen as seen during puberty, pregnancy, and while taking birth control pills increase your risk.
- Are obese. Extra weight puts pressure on the veins and causes them to swell.
- Work in a profession that requires long periods of standing, lifting weights, or sitting with legs bent.

Besides the discomfort and an unpleasing cosmetic appearance, varicose veins are usually not dangerous. Occasionally, however, you might see one of these complications:

Thrombophlebitis: a varicose vein on the surface of the skin can become inflamed; this is due to a blood clot which formed due to the poor circulation in the area. Symptoms include:

- Painful swelling
- Warmth to the touch
- Redness (sometimes along the line of the vein).
- Tender, hard nodules
- Itching
- Fever

Basic treatment involves moist warm compresses and anti-inflammatory medicine for discomfort and fever. Elevation of the affected extremity may be useful. Elastic support hose is helpful while performing activities of daily living. Although most cases of thrombophlebitis are not due to infection, antibiotics are occasionally needed. Cephalexin

(Keflex) is known to have activity against Staphylococcus, the most common bacterial cause.

As an aside, hemorrhoids are a type of superficial thrombophlebitis. They are discussed in the next chapter.

Deep vein thrombosis (DVT): A blood clot that forms in a deep vein. The patient will experience a "full" or "firm" feeling, usually in the calf area. This will be accompanied by pain, heat, swelling, and redness as in superficial thrombophlebitis.

While many people may present with no symptoms at all, a DVT can be dangerous if the blood clot dislodges and makes it way to the lungs or other vital organs. Indeed, shortness of breath may be the only symptom noticed. This is referred to a "**pulmonary embolism**" and is possibly life-threatening. Other signs and symptoms may include breathlessness, chest pain, a fast heart rate, panting, and/or bloody phlegm.

In addition to compresses and pain relief, patients with deep vein thrombosis may require blood thinners; Salicin from the under bark of willows, poplars, and aspens is a natural alternative if the pharmaceuticals have run out. The amount given using this method will, however, always be uncertain. Each tree may have variable amounts of Salicin. Do not attempt this treatment on someone on anticoagulant medications such as Coumadin.

If your patient has varicose veins, have them stock up on compression stockings or support pantyhose. If the resources are there to deal with this issue in normal times, consider doing so. Surgical removal is indicated in some cases. Encourage your patients at risk to:

- Exercise their legs to improve tone; this will provide support to the blood vessels.
- Avoid standing for long periods of time. Shift their weight from foot to foot often and take a short walk if they sit all day.
- Keep their weight down to avoid putting strain on their legs.
- Elevate their legs above the level of the heart for a half hour daily, and during sleep.
- Wear support stockings.

- Avoid wearing high heels for long periods (probably not an issue in the aftermath of a disaster).
- Eat a low-salt diet. Less salt consumption can help with the swelling that you see with varicose veins.
- Prevent spider veins by wearing sunscreen; this will help people with fair complexions.

The herbal remedy most quoted to treat varicose veins is the horse chestnut (Aesculus hippocastanum. Horse chestnuts contain a substance called aescin, which appears to block enzymes that damage capillary walls. Take 300 mg of horse chestnut seed extract (usually contains 50 mg of aescin) by mouth twice daily. For external use only, rub a mixture of 4 parts witch hazel with 1 part tincture of horse chestnut and rub on affected varicosities. Not for those with liver or kidney disease. Horse chestnut can be fatal if eaten raw.

HEMORRHOIDS

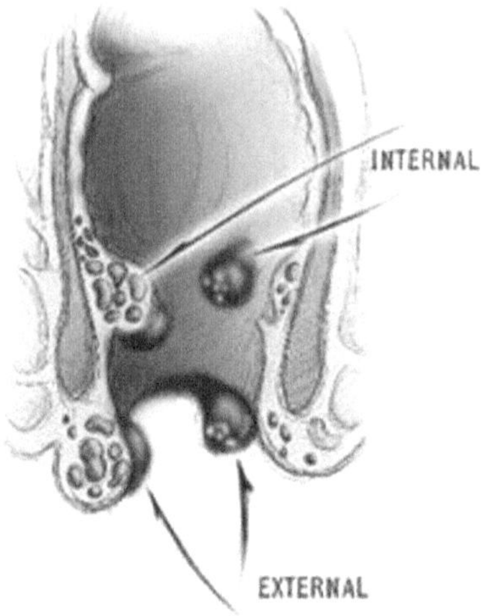

HEMORRHOIDS

Hemorrhoids are painful, swollen veins in the lower portion of the rectum that often protrude from the anus. They are thought to be caused from pressure due to the fact that humans stand on two legs; animals that walk on four legs rarely get them. Another likely cause is a low fiber diet causing excessively hard stool. This causes straining during bowel movements which may increase the risk of hemorrhoids.

Hemorrhoids are extremely common during pregnancy and are usually asymptomatic unless they develop a clot (a "**thrombosis**") and become inflamed. Once they become thrombosed, they cause a constant pain that will make it difficult to carry out activities of daily survival (or even sit down).

Hemorrhoids may be internal or external. Symptoms of hemorrhoids include:

- Anal itching.
- Bleeding, usually seen on toilet tissue.
- Pain, worse in the sitting position.

- Pain during bowel movements
- Painful bumps near the anus.

Diagnosis is easily made simply by looking at the area. They will appear as a bluish lump at the edge of the anal opening. Some hemorrhoids develop inside the anal canal, and may be difficult to spot. A rectal exam with a gloved finger will make the diagnosis in this case.

Hemorrhoids only require treatment when symptomatic. Treatments for hemorrhoids include:

- Mild corticosteroid creams such as Anusol-HC or wipes such as Tucks pads to help reduce pain and swelling
- Stool softeners to decrease further trauma to the inflamed tissue.
- Witch Hazel compresses to reduce itching.
- Warm water baths (known as "Sitz baths") to reduce general discomfort.

Even painful hemorrhoids will usually go away by themselves over a few weeks, but sometimes the discomfort is so severe that you may be required to remove the clot from the swollen vein. This is performed by incising the skin over the hemorrhoid and draining the clotted blood.

A #11 or #15 scalpel may be used (preferably under local anesthesia) to incise the hemorrhoid after cleaning the area thoroughly with Betadine. Cut just deep enough to evacuate the clot. The patient should experience quick relief as a result Gauze pads should be placed at the site to absorb any bleeding. Be prepared to suture the incision site if the bleeding is heavy.

It should be noted that this procedure is not the best way to remove a hemorrhoid, as simple incision does not remove it in its entirety. It may come back at a later time. Modern procedures, such as placing bands around the hemorrhoid, are less traumatic and more permanent in their results, but will not be an option off the grid.

SECTION 8

✚ ✚ ✚

OTHER IMPORTANT MEDICAL ISSUES

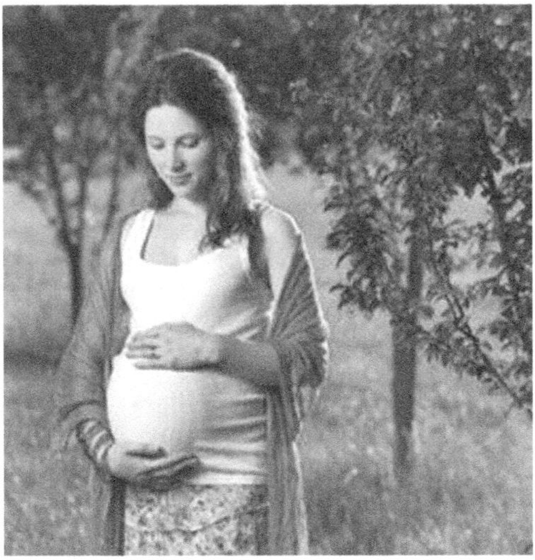

CPR IN AN AUSTERE SETTING

Most medical books start off with a chapter on CPR (**Cardio-Pulmonary Resuscitation**), so you might wonder why this subject has not been given significant coverage so far in this book. The answer is based on hard realities that we must confront in a survival scenario.

Although CPR is an important skill that everyone should know, there are fewer situations in a collapse scenario where CPR will return a victim to normal function. There are only a small number of circumstances where a patient goes from being a patient in need of resuscitation to a person who is back to normal.

CPR is best used as a stabilization strategy. You want to get the heart pumping and breathing supported so that you can get your patient as quickly as possible to a facility where there are ventilators, defibrillators, and other high technology. But what about a situation where this technology is no longer available?

There won't be cardiac bypasses for your patient who has had a heart attack. There won't be surgical suites for your patient with a shotgun blast to the abdomen or chest. The sobering truth is that many of these injuries will be "**mortal**". This means that death is the inevitable end result, no matter what you try to do. The poor prognosis for these people in hard times is tragic; it makes you truly appreciate the benefits of modern medicine.

There are still instances, however, where CPR may actually restore a gravely ill person to normal function. Airway obstruction with a foreign object can be dealt with by using the Heimlich maneuver. Environmental conditions such as hypothermia, heat stroke, or smoke inhalation will often respond to resuscitative efforts with complete recovery. Anaphylactic reactions may require CPR until the patient responds to Epinephrine and resolves the attack. Rarer events such as lightning strikes or near-drowning may require resuscitation to revive the victim.

We chose not to put a large number of illustrations or write an entire course on how to do CPR in this book. There is no substitution for learning it in person by taking a hands-on course. We don't want you to think that you shouldn't take a course just because you read this book. Your responsibility as medic is to get training; this is mandatory for anyone that expects to be a caregiver in a long-term survival scenario.

Airway Obstruction

One situation where you can save a life by knowing how to perform a simple maneuver is in the case of an airway obstruction. This most commonly occurs as a result of a bite of food lodging in the back of the throat and cutting off respiration. This is a relatively common way to die, even in modern times, and it really shouldn't be.

If you see a conscious adult in sudden respiratory distress, ask quickly: Are you choking? If they can answer you, there is still air passing into their lungs. If it's a complete blockage, they will be unable to speak. They'll probably be agitated and holding their throat, but they will hear you and (frantically) nod their head "yes". This is your signal to take action.

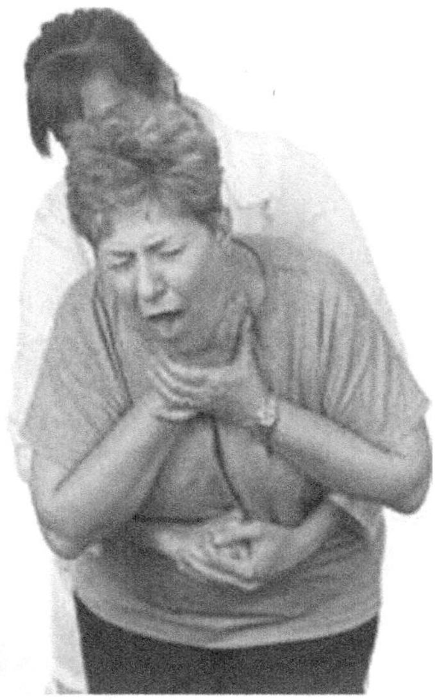

Heimlich Maneuver

Tell the victim that you're there to help them and immediately get into position for the **Heimlich maneuver**, otherwise known as an "abdominal thrust" (see figure above). Get behind the victim and make a fist with your right hand. Place your right fist above the belly button; then, wrap your left arm around the patient and grasp the fist. Make sure your arms are positioned just below the ribcage. With a forceful upward motion, press your fist abruptly into the abdomen. You might have to do this multiple times before you dislodge the foreign body.

If you are unable to dislodge the obstructive item, your patient will eventually lose consciousness due to lack of air. Place the patient in a supine position and straddle them across the thighs or hips. Open their mouth and make sure that the object can't be removed manually. Give several upward abdominal thrusts with the heels of your palms above the belly button (one hand on top of the other). Check again; you might have partially dislodged the offending morsel.

In old movies, you might see someone slap the victim hard on the back; this is unlikely to dislodge a foreign object and will waste precious time. An exception to this is in an infant: place the baby over your forearm (facing down) and apply several blows with the heel of your hand to the upper back.

Tracheotomy

An extreme method that can be used to open an airway is called "**tracheotomy**". This procedure, also called a cricothyroidotomy, involves cutting an opening in the windpipe below the level of an obstruction. Tracheotomy should be performed only when an airway obstruction completely prevents the ability to breathe after multiple Heimlich maneuvers have been attempted unsuccessfully.

To perform a tracheotomy, you will need a sharp blade and some sort of tube, such as a straw. Of course, a good first aid kit would be very helpful. Don't worry about antiseptics for now; you are performing this procedure because someone may die in the next few minutes.

The procedure goes as follows:

- Start at the Adam's apple, also called the thyroid cartilage. Move about 1 inch down the neck until you feel a bulge. This is the cricoid cartilage.
- Make a horizontal incision with your knife or a razor blade in the crease between the Adam's apple and the cricoid cartilage. This incision can be an inch or so long.
- Incise downward a half-inch deep or so. There shouldn't be a lot of blood.
- Below the incision, you'll see the yellow-gray crico-thyroid membrane. Make an incision through it; this should allow passage of air into the lungs. Be careful not to cut too deeply.
- Place something hollow in the opening, to maintain a clear airway. A straw would do in a pinch. Try to get it a couple of inches down the windpipe; doing this makes it less likely to fall out.
- If the patient fails to breathe on their own, you may need to perform CPR, including rescue breaths through the tube you inserted.

Notice that we didn't tell you to "prep" the area with Betadine or other antiseptic. Although not a bad idea, you just don't have the time. we don't have to tell you that this is a dangerous procedure. A lot can go wrong, but the patient is dying and it may be your last resort. Only consider it when help is not on the way, and you have tried every other option first.

CPR In The Unconscious Patient

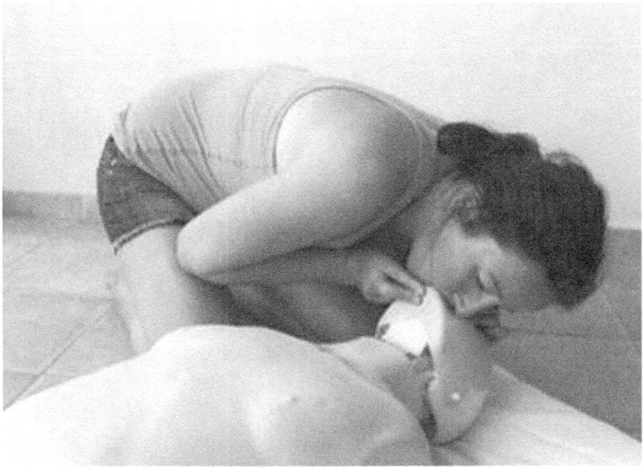

Rescue Breath (only if CPR-trained)

If you come across someone who is apparently unconscious, be certain to first verify their mental status. Simply ask them loudly: "Are you OK?" No answer? Grasp the person's shoulders and move them gently while continuing to ask them questions. If they are still unresponsive (which you should be able to determine in seconds), check their pulse and respirations. If they aren't breathing or no pulse is felt, it's time to start resuscitative efforts. Place your patient in a position so that they are lying flat on their back.

You will begin chest compressions by placing the heel of your hand in the middle of the chest; Place it, palm down, over the lower half of the breastbone at the level of the nipple. Place your other hand on top and interlace your fingers. Keeping yourself positioned directly above your hands (arms straight), press downward in such a fashion that the breastbone (also called the "sternum") is compressed about 2 inches. Allow the chest to recoil completely and then perform 30 compressions, at a rate of at least 100 compressions per minute.

This works well for adults but you would want less pressure in a child. Be certain to avoid the rib cage, as broken ribs are a common complication of the procedure.

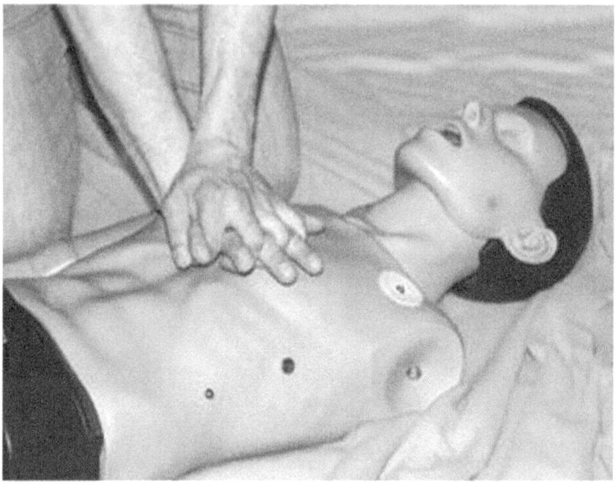

Chest Compressions

After 30 chest compressions, evaluate the victim for breathing and clear the airway. Look quickly inside the mouth for a foreign object. If there is none, place the patient's head in a position that will allow the clearest passage for air to enter the body. This is called the "**Chin-Lift**". Tilt the head back (unless there is evidence of a neck injury) and grasp the underside of the chin and lower jaw with one hand and lift. Using this method, the tongue and other throat structures are placed in a position that helps the patient take in air. A useful medical item is a plastic "airway". There are both rigid oral and flexible nasal versions that help keep the airway open.

If you aren't trained in CPR, just continue compressions. If you *do* know CPR, you may give 2 long breaths mouth-to-mouth (3 seconds between each one). These are called "rescue breaths". Pinch the nose closed to prevent the escape of air that needs to get into the lungs.

You can determine the effectiveness of your efforts by watching the patient's chest rise as you give the breaths. Continue giving 30 compressions, then 2 rescue breaths for 5 cycles or two minutes. Then, check your patient's status. If no luck, repeat the process all over again.

Many people are reluctant to perform rescue breaths due to concerns about contagious disease. If this is an issue, take a nitrile glove and cut the ends off of the two middle fingers. Place over the victim's mouth (cut glove fingers down) as you breathe for them. This provides a barrier that still allows air flow. Commercially-produced protective CPR masks are also available to keep with your first aid kit.

Another useful item for your medical supplies is a bag valve mask, otherwise known by the brand name "Ambu-Bag". This can be placed on the patient's mouth to form a seal through which you can ventilate them by pressing on the air-filled "bag". This provides pressure to force air inside the respiratory passages.

To review: if you are the lone resuscitator and have training, perform 30 compressions and then deliver 2 rescue breaths as described above. Try for a compression rate of 100 beats per minute. Perform several cycles of the above; then re-evaluate the patient's pulse and respirations. If you don't have training, simply perform chest compressions at a rate of 100 per minute until a trained helper arrives. Once you have started CPR, don't stop until the patient has responded or it is clear that they will not.

After 30 minutes of CPR without result, the pupils of the patient's eyes will likely be dilated and will not respond to light. At this point, your patient has expired and you can cease your efforts. Some may feel this is not long enough; in truth, however, just a few minutes without oxygen is enough to cause irreversible brain damage. In a grid-down situation, you will not be equipped to provide long term chronic care to someone who no longer has brain activity.

There are units known as **defibrillators** available that, though quite expensive, are very useful in a cardiac arrest. These machines produce an electric shock to the heart and sometimes can restart a pulse that has stopped. If caused by a heart attack, a cardiac arrest without defibrillation will have a very low survival rate. It would be wise for your survival group to chip in and purchase a unit. "Home" defibrillators can be found online and are surprisingly easy to use.

To begin, turn the unit on and connect the electrodes per the instructions. Place one electrode pad on the right chest above the nipple and below the collarbone. Place the other on the left chest outside the nipple and several inches below the armpit. The unit will analyze the heart rate (or lack of one) and tell you, believe it or not, whether a shock is necessary. If one is indicated, clear everyone away from the patient and press the button to activate the electric shock. Recheck vital signs and begin chest compressions as needed.

Let's say that you are successful in establishing a pulse and breathing in your unconscious patient. If you must, for some reason, leave them, position them so that they will not vomit and possibly aspirate stomach acid into the lungs (see image below). This is known as the "**recovery position**".

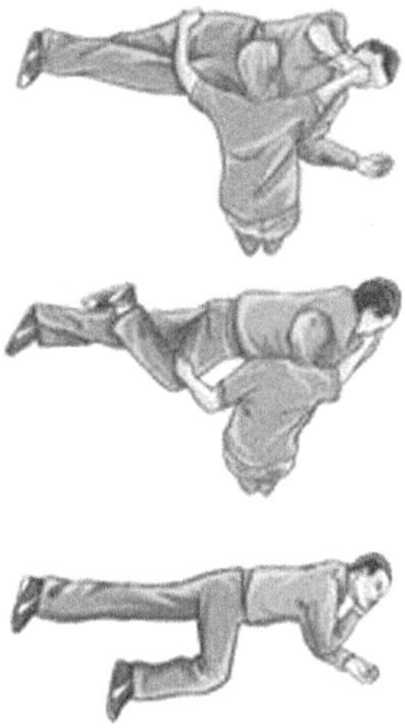

The Recovery Position

In some cases, the actual injury or illness that caused unconsciousness may not be fatal, but the resulting regurgitation of stomach acid into the lungs ("**aspiration pneumonia**") will be. Many alcohol, pill, or recreational drug overdoses cause death in this manner.

To achieve the recovery position:

- Kneel on one side facing the supine patient.
- Position the patient's arm (the one closest to you) perpendicular to the body.

- Flex the elbow.
- Position the other arm across the body.
- Bend the leg that is farthest from you up; reach behind the knee and pull the thigh toward you.
- Use your other arm to pull the shoulder farthest from you while rolling the body toward you.
- Maintain the upper leg in a flexed position so that the body is stabilized.

Although CPR will be of limited use when modern medical facilities are not available, it is still important to know. Take a hands-on class, which is a much better way to learn it than just reading about it. A survival community medic should not only be skilled in performing CPR, but should also teach it to every group member.

HEADACHE

Headaches are one of the most common medical symptoms that you will see in your role as medic. The brain matter itself doesn't have pain receptors; there are several structures around the brain, however, that do. Muscles, blood vessels, and sinuses are just some examples.

Nerves associated with blood vessels and muscles are activated and send pain signals to the brain. Headaches that occur suddenly may be related to infection or colds/flus, but may also be the herald of a life-threatening event such as a stroke. Ear and sinus infections are particularly likely to cause headaches.

Many consider headaches to be, well, more of a headache than an actual danger, but headaches can be associated with a large number of medical conditions, not to mention traumatic injuries.

There are almost more causes for headaches than you can reasonably write down; in a collapse, however, common causes will be:

- Hunger
- Dehydration
- Stress
- Infections
- Fevers
- Elevated blood pressures
- Caffeine or Alcohol withdrawal
- Fumes

Headache Types

Tension Headache

By far, the most frequently-seen type of headache is the **tension headache**. This is caused by spasms of the muscles of the neck and head. Tension headache is usually seen bilaterally (on both sides) and/or the back of the head and neck. They may be related to stress, anxiety or depression, a head injury, or even just time spent with the head or neck in an abnormal position. Lack of sleep, teeth grinding, and poor posture are also factors.

Tension headaches may last a half hour or they can last a week. A sensation of pressure or tightening is the most common symptom. This type of headache may be improved by massaging the back of the neck and temples. Ibuprofen and Acetaminophen are old standbys as treatment. Identifying the situation that triggers the headache may help avoid future episodes.

Sinus Headache

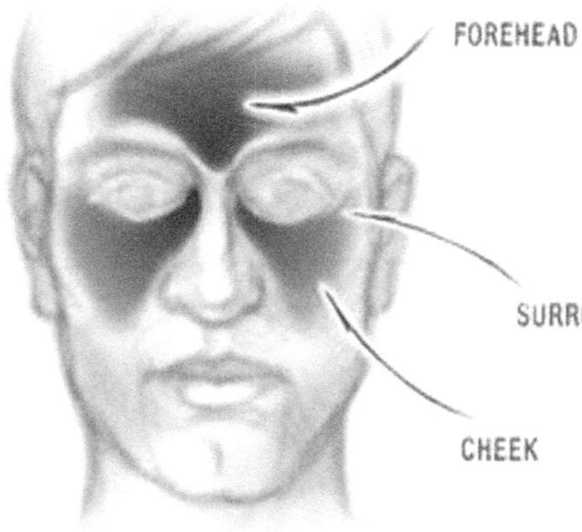

SINUS HEADACHE

Your **sinuses** are a group of several air-filled spaces in the skull that surround the nose. Sinus headache can be caused by infection or may be related to allergies. Besides pain, additional signs include thick mucus congestion (sometimes green or yellow in color), low-grade fever, and cough.

Pain may be localized over the particular sinus infected, such as the cheek or forehead. It may worsen when lying down or bending over. Discomfort is often one-sided, which may help you make the diagnosis.

Antibiotics may be helpful to treat the infections that can cause this type of headache. Amoxicillin (Fish-Mox Forte) 500mg three times a day for a week is a reasonable first choice. If you are allergic to Penicillin family drugs, consider Trimethoprim-Sulfamethoxasole (Bird-Sulfa) 160mg/800mg twice daily. Nasal decongestants such as Pseudoephedrine (Sudafed) may give some relief; so may sterile saline nasal irrigation.

Migraines

Another common cause of headache is the **migraine**. The exact cause of migraines is uncertain. It is thought by some to be related to spasms in the blood vessels. Migraines may be genetic in nature, as they seem to run in families. Women are more susceptible than men.

A specific pattern of symptoms is seen in this variety of headache:

- Pain behind the eye (usually one-sided)
- Sensitivity to light, noise, or odors
- Nausea and vomiting (causing loss of appetite or stomach discomfort)
- Vision changes (blurring, lights and color phenomena)

Bed rest in the dark will be helpful here, as well as Ibuprofen and/or Acetaminophen. Some migraine medications use caffeine, and are thought to be effective. Tea and Coffee might be alternatives in an austere setting. If you are a chronic migraine sufferer, ask your physician for Sumatriptan (Imitrex), a strong anti-migraine medication, to stockpile.

Other Headache Causes

In women, hormonal changes may be responsible for headaches. Pregnancy, menopause, menstruation, and the use of birth control pills have all been implicated as risk factors. Cranberry juice and other natural diuretics eliminate excess fluid from the body and may be helpful to limit swelling. Limiting pre-menstrual salt intake may also help.

Headache caused by dehydration will be rampant in a long-term survival situation. This variety will also present bilaterally and is commonly made worse by standing up rapidly from a lying position. These patients need fluids, which will gradually improve their symptoms.

Less common causes of headache would include an infection of the central nervous system called "**meningitis**". Along with headaches, meningitis presents with a stiff neck, fever, and possibly a rash. This very serious condition may be caused by bacteria or viruses. Without modern medical facilities and labs, you could attempt to treat this condition with antibiotics and antivirals; expect variable results.

Uncontrolled high blood pressure or a burst blood vessel in the brain may cause a stroke (previously discussed elsewhere in this book). Besides the sudden onset of a severe headache, you will notice that your patient has lost strength in the arm and leg on one side; you will also note decreased motion on one side of the face and absent or slurred speech. Loss of vision is sometimes seen.

Natural Headache Relief

If you would like a strategy to deal with a headache without drugs, try the following:

- Place an ice pack where the headache is.
- Have someone massage the back of the patient's neck.
- Using two fingers, apply rotating pressure where the headache is.
- Lie down in a dark, quiet room. Get some sleep if at all possible. If your blood pressure is elevated, lay on your left side (pressure is usually lowest in this position).
- Track what you were doing or, perhaps, what you ate before the headache started; avoid that activity or food if possible.

A number of herbal remedies are available that might help headache. Feverfew is an herb that stops blood vessel constriction and is anti-inflammatory. This can be taken on a daily basis (1-2 leaves) for those with chronic problems (warning: Feverfew should not be ingested during pregnancy or nursing). Gingko Biloba has a similar action.

The pain of tension headaches can be relieved if you utilize herbs that have sedative and antispasmodic properties. Teas made from Valerian, skullcap, lemon balm, and passion flower have both. Herbal muscle relaxants may also help: Rosemary, chamomile, and mint teas are popular options.

For external use, consider lavender or rosemary oil. Massage each temple with 1-2 drops as needed.

EYE CARE

By picking up this book, you have demonstrated that you have excellent foresight. Unfortunately, that doesn't mean that you necessarily have excellent eyesight. Ask anyone on the street which of the five senses they would least be willing to sacrifice. They probably will tell you that their vision is the sense they would most want to preserve. Human beings aren't perfect, and one of our most common imperfections is that of being nearsighted (also known as "**myopia**") or farsighted (also known as "**hyperopia**").

Most of us correct our eye issues with eyeglasses or contact lenses. In a collapse setting, these vision aids become more precious than gold, but most people haven't made provision for multiple replacement pairs of contact lenses or (better) spare eyeglasses.

Imagine what would happen off the grid if your contact lenses dry out or one of your children steps on your glasses. We can't think of anything scarier than being on your own and not be able to see. Having a few pairs of *reading* glasses in your storage will be helpful as well; everyone reaches an age when eyesight naturally changes. It's important to realize that there won't be anyone manufacturing eyewear after a true long-term disaster.

Protective eyewear is another required item. Many with perfect vision will be negligent about wearing eye protection when they chop wood or other chores likely to be part of normal off-grid living. Without eye protection, the risk of injury when performing strenuous tasks will be much higher. Whenever you are doing chores outdoors, you should ask yourself why you *shouldn't* use eye protection.

Early in this book, we mentioned that you should deal with your medical issues before a collapse occurs. Bad eyesight might be one of those issues. One option you may not have considered is having your eyesight corrected to 20/20 with **LASIK** surgery. Lasik surgery uses pinpoint lasers to change the shape of your retina so that you are less nearsighted or farsighted. It's a quick procedure and your eyesight will improve immediately. At most, you might feel like there's a grain of sand in your eye for a day or two. LASIK surgery has been routinely available for years now, and is one of the safest surgical procedures in existence. It will give you a tangible benefit that will increase your chances for survival.

Most don't consider sunglasses to be a medical supply item, but they are. Even if you are just taking a hike outdoors, sunglasses provide eye protection from ultraviolet light. Ultraviolet (UV) light causes, over time, damage to the retinal cells which can lead to a clouding over of your eye's lenses (also called "**cataracts**"). This condition can only be repaired by surgery that will not be available in a collapse. Protection from ultraviolet (UV) light will help prevent long-term damage.

In cold weather conditions, failure to use sunglasses can cause a type of vision loss known as "**snow blindness**". Snow blindness is painful and dangerous in the wilderness. Goggles can be improvised by carving slits into a piece of bark or even cardboard. Luckily, snow blindness will improve on its own with eye patching.

Infections Of The Eye

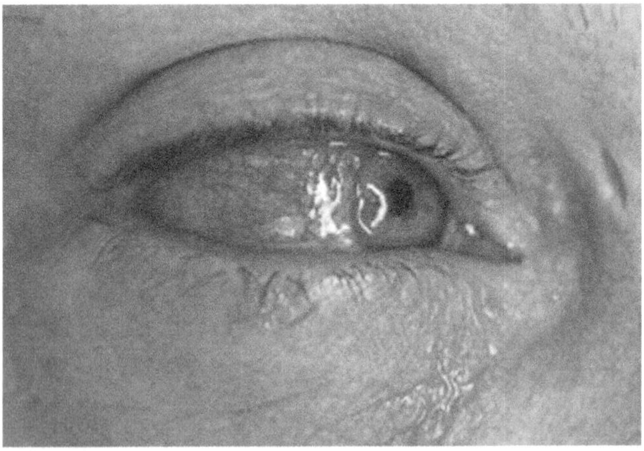

Conjunctivitis or "Pink Eye"

There are various eye conditions that will be more common in a grid-down situation. The most common will be "**conjunctivitis**". The conjunctiva is the thin membrane that covers the white of your eye. Conjunctivitis is an inflammation which causes the affected eye to become red and itchy, and you may note a milky discharge. It can be caused by chemical irritation (soap in your eyes, for example), a foreign body, an allergy, or an infection.

An eye infection is also called "Pink eye" and is highly contagious among children due to their rubbing their eyes and then touching other people or items. Studies have shown that people commonly touch their faces and eyes with their (often dirty) hands throughout the day. Observe any family member for a half hour and you'll see that this is true.

Irritated, teary red eyes may also be seen in allergic reactions, which can be treated with antihistamines orally or antihistamine eye drops. Eye allergies can be differentiated from eye infections: Allergic reactions are less likely to have a milky discharge associated with them.

To avoid spreading the germs that can cause eye infections:

- Wash your hands regularly.
- Don't share eye drops with others.
- Don't touch the tip of a bottle of eye drops with your hands or your eyes because that can contaminate it with germs. Keep the bottle two or three inches above your eye.
- Don't share eye makeup with others.
- Never put contact lenses in your mouth to wet them. Many germs are present in your mouth that could easily infect your eyes.
- Change your contacts often, the longer they stay in your eyes, the higher the chance is that your eye can get infected or be traumatized.
- Any time you have an eye examination, ask the doctor if he/she has any samples of medicated eye drops to give you, in case of emergency.

Antibiotics like Doxycycline 100mg twice a day for a week or less will relieve infectious conjunctivitis. Herbal treatment may also be of benefit. To treat pinkeye using natural products, pick one or more of the following methods:

- Apply a wet Chamomile or Goldenseal tea bag to the closed, affected eye, for 10 minutes, every two hours.

- Make a strong Chamomile or Eyebright (*Euphrasia officinalis*) tea, let cool, and use the liquid as an eyewash (using an eyecup) three to four times daily.
- Use 1 teaspoon of baking soda in 2 cups of cool water as an eyewash solution.
- Dissolve 1 tablespoon of honey dissolved in 1 cup hot water; let cool, and use as an eyewash.

Use the above tea, baking soda liquid, or honey solution on gauze or cloth, and then apply a compress to the affected eye for 10 minutes, every two hours. For relief from the discomfort of conjunctivitis, a slice of cucumber over the eyes will be effective due to its cooling action.

Styes

A stye (or sty) is a bump on the eyelid. It presents as a pimple that can be outside or inside. Styes are caused by a blocked gland near an eyelash due to an accumulation of bacteria called Staphylococcus aureus (Staph).

Luckily, styes do not affect vision unless they become very large, which is a rarity. Normally, they tend to grow, "pop" and drain, and go away after a few days. Despite this, there is often a sense of urgency to deal with it, due to discomfort and cosmetic appearance.

Symptoms of a stye include:

- Swelling, often with a yellowish bump at the level of the skin
- Redness
- Warmth
- Discomfort
- Discharge and crusting

A stye is sometimes confused with another condition called a "chalazion" A chalazion is caused by the blockage of eyelid gland ducts that excrete an oily substance that lubricates the eye. Styes develop quickly, but a chalazion forms over a longer time (sometimes in the area of a previous stye). Unlike styes, a chalazion is painless, but just as disfiguring. Like styes, they might resolve on their own, although it may take months.

The simplest way to deal with a stye is to apply warm moist compresses for, say, 10 minutes twice or three times a day. This helps the stye drain faster and go away. In between, clean gently with a cotton swab or ball in warm water. Antibiotic eye solutions and ointments are also available that will help to speed recovery. Use Acetaminophen or Ibuprofen for pain relief.

If you get styes often, it's time to evaluate your hand washing regimen. Most people don't wash their hands as often as they should, and this can cause infections like styes or "pink eye", also called conjunctivitis. This is especially an issue for those who wear contacts. A good method of prevention is to perform eyelid scrubs regularly with a warm moist cotton ball and a small amount of baby shampoo.

Many people will try to squeeze the stye like any other pimple, but this can traumatize the area and cause worse problems like infection of surrounding tissues. This is called "cellulitis" and is discussed elsewhere in the book. If the cellulitis spreads to the face, you should give your patient oral antibiotics in the penicillin, erythromycin, or cephalosporin families.

Natural remedies include:

- Warm saline solution washes several times a day
- Coriander or tamarind seed washes may reduce swelling. Soak seeds in warm water, then strain and use the water as a wash for your eye.
- Apply warm tea bags to the area; the tannic acid in teas may be helpful.

Eye Trauma

The human body is truly a miracle of engineering. The conformation of your skull is such that your eyes are slightly recessed in bony sockets, which helps protect them from injury. Despite this, there are many different activities of daily living that can be traumatic to your eyes.

Here are just a few of the ways you can injure your eyes:

- Accidents while using tools
- Splatter from bleach or other household chemicals
- Hedge clippers or lawn mowers
- Grease splatter from cooking
- Chopping wood
- Hot appliances near your face, such as curling irons or hair dryers

The list goes on and on; you could damage your eye by popping a cork on a bottle of champagne (if you could find champagne in a collapse). The grand majority of these injuries are avoidable with a little planning. Despite this, it is likely you will come upon an eye injury at one point or another.

Foreign Objects

If there's a foreign object in the eye, there will be immediate symptoms, such as:

- Eye pain or pressure
- Tearing up
- Light sensitivity
- Frequent blinking
- Redness (a "bloodshot" eye)

The patient will tell you that they feel something in their eye. The most common location will be under the upper eyelid.

The most important thing to do when anyone presents to you with eye pain is a careful examination. Use a moist cotton swab (Q-tip) to lift and evert the eyelid. This will allow you to effectively examine the area. An amount of clean (drinkable) water can be used as irrigation to flush out the foreign object. Alternatively, touch lightly with the Q-tip to dislodge it.

It will be rare for a foreign object to actually impale the eye. You'll need a high-speed impact for this to happen, mostly seen in explosions. This will be difficult to remove, and, even in the best of circumstances, there will be some scarring and some loss of vision if it's on the cornea or pupil.

Let's say you looked, and there's no foreign object. Take a close look at the "**cornea**". The cornea is a clear layer of tissue over the colored part of the eye (the '**iris**") which exists for purposes of protection and to help with focusing. When this layer of tissue is scratched or damaged, it's called a "**corneal abrasion**". This type of injury is relatively common, especially in those who wear contact lenses. The patient will probably complain to you that they still feel as if there's a grain of sand in their eye. Abrasions on the cornea may be hard to see without special fluorescein dye eye drops.

The abraded eye needs to rest and heal. After cleaning it out with water and using antibiotic drops (if available), cover the closed eye with an eye pad and tape. Many recommend covering both eyes, as the open eye will move around and the closed eye will follow its movements. Ibuprofen is useful for pain relief. Over the next few days, the eye should heal by itself.

For prevention of corneal damage, consider the following:

- Wear eye protection whenever you're performing any activity that could possibly cause an eye injury, such as shop work, target shooting, or using power tools. Anyone who is close to you when you're doing these activities should also wear protective gear.
- When working in the yard, watch for low hanging branches; before mowing the yard, remove loose objects in your path. Make sure that your kids never point water under force (say, from a garden hose) at someone's face.
- Put in your contact lenses carefully; don't sleep in them.
- Keep fingernails trimmed short.
- Use a grease shield when you're using your frying pan.

Occasionally, blunt trauma to the eye or even simple actions like coughing or sneezing may cause a patch of blood to appear in the white of the eye. This is called a "subconjunctival hemorrhage" or "**hyphema**", and certainly can be alarming to the patient. Luckily, this type of hemorrhage is rarely dangerous, and will go away on its own without any treatment.

If there is a loss of vision associated with the hyphema, however, there is more cause for concern. Evaluate this injury as described for abrasions.

Keeping the patient's head elevated will allow any blood to drain to the lower part of the eye chamber. This strategy may help preserve vision. Cool compresses applied to the affected eye are also recommended, perhaps using the natural substances mentioned earlier.

NOSEBLEEDS AND NASAL TRAUMA

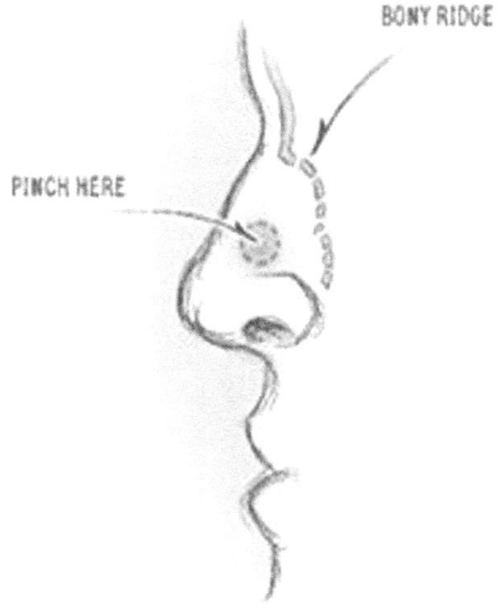

NOSE BLEED

It's a rare individual who has never had a nosebleed. The nose has many tiny blood vessels and is situated in a vulnerable position as it protrudes from the face. Nosebleeds can occur at any age, but are seen mostly in children and the elderly.

Nosebleeds can occur from outside causes, such as trauma to the face. It can also be caused by factors that affect the inside of the nose, such as excessive "picking" or irritation from upper respiratory infections. Environmental factors such as cold or dry climates may also play a role. In rare cases, underlying illness such as faulty blood clotting may be implicated as the cause.

To effectively stop a nosebleed:

- Sit upright with the head tipped slightly forward. Although you may have been taught to tilt your patient's head backward, this may just cause blood to run down the back of the throat.
- Breathe through your mouth.

- Spit out blood in the mouth and throat instead of swallowing it. Blood may irritate the stomach.
- Spray the nose with a medicated nasal spray such as oxymetazoline hydrochloride, 0.05 percent (Afrin) into the affected nostril.
- Using your thumb and index finger, firmly pinch the soft part of the nose just below the bone. Push towards the face.
- Apply an ice pack to the affected side. Cold constricts the blood vessels and may help stop the bleeding.
- Apply pressure for 5-10 minutes. Be patient.
- Check to see if your patient's nose is still bleeding after 10 minutes. If still bleeding, hold it for 10 more minutes.
- Place a little petroleum jelly inside the nose.

In prolonged cases, cut a strip from Celox or Quikclot powder-impregnated gauze and carefully place with a blunt tweezers or Kelly clamp. Alternatively, the bleeding nostril can be flushed with sterile saline; then, gently introduce a thin strip of cloth drenched in epinephrine (from an Epi-pen or other anaphylactic shock kit) and pack gently into the nostril. Do not remove the packing for several hours. Whether the bleeding is due to trauma or not, blowing the nose to eject blood and clots should be avoided, as it may restart the bleeding.

Commercial products such as Nasalcease or Woundseal are available and thought to be effective; you might consider them as medical storage items. A natural hemostatic agent is geranium oil. A few drops on a strip of gauze could be placed in the bleeding nostril with good results in many cases.

In patients with frequent nosebleeds, chronic irritation of the walls of the nostril may be at work. Protect this area by applying small amounts of petroleum jelly gently inside the nose. Admonish children to avoid "picking" their nose and monitor the use of aspirin, which could cause bleeding due to its anticoagulant effect.

The "Broken" Nose

Trauma to the nose can result in damage to the bone or cartilage. If there is a nasal fracture, the patient will have swelling and any pressure on the nose is very painful. This may cause deformity and difficulty breathing due to swelling. Usually, few major medical problems will result from this type of injury. If the patient can breathe through their nose and there is no major deformity, you may choose to observe the situation. Swelling will go down with ice packs over 48 hours and give you a better picture of what's happening. An instrument known as a "nasal speculum" will allow you to spread the nostrils to look for hematomas and other abnormalities.

In a survival setting, you may choose to "straighten" a deformed nose. It will not straighten out by itself. In an austere setting, it is often performed using the thumbs to realign to a normal position. Be aware that this may cause further damage and should not be done if modern medical care is available. Physicians use instruments like nasal elevators and special materials to manipulate, pack, and "cast" the nose. Most of these items are unlikely to be in your medical kit. Attempts at reduction of a nasal fracture should not be done after two weeks have elapsed.

If you chose to act and were successful in reducing the deformity, you might then consider placing some moist gauze packing and taping the nose in position. The packing should not be removed for two or three days. Early on, place cold packs over the nose for periods of 20 minutes intermittently throughout the day. This will be useful only for the first 48 hours, but will help reduce swelling and discomfort. Acetaminophen and Ibuprofen will also be helpful for pain relief. Swelling in nasal passages may be improved with a nasal decongestant.

EARACHE

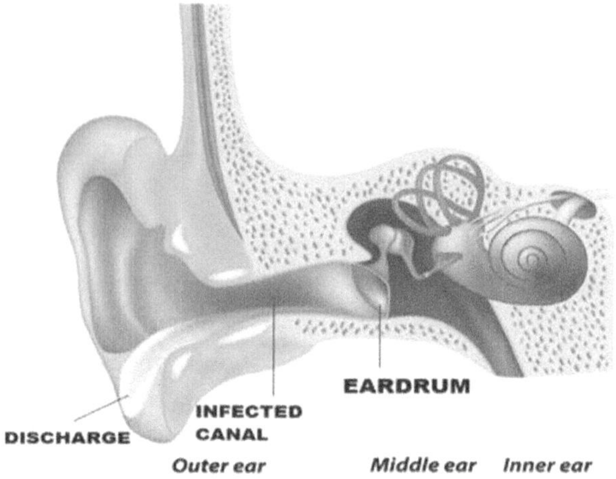

It's a rare parent who hasn't had to deal with this problem at one point or another. In some cases, it's a chronic problem that affects the quality of life of an otherwise healthy child. The most common symptom you'll see relating to the ear is pain, usually due to an infection.

The ear is divided into 3 chambers, the outer, middle and inner ear. Inflammation of the ear is called "**otitis**". The most common ear infections will be in the external and middle ear chambers.

The easiest way to prevent this is to carefully use cotton swabs moistened with rubbing alcohol to dry the ear canal after swimming or excessive sweating. Forceful use of a cotton swab, however, is to be avoided; it is, indeed, the next most common cause of ear pain. Normally, you shouldn't place anything in the ear canal sharper than your elbow.

Ear Infections

Otitis Externa

Otitis Externa, also known as "**Swimmer's Ear**" is an infection of the outer ear canal, and most commonly affects children aged 4 -14 years old. Cases peak during summer months, when most people go swimming. Bacteria will accumulate and multiply in water or sweat. Once caught in the ear canal, inflammation and discomfort ensue.

Symptoms of Otitis Externa include:

- Gradual development of an earache or, possibly, itching
- Pain worsened by pulling on the ear
- Ringing in the ears (**tinnitus**) or decreased hearing
- A "full" sensation in the ear canal with swelling and redness
- Thick drainage from the ear

Standard treatment may include a warm compress to the ear to help with pain control. An antibiotic/steroidal ear drop will be useful, and should be applied for 7 days. In order to get the most effect from the medicine, place the drops in the ear with the patient lying on their side. They should stay in that position for 5 minutes to completely coat the ear canal. Severe cases may be treated with oral antibiotics (such as Amoxicillin) and ibuprofen.

Otitis Media

The most common cause of earache is an infection of the middle ear, called "**otitis media**". Normally, the eardrum is shiny and grayish. When there is an infection in the middle ear canal, the eardrum will appear dull. This is because there is pus or inflammatory fluid behind it. Standard treatment often includes oral antibiotics and ibuprofen, especially in adults with the infection.

Otitis media is most common, however, in infants and toddlers. This is why mothers are always cautioned against bottle or breast-feeding with their baby lying flat. You can expect otitis media to present with one or more of the following:

- Pain, more so when lying down
- Difficulty sleeping
- Crying and irritability
- fever
- loss of appetite

- Loss of balance
- Holding or pulling the affected ear
- Drainage of fluid from the affected ear
- Difficulty hearing from the affected ear

A number of natural remedies are available for earache. Follow this procedure:

- Mix rubbing alcohol and vinegar in equal quantities, or alternatively, 3% hydrogen peroxide.
- Place 3-4 drops into affected ear.
- Wait 5 minutes; then, tilt head to drain out the mixture.
- Next, use either plain warm olive oil, or add 1 drop of any one of these essential oils to 2 ounces of the olive oil: tea tree, eucalyptus, peppermint, thyme, lavender, garlic, or mullein.
- Warm the olive oil slightly and place 2-3 drops into the ear canal. This does not have to be drained or removed.
- A cotton ball with 2 drops of eucalyptus oil may be secured to the ear opening during sleep.

Some patients find a heat source soothing to a painful ear. If you are in a collapse situation, dip a sock or other absorbent material into heated water. Wring it out and place it on the outside of the affected ear.

Other Ear Problems

Inner ear canal issues often cause dizziness, also known as "**vertigo**". Oftentimes, it is caused by an inflammation known as **Otitis Interna**. These patients commonly feel nauseous as well as dizzy. Treatment with diazepam (Valium) or Dimenhydrinate (Dramamine) can help with symptoms. Amoxicillin (veterinary equivalent: Fish-Mox Forte) 500mg three times a day for 7 days (adults) is an appropriate antibiotic therapy if the otitis was caused by an infection.

Ear wax, also known as "**cerumen**" is a chronic problem for certain people. Cerumen is normal and protective in healthy ears. It traps dust particles before they can reach the ear drum.

Normally, people use cotton swabs to remove ear wax, but this method often pushes ear wax further in. Cleaning the opening of the ear canal with a twisted moist washcloth is safer.

When, for whatever reason, cerumen is lodged against the eardrum, it can affect hearing. Other symptoms include:

- Earache
- Hearing loss
- Itching
- Odor or discharge
- Ringing in the ear (also called "**tinnitus**")

Commercial ear rinses with special syringes are available for treatment. Standard home remedies involve a few drops of mineral or baby oil in the ear. This softens the wax, which can then be flushed out with 3% hydrogen peroxide. Some just use the hydrogen peroxide by itself.

Using An Otoscope

Evaluation of the ear canal and eardrum is performed with a special instrument known as an "**otoscope**". Always hold the otoscope in the left hand if you're looking in the left ear, the right hand for the right ear. Holding the otoscope like you would a hammer seems to work best, as it allows you to gently rest your knuckles against the side of the head. Alternatively, you could hold the otoscope as you would a pencil.

The external ear canal is about 2-5cm long in adults, shorter in kids. In children, it's relatively straight; in adults, it is not, so you will need to pull the fleshy part of the ear (the "**pinna**") upwards and backwards to get a better view of the ear drum (also known as the "**tympanic membrane**").

If using the otoscope on a child, always start by explaining what you're doing, and that it might feel "weird", but shouldn't hurt. Choose an otoscope end attachment (called a "speculum") of appropriate size for a child. They often come in sets of different sizes.

Examine the normal ear first. This will allow you to see what the normal anatomy looks like and also will prevent your transferring the infection from the infected ear to the healthy one. Be sure to have the light at high intensity.

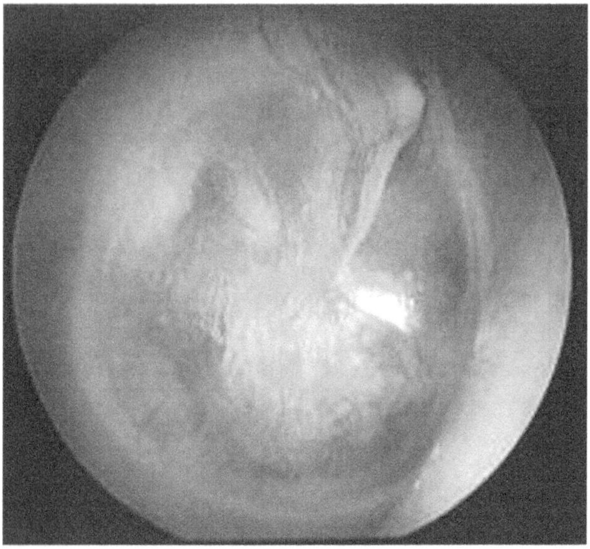

Normal Eardrum Viewed with an Otoscope

You will first see the external canal wall. Is there redness or swelling compared to the normal ear? Is there debris, excessive wax, or even a foreign object? Don't be surprised if you see hair; this is normal.

Now look at the eardrum at the end of the canal. A normal eardrum will appear pearly gray, shiny, and translucent. A dull yellowish color usually indicates fluid behind it; in the worst cases, the eardrum will appear to bulge out towards you due to pressure from within.

BIRTH CONTROL, PREGNANCY, AND DELIVERY

It's a rare individual that doesn't have a wife, girlfriend, mother, daughter or granddaughter that isn't of childbearing age (say 13 to 50 years old). Even if they aren't related to you personally, they could be in your survival group. Remember that, even if you have a daughter that's only 5 years old now, one day she will come of reproductive age.

In a collapse situation, society will be unstable and organized medical care will be spotty at best and nonexistent at worst. If we reach the point that we lose our access to modern healthcare, one of the least welcome events might be one that is ordinarily considered a blessing: a pregnancy.

In a long-term survival scenario, the normal view would be that we have the responsibility to repopulate the world. This is absolutely true further down the road, but first your family must survive. Until things settle down, a pregnancy and the possible complications that accompany it will be a burden.

So why is it important to prevent pregnancies in the early going of a societal collapse? The death rate among pregnant women (also known as the Maternal Mortality Rate) at the time of the American Revolution was about 2-4% *per pregnancy*. Given that the average woman in the year 1800 could expect 6-10 pregnancies over the course of her reproductive life, the cumulative Maternal Mortality Rate easily approached 25 per cent. That means that 1 out of 4 women died due to complications of being pregnant, during the childbirth, or even soon after a successful delivery.

If a major disaster occurs, women might face unacceptable levels of risk. There won't be either medicine or medical supplies in which to treat pregnancy and childbirth complications. Deaths may happen simply because there are no IV fluids or medications to stop bleeding or treat infection.

These tragedies would happen at a time when we will need every member of our survival group to be productive individuals. Growing food, managing livestock, perimeter defense, and caring for children will take the energy of all involved. When a pregnancy goes wrong, it takes away a valuable contributor from the survival family (sometimes permanently) and places an additional strain on resources and manpower.

Pregnancy And Childbirth Complications

Let's discuss some of the reasons that women could cease to become productive group members (or even die) during pregnancy or childbirth:

Hyperemesis Gravidarum

Simply put, **Hyperemesis Gravidarum** is medical-speak for excessive vomiting during pregnancy. Almost every woman will experience nausea and vomiting in the early stages. A small percentage of them, however, have an exaggerated response to the hormones of pregnancy that causes them to vomit so much that they become dehydrated. Since they can't maintain a reasonable oral fluid intake, intravenous hydration is required. Without it, severe dehydration could be life-threatening.

How many survival groups will have access to IV equipment and the know-how to institute IV fluid therapy? One of our hobbies is collecting old medical books, most of them from at least 100 years ago (in other words, where we will be medically if a collapse occurs). When these books discuss Hyperemesis Gravidarum, they relate death rates in 10% to 40% in severe cases.

Miscarriage

The human race is not perfect, and we don't always produce perfect pregnancies. Approximately 10% of all pregnancies end in miscarriage. When a woman miscarries, many times she will not pass all of the dead tissue relating to the pregnancy. On occasion, this tissue will become infected or cause excessive bleeding.

The treatment in this case would be something called a **dilatation and curettage** (D & C), which is a procedure that uses scrapers called curettes to remove the retained tissue. This will stop the bleeding and prevent infection. Again, how may survival groups have the ability and knowledge to perform this procedure or have access to the antibiotics necessary to treat possible infection?

Hypertension

There is a condition known as Pregnancy-Induced Hypertension that is relatively common. When a woman reaches the last month of a pregnancy (usually her first), she might begin to have elevated blood pressures that cause extreme swelling (edema). Normal pregnancy causes swollen ankles, but pregnancy-induced hypertension swells up the entire body, including the face. Left untreated, this condition can lead to seizures and become life-threatening. Off the grid, the only treatment available would be bed rest, which at best takes away a productive member of your group, and at worst may fail to prevent a worsening of the condition.

Childbirth Complications

Let's say the pregnancy itself was uncomplicated. The birth process, while usually perfectly natural and routine, could also present some dangers. Every childbirth, for example, involves some bleeding. It could be a little; it could be a lot. It could be caused by lacerations from the passage of the infant through the vaginal canal or from a stubborn **placenta** (afterbirth) that does not expel itself spontaneously.

When childbirth is associated with excessive bleeding, certain procedures and maneuvers are performed by trained midwives or obstetricians to stop the hemorrhage. When hemorrhage occurs and no trained individuals are present at the birth, the bleeding may not stop before major damage has been done to the mother.

In some cases, it's necessary to actually reach into a woman's uterus, grab the placenta and remove it. This procedure is performed when part of the placenta is "retained". If a portion of the placenta is not spontaneously expelled after birth, this tissue will prevent the uterus from contracting. Uterine contractions are the natural way that bleeding stops. Therefore, excessive bleeding may occur.

Of course, retained tissue could become infected, also. Every medic must have the knowledge, equipment, and medications that might be needed to safely get female group members through childbirth.

Complications after childbirth

Conditions in the delivery room after a disaster could be conducive to the development of infections, even if the delivery goes without a hitch. This was a major cause of maternal mortality before modern medical care and antibiotics became available.

Other problems may manifest themselves in the "**postpartum**" period, the first days to weeks after the baby is born. For example, a woman who has a hemorrhage during childbirth could be so weakened by loss of blood that she is unable to return to normal activities for a very long time. Some women will undergo a period of depression for a time ("postpartum depression") and have difficulty being productive.

We don't want anyone to think that all women will die during, or right after, their pregnancy. We're only saying that not all survival groups have prepared to obtain the knowledge, resources, and ability to deal with the complications that could occur. The question is: If people are rioting in the streets and your garden isn't doing so well yet, do you really need to add a newborn baby to your list of responsibilities?

How To Prevent Pregnancy

So, what's your plan? Even long-time Preppers haven't spent much time figuring out what birth control method they will use if a catastrophe takes them off the grid. Have you included condoms or other birth control method in your bug-out bag? The majority have not, so congratulations if you did. That means you've thought about more than just beans and bullets.

It's important to have **condoms** in your storage, but condoms can break; even if they don't, they won't last forever. With spermicide, condoms expire after 2 years; without spermicide, perhaps at most 3-5 years. **Diaphragms**, another common method in which a woman places a rubber or latex barrier over her cervix, require chemical spermicides and will also become brittle over time.

Some women use IUDs (**intrauterine devices**) to prevent pregnancy. Some of these use hormones that wear off over time. They must be inserted into the body of the uterus, something best done by someone with experience to prevent injury. Poor technique could perforate the uterine walls.

Birth control pills are useful, but it's difficult to get more than a few months' supply at any one time. Insurance companies tightly control when women can get their next pack of pills. Even if you could get them, they cost a bundle if purchased outside of insurance plans. The cost of stockpiling several years' worth can be difficult for the average person.

Natural Birth Control Methods

Some advocate the use of lemon or lime juice as a douche prior to intercourse. The high acid content is thought to be lethal to sperm. Others consider using an actual slice of lemon or lime as a "cap" in the vagina during the act of intercourse.

It's important to know that these methods are *not* effective if used after the sexual act, as multitudes of sperm have already entered the cervix and are well on their way to performing their duty. Be aware that some women will experience some irritation preventing pregnancy in this manner.

There is no commercial or even herbal contraceptive that is 100% effective and is guaranteed to have no side effects. Therefore, the best strategy is to predict, as accurately as possible, fertile parts of the cycle and plan to be abstinent or especially careful during these times.

To make these predictions, we will have to go back to a traditional form of birth control: **Natural Family Planning** (the modern version of the Rhythm Method). Although not as effective in preventing pregnancy as the Pill, it is up to 90% effective if implemented correctly. There is no need to put hormones into your system and no side effects. Natural Family Planning is a time-honored method to prevent pregnancy that fits in well with any collapse strategy.

Natural Family Planning involves trying to figure out your fertile period and avoiding unprotected intercourse during that time. This method works best on women who have relatively regular cycles. Cycles are predictable if a woman releases an egg for fertilization (this is called "**ovulation**") on a monthly basis.

If you or your partner has 28 day menstrual cycles, you can bet that ovulation is occurring. A pregnancy is likely in any couple having regular sexual relations. So likely, in fact, that 80-85% of couples can expect a pregnancy within the first year of a collapse if not careful. The egg will disintegrate in 24-48 hours, however, if not fertilized.

You can tell the day that you or your partner is ovulating by doing a little research. This involves, in part, taking your temperature with a thermometer daily for a cycle or two. There are actually special thermometers that are used for this purpose called **Basal Body Temperature** Thermometers, although I would think that any thermometer that goes up by 1/10 degree increments would suffice (e.g., 98.1, 98.2, 98.3 degrees Fahrenheit). Make certain to take temperatures daily at the same time, preferably before you get out of bed in the morning. This might be problematic during a survival situation, so consider performing this calculation prior to a catastrophe occurring.

When you ovulate, your basal body temperature goes up about half a degree and stays up until the next period. Make a graph or chart of the daily temperatures and you'll see a pattern develop. Always count Day #1 as the first day of menstrual bleeding to start with.

Once you've done this for a few cycles, you will have a good idea about when you or your partner is at risk for getting pregnant. A common physical symptom that goes along with this: Many women will notice some one-sided discomfort in the lower abdomen when they ovulate.

Let's say that you or your partner has 28 day cycles and that the temperature rise occurs around day 14. You should avoid having unprotected sexual intercourse from about day 10 - day 18 (a few days prior and a few days after the likely day of ovulation). If ovulation occurs later, say day 16, just move the "danger" period over to day 12 - day 20. Ovulation may occur a couple of days earlier or later in any one cycle, so you want to have a margin of error in determining the time period eligible for fertilization.

Observing the cyclical changes in cervical mucus is a useful adjunct. The **cervical mucus method** is based on observation of the character of cervical mucus during the course of the menstrual cycle. To use this method, it's important to understand how cervical secretions change during a typical menstrual cycle. Generally, you'll see:

- Little or no cervical secretions for several days after each period.
- Sticky, thick secretions for the next few days.
- Clear and watery mucus as ovulation occurs.
- Thicker and less quantity of cervical secretions until the period begins.

You can obtain a sample of cervical mucus by gently placing two gloved fingers into the vagina all the way to the cervix (the neck of the womb). It will feel like a firm projection at the end of the vagina. Examine the mucus: Cervical mucus when not ovulating will be thick; spreading your fingers will cause it to snap. During ovulation, spreading two mucus-laden fingers will cause the watery mucus to stretch significantly before breaking.

Make sure you have washed your hands thoroughly before the exam and have an ample supply of gloves. Nitrile gloves are preferable to avoid reactions in those women allergic to latex.

Performed correctly, the Natural Family Planning method is an effective and completely natural way to prevent pregnancy. In survival scenarios, it will allow you to decide when things are stable enough to bring a newborn into the world.

Pregnancy Care Basics

Despite all the best efforts made to prevent pregnancy, the best laid plans of mice and men sometimes go awry. Whether by accident or on purpose, you may find yourself responsible for the care of a pregnant woman. It will be important to know how to support that pregnancy and, eventually, deliver that baby.

You won't have access to ultrasound technology to take a look at the fetus; whether it's a boy or a girl will once again become a mystery only solved at birth. Even twins might be a surprise.

Without prenatal mega-vitamins, babies will be smaller at birth. This may not be so bad, since Caesarean Section will no longer available. It's less traumatic for the mother to deliver a 6 or 7 pound baby than a 10 pounder.

Despite all the possible complications that we mentioned in the previous section, pregnancy is still a natural process. It usually proceeds without major complications and ends in the delivery of a normal baby. Although your pregnant patient will not be as productive for the survival group as she would ordinarily be, she will probably still be able to contribute to help make your efforts a success. To make a pregnancy a success, the medic will need to have a little knowledge of the subject and an idea of how to deliver the fetus.

We are, of course, fortunate to have simple tests that can identify pregnancy almost before your patient misses a period. What if these tests are no longer available? You will have to rely on the following tried and true signs and symptoms to identify the condition:

- Absent menstruation
- Tender Breasts
- Nausea and vomiting
- Darkening of the nipples
- Fatigue
- Frequent Urination
- Backache

These symptoms, in combination, are indicative of pregnancy. The timing of each will be variable; some will be noticed earlier than others. It should be noted that this investigation will likely be necessary only in those women experiencing their first pregnancy. Once you have been pregnant, you will most likely know when it happens again.

Of course, as time goes on, the abdominal swelling associated with uterine and fetal growth will be undeniable. Stretch marks come later, as do hemorrhoids, backache, and varicose veins (all very common but not universal). These changes are part and parcel of the average healthy pregnancy. Most of the above will improve after the pregnancy is over, but may not disappear completely.

So, what's the due date? This is the question everyone will want answered once a pregnancy is identified. A human pregnancy lasts 280 days or 40 weeks from the first day of the last menstrual period to the estimated date of delivery. This used to be called the "**estimated date of confinement**" because, yes, they confined women to their beds as they approached it.

This date is simple to calculate if you have regular monthly periods. To get the **due date**, subtract 3 months and add 7 days to the first day of the last period. Example: If the first day of last menstrual period (LMP) is 9/7, then the due date is 6/14.

If the woman does not know when her last cycle started, you can still estimate the age of the pregnancy by physical signs. When you gently press on the woman's abdomen, you will notice a firm area (the uterus) and a soft area (the intestines). Identify the uppermost level of firmness, and you will able to estimate the approximate age of the pregnancy.

If the "lump" is peaking just over the pubic bone, you're at 12 weeks. Halfway between the pubic bone and the belly button is 16 weeks. At the belly button is 20 weeks. Each centimeter above the belly button adds a week, so have a measuring tape handy. A term pregnancy will measure about 40 centimeters (give or take) from the pubic bone to the top of the uterus.

Twins, as you might imagine, will throw all of these measurements out the window. They will occur in 1 in 60 births, more often if there is a family history. Don't worry about triplets: They occur in only 1 in 7,000 births unless you use fertility drugs.

Once you have identified the pregnancy, you should make every effort to assure that your patient is getting proper nutrition. Deficiencies can affect the development of the fetus, so obtaining essential vitamins and iron through the diet will give the best chance to avoid complications. If you have stockpiled prenatal vitamins, use them.

Common early pregnancy issues will include **hyperemesis**, as described in the last section. Be sure to ask your physician for prescriptions for Zofran (ondansetron) and/or other anti-nausea medications to add to your stockpile. Hyperemesis will disappear in almost all women as they advance in the pregnancy. Dry bland foods, like crackers, are helpful in getting a woman through this stage. Ginger tea is a time-honored home remedy to decrease "**morning sickness**".

Another early pregnancy issue is the **threatened miscarriage**. This will be characterized by bleeding or spotting from the vagina, along with pain that simulates menstrual cramps. As 10% of pregnancies end in miscarriage and a higher percentage threaten to, this will be an issue that you must know how to deal with.

Other than placing your patient on bed rest, there will not be much you'll be able to do in this circumstance. Some of these pregnancies don't continue because the fetus is abnormal, and no amount of rest will stop many of these pregnancies from ending very early. The good thing is that a single miscarriage generally does not mean that future pregnancies will be unsuccessful.

Keep a close eye out for evidence of infection, such as fever or a foul vaginal discharge, after a miscarriage. Women with these symptoms would benefit from antibiotic therapy.

Pregnant women should be evaluated periodically to see how the fetus is progressing. Besides verifying progressive growth in the size of the uterus, the fetal heartbeat should be audible via stethoscope at around 16-18 weeks, or much earlier if you have a functioning battery-powered fetal heart monitor (also called a Doppler ultrasound). These are available for sale online. Your exams should be more frequent as the pregnancy advances, weekly once your patient reaches 35 weeks.

Weight gain is desirable during pregnancy. An average weight gain would be 25 pounds or so. Blood pressure should be taken regularly to rule out pregnancy-induced hypertension. Elevated blood pressures behoove you to place your patient on bed rest. Lying on the left side will keep her blood pressure at its lowest. Check for evidence of edema (swelling of the feet, legs and face) as well as excessive weight gain.

Labor

As the woman approaches her due date, several things happen. The fetus begins to "drop", assuming a position deep in the pelvis. The patient's abdomen may look different, or the "**fundus**" (the top of the uterus) may appear lower. As the neck of the uterus (the **cervix**) relaxes, the patient may notice a mucus-like discharge mixed with a little blood. This is referred to as the "**bloody show**" and is usually a sign that labor will occur soon, anywhere from the next few hours to a week or so.

If you examine your patient vaginally by gently inserting two fingers of a gloved hand, you'll notice the cervix is firm like your nose when it is not ripe, but becomes soft like your lips when the due date is approaching. This softening and thinning out of the cervix is called "**effacement**".

Effacement is measured in percentages. When 50% effaced, the cervix is half its normal thickness and length. At 100% effacement ("completely effaced"), the cervix is paper-thin. Effacement usually occurs before any significant opening of the cervix (also called "**dilation**")

Dilation of the cervical opening will be very slow at first, but speeds up once your patient reaches about 3-4 cm. At this level of dilation, you will be able to place two (normal-sized) fingertips in the cervix and feel something firm; this is the baby's head. Frequent vaginal exams are invasive, however, and not necessary in most cases.

Contractions will start becoming more frequent. To identify a contraction, feel the skin on the soft area of your cheek, and then touch your forehead. A contraction will feel like your forehead. False labor, or **Braxton-Hicks contractions**, will be irregular and will abate with bed rest (especially on the left side) and hydration. If contractions are coming faster and more furious even with bed rest and hydration, it's likely the real thing!

A gush of watery fluid from the vagina will often signify "**breaking the water**", and is also a sign of impending labor and delivery. The timing will be highly variable, however, and sometimes urine leakage may confuse the situation. A product called nitrazine paper, will turn a bright blue when it touches amniotic fluid due to its high Ph. A bright blue result (nitrazine positive) usually verifies that the bag of water is broken. If you have a microscope in the hospital tent, a little amniotic fluid on a slide will reveal fern-like crystals. This is called "ferning" and is more solid proof of membrane rupture than nitrazine positive tests.

Delivery

Dilation to 10 cm, otherwise known as "complete dilation" should be achieved before any concerted efforts to push the baby out. The delivery of a baby is best accomplished with the help of an experienced midwife or obstetrician, but those professionals will be hard to find in survival settings. If there is no chance of accessing modern medical care, it will be up to you to perform the delivery.

To get ready for delivery, wash your hands and put gloves on. Then, place clean sheets so that there will be the least contamination possible. Tuck one under the mother's buttocks and spread it on your lap so that the baby, which comes out very slippery, will land on the sheet instead of the floor if you lose your grip on it. Place a towel on the mother's belly; this is where the baby will go once it is delivered. It will be very important to dry the baby and wrap it in the towel, as newborns lose heat very quickly.

As the labor progresses, the baby's head will move down the birth canal and the vagina will begin to bulge. When the baby's head begins to become visible, it is called "**crowning**". If the water has not yet broken (which can happen even at this late stage), the lining of the bag of water will appear as a slick gray surface. Some pressure on the membrane will rupture it, which is okay at this point (controversial to some). It might even help the process along.

To make space, place two gloved fingers along the edge of the vagina by the "**perineum**". This is the area between the vagina and anus. Using gentle pressure, move your fingers from side to side. This will stretch the area somewhat to give the baby a little more room to come out. Although not advocated by all, "perineal massage" might decrease the risk of lacerations caused by the delivery of the baby.

With each contraction, the baby's head will come out a little more. Don't be concerned if it goes back in after the contraction. It should make steady progress and more and more of the head will become visible over time. Encourage the mother to help by taking a deep breath with each contraction and then pushing while slowly exhaling.

On occasion, a small cut is made in the bottom of the edge of the vagina to make room for the baby to be delivered. This is called an "**episiotomy**". We discourage this if at all possible, as the cut has to be sutured afterward. The decision should be made as the head is crowning; You should only perform an episiotomy if you believe a very large, jagged tear will occur that would damage the anal sphincter or rectum.

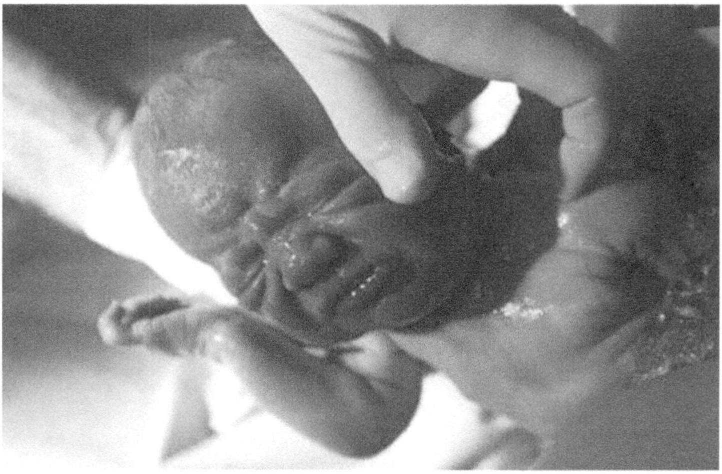

As the baby's head emerges, it will usually face straight down or up, and then turn to the side. The cord might appear to be wrapped around its neck. If this is the case, gently slip the cord over the baby's head. In cases where the cord is very tight and is preventing delivery, you may choose to doubly clamp it and cut between. This will release the tension and make delivery easier.

Next, gently hold each side of the baby's head and apply gentle traction straight down. This will help the top shoulder out of the birth canal. Occasionally, steady gentle pressure on the top of the uterus during a contraction may be required *if* the mother is exhausted. Many times, however, little if any help will be needed for the baby to deliver, (especially in a woman who has had children before). Once the shoulders are out, the baby will deliver with one last push. The mother can now rest.

Put the baby immediately on the mother's belly and clean out its nose and mouth with a bulb syringe. It will usually begin crying, which is a good sign that it is a vigorous infant. Spanking the baby's bottom to get it to cry is rarely needed, and is more of a cliché than anything else. A better way to stimulate a baby to cry is to rub the baby's back.

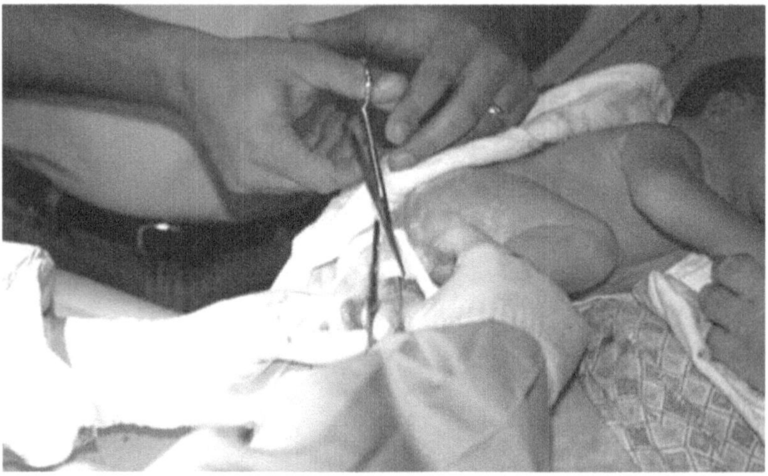

Dry the baby and wrap it up in a small towel or blanket. At this point, you may clamp the cord twice (2 inches apart) with Kelly or Umbilical clamps, and cut in between with a scissors. There is usually no hurry to perform this procedure. The items needed are available in commercially-produced delivery kits.

Once the baby has delivered, it's the placenta's turn. Be patient: In most cases, the placenta will deliver by itself in a few minutes. Avoid pulling on the umbilical cord to force the placenta out. Breaking the cord due to excessive traction will require your placing your hand deep in the uterus to extract it. This is traumatic and can introduce infection. You can ask the mother to give a push when it's clear the placenta is almost out.

If traction is necessary for some reason, place your fingers above the pubic bone and press as you apply mild traction. This will prevent the uterus being turned inside out (a potentially life-threatening situation) if the placenta is stubborn. A moderate amount of bleeding is not unusual after delivery of the afterbirth.

Once the placenta is out, examine it. The "fetal" surface is grey and shiny; turn it inside out and you will see the "maternal" surface, which look like a rough version of liver. The fetal surface is separated into sections called "**cotyledons**". If a portion of the placenta remains inside, you may have to extract it manually.

The uterus after delivery contracts to control bleeding. The fundus is now felt around the level of the belly button. In a long labor, the uterus may be as tired as the mother after delivery, and may be slow to contract. As a result, this may cause excessive bleeding. Gentle massage of the top of the uterus will make it firm again and limit blood loss. You may have to do this from time to time during the first 24 hours or so after delivery.

Monitor the mother closely for excessive bleeding over the next few days. In normal situations, the bleeding will become more and more watery as time progresses. This is normal. Also, keep an eye out for evidence of fever, foul discharge or other issues.

Place the baby on the mother's breast soon after delivery. This will begin the secretion of "**colostrum**", a clear yellow liquid rich in substances that will increase the baby's resistance to infection. Suckling also causes the uterus to contract, which decreases blood loss. It's also important to recognize the bonding element between mother and baby when breastfeeding.

It should be noted that there are different schools of thought regarding some of the above. Remember that your goal is to have an end result of a healthy mother and baby, both physically and emotionally.

ANXIETY AND DEPRESSION

In a natural or man-made disaster, it goes without saying that we will experience epidemics of both anxiety and depression. The stress of living off the grid will be, for most, an emotional roller-coaster. As such, an effective medic will have to be skilled in identifying those that need help, and doing everything possible to support and treat them.

The stability of your survival community is dependent on the stability of its members. Be mindful of group dynamics, and work to foster a sense of common purpose and caring. Those medics who can accomplish this goal will have patients that may have medical issues but not psychological ones.

Anxiety

It is a rare individual who will not experience significant anxiety when deprived of the benefits of modern civilization. Even in normal times, anxious people think catastrophically: That is, they are always assuming the worst. In most cases, things are rarely as bad as they seem but, after a disaster, their concerns may be completely realistic. Anxiety is similar to the "fight or flight" response, something useful in an emergency. Unfortunately, anxiety may be constant whether or not there is an immediate danger.

Anxiety is more than just an uneasy mind, and one sufferer may present to you quite differently from another. The symptoms can be mostly emotional, mostly physical, or some combination of both. You may note:

Emotional Symptoms:

- Irrational fear
- Difficulty concentrating
- Jumpiness
- Extreme pessimism
- Irritability
- Mental "paralysis" or inability to act when needed
- Inability to stand still

Physical Symptoms:

- Shortness of breath
- Palpitations (rapid pulse)
- Perspiration
- Upset stomach/diarrhea
- Tremors/tics/twitches
- Tense muscles
- Headache
- Insomnia

Acute anxiety attacks, also known as "**panic attacks**", may occur without warning and are characterized by intense feelings of fear and impending doom. These episodes are usually short-lived but severe enough that a person may feel what they believe to be physical chest pain. Their breathing may become so rapid that they faint.

Panic attacks occur most commonly in young adults. Classic complaints include:

- Chest pain
- Choking sensation
- Feeling they are in an unreal or surreal environment
- Feeling the walls "close in" on them ("claustrophobia")
- Nausea or strange "pit of the stomach" feelings
- Hot flashes (sensations of heat and flushing)

After making certain that there is no physical problem causing the above symptoms, you should closely observe the patient. Panic attacks rarely last more than an hour, and a single episode will usually resolve without medication. Your support and assurance may be all that's needed.

Those who experience frequent attacks may benefit with more intervention. From a treatment standpoint, this may involve a combination of medications and supplements.

Unless your patient had a history of anxiety in normal times, you won't have stockpiled many anti-anxiety medications like Alprazolam (Xanax). As such, you must look to your medicinal herb garden for plants that may have an effect on mood. There are many herbs that claim to relieve anxiety. Most of these have a mild sedative effect and can be easily made into teas (also called infusions). They include:

- Valerian: 1 teaspoon dried root in 1 cup water
- Hops: 1 teaspoon female flowers in 1 cup water
- Lemon Balm: 1 teaspoon dried leaf or 5-6 fresh leaves in 1 cup water
- Passion flower: 1 teaspoon dried herb (avoid roots) in 2 cups water
- Skullcap: 1 tablespoon dried leaves in 1 cup water
- Chamomile: 1 teaspoon dried flowers in 1 cup water
- Catnip: 1 teaspoon dried leaves in 1 cup water
- Green tea: 1 tea bag in 1 cup water
- Kava: 1-2 teaspoons of dried root in 1 cup water

Some should be strained before drinking or have raw honey or lemon added for flavor. It should be noted that Kava may be dangerous in those with liver and other medical problems.

Essential oils of lavender, frankincense, chamomile, citrus, and others are versatile and can be used as aromatherapy, direct inhalation therapy, or for topical use. Rub the oil between your hands and bring them up to your nose and slowly inhale. For topical use, mix with a 50/50 mixture of essential oil and carrier oil (such as olive). Apply small amounts on temples, neck, and shoulders twice a day.

Perhaps the most important tools to aid the anxious patient are your counseling and communication skills. When you talk to your anxious group member, listen calmly and attentively. Ask them to tell you exactly what they're worrying about; acknowledging their fears will help you build rapport and trust.

One useful method of dealing with anxiety is to have your patient write their concerns down on paper. Sometimes just seeing them in black and white will have a positive effect. In one study, students were asked to write down their fears about an upcoming final exam. Those who put them down on paper did better on the exam than those that didn't.

Convince your patient to set aside just a short part of their day to concentrate on their worries with their list in hand. Keep that time period limited to 20 minutes or so. They might think less of their fears the rest of the day and become more productive.

In a survival setting, the items on their list will relate to the uncertainty of their current situation. Let them know that there is always some uncertainty in life, both in good times and bad times. Try to convince them that dwelling on those issues will not make things any less uncertain, but *will* prevent them from dealing successfully with them.

Work to improve your patient's quality of life. You can do this by:

- Assuring good nutrition
- Reducing substances such as nicotine, caffeine, and alcohol
- Encouraging exercise and constructive activities
- Promoting rest breaks and good hygiene and sleep habits
- Instituting sessions for relaxation therapy (examples include meditation, massage, and deep breathing)

Depression

Many people with anxiety disorders also suffer from depression. Since depression makes anxiety worse (and vice versa), it's important to have strategies to treat both conditions. In a collapse, things may be so bad that everyone is depressed to one degree or another.

This response to the strain of a survival situation is understandable, and is referred to as "**situational depression**". Their circumstances are what have made them depressed, not some biochemical misfire of brain cells. Depression may be cyclical, relating to, for example, a woman's menstrual cycle or the time of the year.

Like anxiety, there are a number of symptoms that are commonly seen in various combinations:

- Feelings of hopelessness or inadequacy
- Apathy

- Change in Appetite
- Weight loss or gain
- Irritability (especially common in men)
- Exhaustion
- Reckless behavior
- Difficulty concentrating on tasks
- Aches and pains (without clear physical cause)

Severe cases of depression are marked by inability to get out of bed in the morning and even thoughts of suicide. Various medications known as "**antidepressants**" are available on the market; these include Prozac, Zoloft, and Paxil, among others. Unfortunately, they will be unlikely to be in your medical supplies unless a member of your group already suffers from chronic depression. As such, you must look to alternatives.

Vitamin supplements like B12, Folic Acid, Tryptophan, and Omega-3 antioxidants may be effective in some sufferers. St. John's Wort has been used with some success, and has even been called "herbal Prozac". It shouldn't be used, however, on pregnant women or children. As with anxiety, you, as healthcare provider, will have to depend on your counseling skills to aid your patient.

In situational depression as will be seen in a collapse situation, you would return to many of the techniques used to treat anxiety:

- Assuring good nutrition
- Reducing substances such as nicotine, caffeine, and alcohol
- Encouraging exercise and constructive activities
- Promoting rest breaks and good hygiene and sleep habits
- Instituting relaxation techniques (meditation, massage, deep breathing)

Additionally, it will be especially important to make sure your people cultivate supportive relationships with each other. People who are depressed often feel very alone. You must work to foster a sense of community; this with provide strength to your emotionally weakened members.

Make sure to accentuate the positive aspects of every situation (if there are any). Encourage each member of your group to share their feelings with the others. Group meetings for this purpose will encourage communication and bonding in the survival group. Incorporate these meetings as a regular event in your community.

You might have read about **Post-Traumatic Stress Syndrome** (PTSD). This condition affects many (perhaps all) who are exposed to stressful events like sexual assault, combat, or natural disasters. Relapses are common and can last for years.

Oftentimes, the patient will re-experience traumatic events mentally; they may become agitated and, sometimes, uncontrollable. Anger, insomnia, decreased work performance, and apathy are common manifestations. Although anxiety is a component of PTSD, anti-anxiety medications do not seem to help as much as anti-depressants. Follow the treatment guidelines previously discussed for depression.

The success of your survival group will depend greatly on your ability to spot emotional issues before the situation deteriorates. Once out of control, these conditions will damage the cohesion necessary to succeed in an adverse environment. Close observation and quick intervention are skills as important to develop as any specific technical skill in a collapse.

SLEEP DEPRIVATION

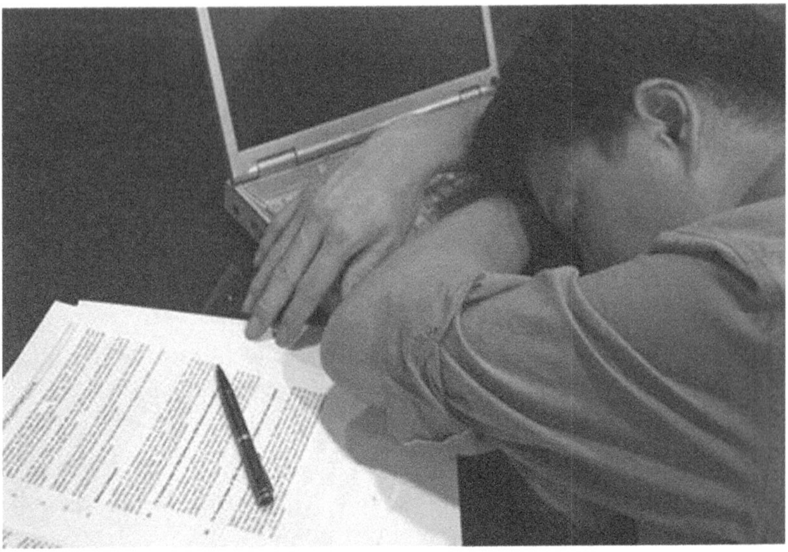

As professionals originally in the field of obstetrics, we can verify that delivering babies at 4 a.m. is not conducive to a good sleep pattern. Lack of sleep is called "**sleep deprivation**", and can be an acute or chronic condition. In a survival scenario, you can imagine the many reasons why you might suffer from not enough sleep: Unfamiliar surroundings, increased responsibilities, fatigue from strenuous activities, and hostile neighbors are just some.

Sleep deprivation can significantly impair your brain's function. There are documented negative effects on performance due to decreased activity in parts of the brain involved in higher thought processes. As a result, you may become incapable of putting events into proper perspective and taking appropriate action.

This impairs your contribution to a survival group. It stands to reason that many car crashes and industrial accidents are, at least in part, caused by lack of sleep. Indeed, over 100,000 serious traffic accidents a year occur in the U.S. become someone fell asleep at the wheel. The British Medical Journal equates 17-21 hours without sleep as the equivalent of a blood alcohol level of .05– 08%.

When you don't get enough sleep, healing is delayed and the increased amount of muscle activity from lack of rest is equivalent to physical overexertion. In a 2004 study that evaluated the performance of medical residents, those getting less than 4 hours of sleep made twice the medical errors than residents who slept 7-8 hours a night. Perhaps the most dangerous thing about the chronically sleep-deprived is that they don't realize that they are functioning at an impaired level.

In addition to what's happening in your brain, the failure to get 7-8 hours of sleep every night causes many of the following signs and symptoms:

- Irritability
- Depression
- Tremors
- Bloodshot, puffy eyes
- Headaches
- Confusion
- Memory loss
- Muscle aches
- Hallucinations and other psychotic symptoms
- Poor control of diabetes and high blood pressure
- Blackouts (sometimes called "microsleeps")
- Weight loss or gain

The lack of deep sleep impairs mood and decreases learning ability. Deep sleep is also important to allow natural enzymes to repair damage caused by "**free radicals**", molecules responsible for aging and tissue damage.

The study also found that lack of rapid eye movement (REM) sleep (dreaming) worsens depression. Depressed patients have depleted amounts of neurotransmitters in the brain.

The best treatment for sleep deprivation involves a concept we'll call "**sleep hygiene**". Good sleep hygiene is adjusts your behavior to maximize the amount of restful sleep you get. Consider:

- Adhering to a standard bedtime (and wakeup time).
- Making your environment as comfortable as possible.

- Avoiding nicotine, caffeine, and alcohol before going to bed.
- Exercising regularly, but not just before going to bed.
- Eliminating as much light as possible in the room at bedtime.
- Staying away from heavy foods for at least 2 hours before going to sleep.
- Keeping your mind clear of stressful issues at bedtime

Some of the above may be difficult during a major disaster. Of course, there are many prescription and over-the-counter sleep aids that might help. Prescription sleep aids include:

- triazolam (Halcion)
- lorazepam (Ativan)
- temazepam (Restoril)
- zolpidem (Ambien)
- zaleplon (Sonata)
- eszopiclone (Lunesta)

In addition, many antidepressants and pain meds have sedative effects. All of above drugs should be used with the utmost caution, due to the potential for addiction and abuse.

Sleeping pills should never be used by those with airway obstruction issues like sleep apnea. It may prevent them from waking up to breathe. "**CPAP**" equipment, which keeps the airway open by air pressure, is more appropriate in these patients, but will an unlikely option in an austere environment.

Over-the-counter sleep aids include the old standby Diphenhydramine, found in medications like Benadryl and Sominex. Usually, diphenhydramine is used for allergic reactions. The 50 mg. dosage, however, is effective in inducing sleep. Be aware that some may experience drowsiness the next day.

Another antihistamine with sedative effects is Doxylamine, also known as Unisom. Other products like Melatonin may be helpful, but work best in those with naturally low levels of the chemical. Be aware that many drugs taken by adults will have the opposite effect on children. Instead of becoming sleepy, they may become agitated.

A better alternative to start with would be some form of natural sleep aid. Some of the common alternative remedies for sleeplessness include the following, usually made into teas:

- Chamomile
- Kava Root
- Lavender
- Valerian Root
- Catnip

Good nutrition is important for general health, but some foods are also thought to be helpful in promoting a good night's sleep. They contain sleep-inducing or muscle-relaxing substances like melatonin, magnesium, or tryptophan:

- Oatmeal – melatonin
- Milk – tryptophan
- Almonds – tryptophan and magnesium
- Bananas – melatonin and magnesium
- Whole wheat Bread – helps release tryptophan

Yoga, massage, meditation, sound machines, and even acupuncture are also alternative methods of dealing with sleep deprivation. Consider making some lifestyle changes now, so that you will be rested and prepared for whatever the uncertain future sends your way.

SECTION 9

MEDICATIONS

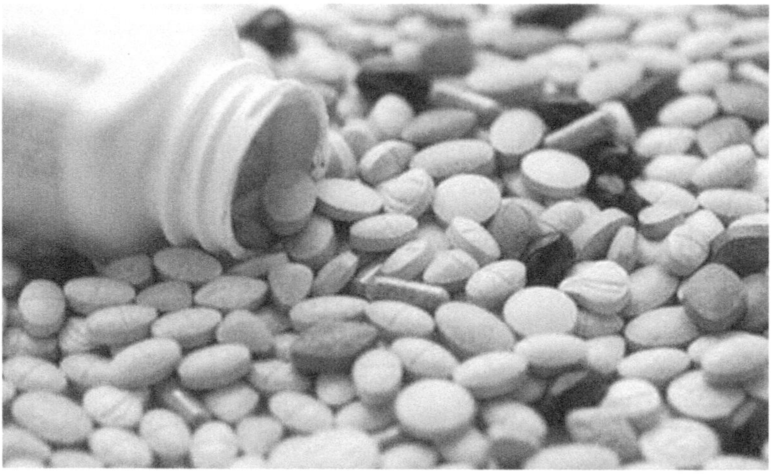

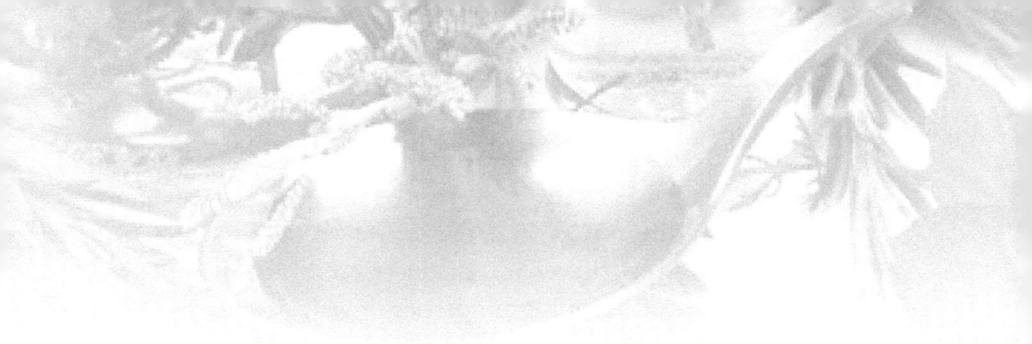

ESSENTIAL OVER-THE-COUNTER DRUGS

Over the counter (OTC) medications deal with a wide variety of problems; indeed, many of them were once only available by prescription. These drugs are highly useful for the survival medic, not just for their effects, but for their ability to be stockpiled in quantity.

Given the complexity of manufacturing pharmaceuticals, most OTC drugs will be nearly impossible to produce after a collapse. Even aspirin, the oldest manufactured drug, won't be available (at least not in a form you'd recognize). Therefore, accumulation of needed medicines should occur *before* a catastrophe hits.

Let's put together a list of what you absolutely must have in quantity as part of your medical supplies. The medications will be listed by their generic names, with U.S. brand names in parenthesis where applicable. Adult doses are also listed. In no particular order, they are:

- **Ibuprofen 200mg** (Motrin, Advil):
  A popular pain reliever, anti-inflammatory, and fever reducer. This medication is useful for many different problems, which makes it especially useful as a stockpile item. It can alleviate pain from strains, sprains, arthritis, and traumatic injury. As well, it can help reduce inflammation in the injured area. Ibuprofen is useful in reducing fevers from infections.

Gastro-intestinal issues are the main side effect. Ibuprofen can be used 1 or 2 every 4 hours, 3 every 6 hours, or 4 every 8 hours.

- **Aspirin, 325mg:** Aspirin has been around since the late 19th century as a pain-reliever, fever reducer, and anti-inflammatory, but it has blood thinning properties as well. It may be all we have to help those with medical issues that require the use of anti-coagulants. It is also useful to treat those with coronary artery disease. If you suspect someone of having a heart attack, have them chew an adult aspirin immediately. 1 baby aspirin (81mg) daily may help prevent coronary artery disease.

  The ingredient in aspirin can also be obtained by chewing on a cut strip of the under bark of a willow, aspen or poplar tree. Take 2 adult aspirin every 4 hours for pain, fever, and inflammation. In a collapse situation, higher doses may be appropriate to replace drugs like Coumadin, but have not been fully researched. Watch for stomach upset.
- **Acetaminophen 325mg** (Tylenol): Another popular pain reliever and fever reducer, it can be used for many of the problems that you can take Ibuprofen or Aspirin for, with the added benefit of not causing stomach irritation or thinning the blood. Unfortunately, it has no significant anti-inflammatory effect. This drug is excellent for treatment of pain and fevers in children at lower doses. Tylenol comes in regular (325 mg) and extra strength (650mg) dosages; adults take 1-2 every 4 hours.
- **Loperamide, 2mg** (Imodium): There's a high likelihood of food and water contamination off the grid, so this medication is essential as an anti-diarrheal. By slowing intestinal motility, less water loss will occur from the body. This decreases the chance of developing dehydration, a known killer in austere settings. Don't take Loperamide if there's a high fever or bloody or black stools.
- **Bismuth Subsalicylate (Pepto-Bismol):** An alternative to loperamide, Bismuth subsalicylate works by reducing inflammation from certain bacteria and viruses. It slows the speed at which fluid moves through your intestines. It also reduces inflammation and keeps certain bacteria and viruses that cause diarrhea from growing in the stomach and intestines.
- **Meclizine 12.5, 25, 50mg** (Antivert): With diarrheal disease, you often have nausea and vomiting, so you will also want to

have Meclizine. Mecilizine is a medication that helps prevent nausea and vomiting and is often used to prevent motion sickness. Meclizine also helps with dizziness, and tends to act as a sedative as well. As such, it may have uses as a sleep aid or anti-anxiety medication. Take 1 25mg tablet 1 hour before boarding a boat or 50-100mg daily in divided doses for dizziness, anxiety or at night before sleep.

- **Antibiotic Ointment** (Neosporin, Bacitracin, Bactroban): When injuries penetrate skin, it puts us at risk for infections which could have life threatening consequences. Triple antibiotic ointment or single drug ointment is applied at the site of injury to prevent this from happening. These products won't cure a deep infection; you would need oral or IV antibiotics for that, but using the ointment immediately after an injury may eliminate the need to use scarce (and precious) supplies. Apply 3-4 times a day.
- **Diphenhydramine 25mg, 50mg** (Benadryl): Diphenhydramine is an antihistamine that alleviates the itching, rashes, nasal congestion and other symptoms of allergic reactions. It also helps drain the nasal passages in some respiratory infections. At the higher 50 mg dose, it makes an effective sleep aid. Use 25mg every 6 hours for mild reactions, 50mg every 6 hours for severe reactions, anxiety or at night before sleep. Diphenhydramine also comes in an ointment for skin eruptions.
- **Hydrocortisone cream (1%):** Highly useful for rashes, this cream is used for various types of dermatitis that causes redness, flakiness, itching, and thickening of the skin. It's a mild steroid which reduces inflammation and, as such, the various symptoms of allergic dermatitis, eczema, diaper rash, etc. Apply 3-4 times a day to affected area.
- **Omeprazole 20-40mg, Cimetidine 200-800mg, Ranitidine 75-150mg** (Prilosec, Tagamet, Zantac, respectively): In a situation where we may be eating things to which we're not accustomed, issues with stomach acid may arise. Antacids will calm heartburn, queasiness, and stomach upset. Calcium Carbonate (Tums) or Magnesium sulfate (Maalox) is available in tablet form that can be stockpiled. These medications are useful for acid reflux and ulcer disease.

- **Clotrimazole, Miconazole cream/powder** (Lotrimin, Monistat vaginal cream): Infections can be bacterial, but they can also be caused by fungus. Common examples of this would be athlete's foot, vaginal yeast infections, ringworm, and jock itch. These conditions will be just as common in times of trouble as they are now, if not more. Apply clotrimazole twice a day externally or miconazole once daily intravaginally. Some vaginal creams come in different strengths. In some, the whole treatment course is over in one day; in others, 3 days or a week.
- **Multivitamins:** In a societal collapse, the unavailability of a healthy balanced diet may lead to deficiencies, not just in calories but in vitamins and minerals. Vitamin C deficiency, for example, leads to Scurvy. To prevent these issues, you should have plenty of multivitamins, commercial or natural, in your medical storage.

  You won't necessarily have to take these on a daily basis; many multivitamins give you more than you need if taken daily. In most cases, you'll just excrete what your body can't absorb in urine or bowel movements. In a collapse, once a week would probably be sufficient to prevent serious problems.

The above lists just some of the over the counter drugs that may aid you in your efforts to keep your people healthy. The Physician's Desk Reference puts out a guide to OTC medications with descriptions, images, risks, benefits, dosages, and side effects. Consider this book for your survival medical library.

The best way to preserve the potency of these medications is to obtain them in pill or capsule form. The liquid versions of any of these medicines just don't remain effective as long. When storing, remember that medications should be stored in cool, dry, dark places. A medicine stored at 90 degrees will lose potency much faster than one stored at 50 degrees.

Over the counter drugs are just another tool in the medical woodshed; accumulate them as well as prescription drugs such as antibiotics. With a good stockpile, you'll have everything you need to keep it together, even if everything else falls apart.

PAIN MEDICATIONS

Old and cranky individuals, such as the authors of this book (some find it charming, we like to think), frequently complain about their various aches and pains. It stands to reason that issues associated with discomfort will be multiplied by the increased workload in survival settings. To get an idea of the kind of workload we're talking about, carry a full 5 gallon bucket of water from the nearest natural water source to your home several times. You'll see what we mean.

Sprains, strains, and worse will be part and parcel of any long-term survival situation. Therefore, those who haven't considered pain issues will be poorly prepared to deal with them. It's a good idea to have a working knowledge of the actions and uses of various pain medications.

Pain is extremely variable; it can be sharp, dull, throbbing, or numbing. Similar injuries may cause varying levels of pain from individual to individual. Pain may be a sign of something else going on that may be serious, or may simply be the result of overexertion.

If we characterize pain by the type of damage caused, we can group it into two or perhaps three categories. Pain is most commonly caused by tissue damage ("**nociceptive**" pain). The damage may be due to trauma or may be due to disease, such as tissue destruction from cancer. Even certain medical treatments such as radiation may cause tissue damage that could lead to pain. This type of pain is often described as "sharp", "stabbing", "achy", or worsens with movement ("it only hurts when I laugh").

Another category is pain caused by nerve damage ("**neuropathic**" pain). Nerves transmit pain signals from the damaged area to the brain. In damaged nerves, the sensation you feel may be very different from what you would expect. This is called a "**paresthesia**". You might feel burning where you touch ice, for example. You might even feel pain in a limb that is no longer there due to amputation.

This type of pain is more likely to be chronic than nociceptive pain from tissue damage. Besides burning, this type of pain can be described as prickling, "pins and needles", or similar to an electric shock.

The third type of pain is "**psychogenic**", or "all in the mind". Although fear, depression, anxiety, and other emotions may play a part in someone's pain, there is most often some physical origin. Although it may be tempting, don't ever dismiss a group member's complaints of pain without fully evaluating them by physical exam.

Pain relief is referred to as "**analgesia**". As pain is variable, there are many different types of drugs available that have different mechanisms of action:

Non-steroidal anti-inflammatories: Also known as **NSAIDS**, these drugs act to decrease inflammation and fever as well as pain. The most popular NSAIDs are Ibuprofen and Aspirin; Naproxen is another other NSAID available without a prescription. For quick relief from pain, the shorter acting Ibuprofen or Aspirin is superior to Naproxen. Naproxen may not have an effect until you have taken a couple of doses, but works well for long-term relief. It should be noted that long-term use of NSAIDS is associated with bleeding and other symptoms related to the gastrointestinal tract.

These drugs are especially useful in injuries associated with swelling or other signs of inflammation. There are various prescription versions of NSAIDS on the market. Are they better than the non-prescription versions? Despite pharmaceutical company claims to the contrary, there is no proven evidence that these expensive medications are much more effective. Your experience may vary.

Acetaminophen: This drug relieves pain by changing the body's sensitivity to things that cause pain (its "pain threshold"), and also lowers fever. This drug is often as effective as other NSAIDs for pain and has fewer side effects. Acetaminophen has no anti-inflammatory action, however; therefore, it may be less effective than some NSAIDs for some conditions, such as arthritis. Not for use in someone with liver disease.

Steroids: Corticosteroids exert their effect upon pain by a very strong anti-inflammatory action. The most common steroids used for inflammation are Prednisone and Cortisone. They can be taken orally or are sometimes injected directly into damaged and inflamed joints. Long-term use of steroids is associated with a whole gamut of side effects and should be avoided unless absolutely necessary. Short courses of steroids are used to deal with inflammation from many different diseases.

Muscle Relaxants: Drugs that relax tense and damaged muscles and also have a sedative effect. A common one is cyclobenzaprine (Flexeril). These are especially helpful for back strains or other injuries (such as dislocations) that cause muscle spasms.

Opioids: Narcotics are used for pain in severe cases, and act by modifying pain signal transmission in the brain. If you have had surgery, you likely have been given these medications for pain relief during recovery.

Opioids and other drugs are classified in "schedules" by the U.S. government. The lower the number, the more restricted the substance. These categories relate to the tendency to cause addiction, have adverse effects, or have no legal medical use. Besides the risk of addiction, narcotics have a strong sedative as well as analgesic effect, and must be used with extreme caution during manual work or driving a vehicle.

The categories are as follows:

SCHEDULE 1 (CLASS I) DRUGS are illegal to possess because they have no accepted medical use, high abuse potential, and clearly unsafe. Heroin is a good example.

SCHEDULE 2 (CLASS 2) DRUGS have a high potential for abuse and dependence but have an accepted medical use, although the addictive potential is high. These drugs include opioids and barbiturates. The common post-op pain med Meperidine hydrochloride (Demerol) falls into this category.

SCHEDULE 3 (CLASS 3) DRUGS have a lower potential for abuse than drugs in the first two categories, accepted medical uses, and mild to moderate addictive potential. These drugs include many steroid, hydrocodone, and codeine-based drugs. Vicodin (hydrocodone and acetaminophen) qualifies to be included here.

SCHEDULE 4 (CLASS 4) DRUGS have a lower abuse potential than Schedule 3 Drugs, accepted medical uses, and less potential for addiction. These include many sedatives and anti-anxiety agents such as Diazepam (Valium) and Alprazolam (Xanax).

SCHEDULE 5 (CLASS 5) DRUGS have a low abuse potential, accepted medical use, and little potential for addiction. These consist primarily of preparations containing limited quantities of narcotics or stimulant drugs for cough, diarrhea, or pain. Lomotil (diphenoxylate/atropine), an anti-diarrheal, is a classic example.

Anti-anxiety and anti-depressant agents: Drugs such as Xanax or Prozac may have an effect on pain by relieving "psychogenic" factors such as anxiety or depression; this allows the patient to better deal with their pain issues. They work by adjusting levels of certain chemicals in the brain tissue.

Anti-Seizure Medication: Some anti-convulsant drugs used to prevent seizures, such as Tegretol, are useful to calm damaged nerves, and are possible options for "neuropathic" pain described earlier.

Combination Drugs: Some pain medications are combinations of different drugs. Percocet, for example, is Acetaminophen and Oxycodone (an opioid). Some are used alternatively during the day; An NSAID, for example, may be prescribed between doses of an opioid.

Most of these drugs are by prescription only, and it will be unlikely that you'll be able to stockpile large quantities of any but the non-prescription versions. As such, it will be important to know about all the natural alternatives you have for pain relief

NATURAL PAIN RELIEF

In a long-term survival situation, your limited supplies of pain meds will eventually run out. This leaves you with natural alternatives from products that you can find in your environments or, perhaps, grow in your garden. Although it's true that the level of pain relief from natural substances will vary, the severity of adverse reactions are usually less, as well. Let's discuss some of these alternatives:

Capsaicin: Capsaicin is an ingredient in chili peppers that decreases pain sensation by deactivating nerve receptors on the skin. This is especially helpful for headache, muscle ache, and arthritis sufferers and those with neuropathic pain (discussed earlier). The most pain relief occurs after regular use. Commercial Capsaicin can be found on the internet.

Salicin: Salicin is the original ingredient in the first pharmaceutical, aspirin, and has been manufactured since the 19th century. Found in the bark of Willow, Aspen, and Poplar trees, Salicin can give pain relief by chewing on strips of green under bark (not outer bark) or making a tea. Like Aspirin, Salicin will help reduce fever, as well.

Arnica: A natural anti-inflammatory, this substance reduces swelling and, therefore, discomfort from injuries to joints and muscles. Normally used as a salve.

Methylsulfonyl-methane (MSM): Derived from sulfur, this substance helps slow down degeneration from joint disease, especially when combined with Glucosamine and Chondroitin. Over the course of time, osteoarthritis sufferers often report significant pain relief. It works by decreasing transmission of pain nerve impulses.

Curcumin: The herb Turmeric contains this substance, which increases the body's defense against inflammation. Less inflammation means less pain.

Ginger Root: A tea made of ginger root is thought to decrease inflammation and provide pain relief generally, but especially works to alleviate gastro-intestinal pain and cramping.

Boswellia: This herb from India produces certain acidic compounds that are touted as useful for chronic pain. It's said to decrease inflammation. Used long term, Boswellia is thought to provide as much pain relief as many NSAIDS.

S-adenosylmethionine (Sam-e): An amino acid, Sam-e seems to reduce inflammation and increase neurotransmitters in the brain that increase the sensation of well-being. Taking this supplement long-term seems to give the best likelihood of obtaining pain relief.

Hops: Isooxygene, an ingredient found in hops, has anti-inflammatory effects; some studies find it comparable to Ibuprofen. Hops may, however, cause a worsening of depressive symptoms in some patients.

Olive Oil: A compound in olive oil known as Oleocanthal works in the same way as many NSAIDS to relief discomfort. Use the "extra virgin" variety.

Quercitin: Flavinoid compounds found in various plants, such as onions, may decrease inflammation. Some researchers believe that vegetarian diets limit the amount of pain experienced by those who adhere to them. Quercitin can also be found in red wine.

Cherries: If eaten when slightly unripe, cherries have antioxidant properties. An ingredient known as Anthocyanin is thought to exert an anti-inflammatory response and may be helpful for various joint diseases.

Fish Oil: Filled with omega-3 fatty acids, fish oil reduces inflammation by releasing chemicals called prostaglandins when digested. It also blocks the production of inflammatory chemicals in the body. Commonly recommended in those with coronary artery disease, larger doses (2000-4000mg/day) are shown in several studies to give significant pain relief from various joint and immune disorders. Be aware that high doses of fish oil can thin the blood.

Many of the above substances are available in supplements that you can find online, many times in combination with each other. The results with regards to pain relief will be variable from patient to patient.

What if your patient has more than slight pain? For major discomfort, here are some well-known (*and illegal*) substances produced from natural substances:

Opium: Derived from the seed pods of poppies, this highly addictive compound exerts significant pain-killing effects. This plant is the source of popular heavy pain medicines such as morphine and codeine. Heroin is another very potent product of the poppy plant.

Cocaine: A well-known derivative of the coca plant from South America, cocaine has natural anesthetic properties and was a popular painkiller for dental procedures not so very long ago. Some local anesthetics like Novocain and Procaine mimic the effect if cocaine.

Curare: Another South American plant, the Pareira vine, contains the compound Curare, which was used by natives on their arrow and spear points to paralyze their prey. This drug is still used today by anesthesiologists to paralyze respiratory action so that they can more easily perform intubations for surgery. Without medications to reverse the effect, the paralysis effect leads to death.

Besides all of the above, consider alternative methods such as aromatherapy, massage, inhalation therapy, yoga, and acupuncture. These options have been used for treatment of pain and some report significant relief.

Be open to every strategy available to deal with a medical issue; there are a lot of tools in the medical woodshed, and you should take advantage of any method that might keep your family healthy in uncertain times.

STOCKPILING MEDICATIONS

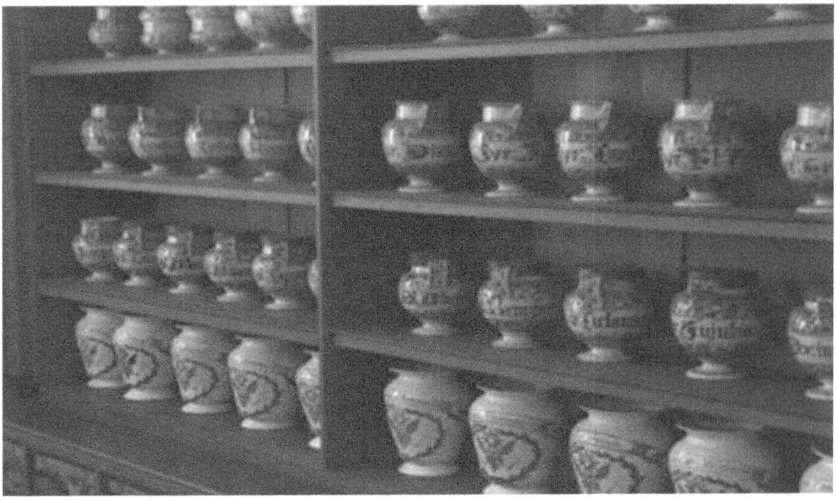

Accumulating medications for a possible collapse may be simple when it comes to ibuprofen and other non-prescription drugs. It will be a major issue, however, for those who need to stockpile prescription medicines. Most people don't have a relationship with a physician who would accommodate a request for large quantities of any medicine. Antibiotics are one example of medications that will be very useful, but very scarce, off the grid.

The inability to obtain antibiotic supplies may cost some poorly prepared individuals their lives in a survival situation. There will be a much larger incidence of infection when people have to fend for themselves and are injured as a result. Any strenuous activities performed that aren't routine in normal times can lead to injuries that break the skin. These wounds will, very likely, be dirty. Within a relatively short time, they'll begin to show signs of infection in the form of redness, heat, and swelling.

Treatment of such infections at an early stage improves the chance that they will heal quickly and completely. However, many rugged individualists are most likely to "tough it out" until their condition worsens and the infection spreads to their blood. The availability of antibiotics would allow the possibility of dealing with the issue before it becomes life-threatening.

The following advice is contrary to standard medical practice, and is a strategy, like many in this book, that is appropriate only when help isn't coming. If there are modern medical resources available to you, seek them out.

Antibiotic Options

Small amounts of antibiotics can be obtained by anyone willing to tell their doctor that they are going out of the country and would like to avoid "Travelers' Diarrhea". If you choose this route, ask them for Tamiflu for viral illness before every flu season, and Amoxicillin, Doxycycline, and Metronidazole to treat bacterial disease caused by skin infections and contaminated water.

This approach is fine for one or two courses of therapy, but a long term alternative is required for the survival caregiver to have enough antibiotics to protect a family or survival group. Concerns about avoidable infection-related death and disease led us to what we believe is a viable option: aquarium and avian antibiotics.

For many years, we have kept aquarium fish and, in ponds, tilapia. We also have parrots as pets. After years of using aquatic medicines on fish and avian medicines on birds, we decided to evaluate these drugs for their potential use in collapse situations. They seemed to be good candidates: All were widely available, available in different varieties, and didn't require a medical license to obtain them.

A close inspection of the ingredients found exactly one: the drug itself, identical to those obtained by prescription at the local pharmacy. If the bottle says FISH-MOX, for example, the sole ingredient is Amoxicillin, which is an antibiotic commonly used in humans. Unless they're listed on the bottle, there are no additional chemicals to makes your scales shiny or your fins longer.

You might be skeptical about considering the use of aquarium antibiotics for humans in a collapse. Those things are for fish, aren't they? Yet, a number of them come in dosages that correspond to pediatric or adult human dosages. Indeed, a surprising number *only* come in human dosages.

The question became: Why should a one inch guppy require the same dosage of, say, Amoxicillin (aquatic version: FISH-MOX FORTE) as a 180 pound adult human? We were told that it was due to the dilution of the drug in water. However, there were few instructions that tell you how much to put in a ½ gallon fishbowl as opposed to a 200 gallon aquarium.

Finally, the "acid test" was to look at the pills or capsules themselves. The aquatic or avian drug had to be identical to that found in bottles of the corresponding human medicine. For example, when we opened a bottle of FISH-MOX FORTE 500 mg and a bottle of Human Amoxicillin 500mg (DAVA pharmaceuticals), we found:

- Human Amoxicillin: Red and Pink Capsule, with the letters and numbers WC 731 on it.
- FISH-MOX FORTE: Red and Pink Capsule with the letters and numbers WC 731 on it.

Logically, then, it makes sense to believe that they are manufactured in the same way that human antibiotics are. Further, it is our opinion that they are probably from the same batches; some go to human pharmacies and some go to veterinary pharmacies.

This is not to imply that all antibiotic medications meet my criteria. Many cat, dog, and livestock antibiotics contain additives that might cause ill effects on a human being. Look only for those veterinary drugs that have the antibiotic as the *sole* ingredient.

Here is a list of the products that meet our criteria and that we believe will be beneficial to have as supplies and are discussed in the next section:

- FISH-MOX (Amoxicillin 250mg)
- FISH_MOX FORTE (Amoxicillin 500mg)
- FISH-CILLIN (Ampicillin 250mg)
- FISH-FLEX (Cephalexin 250mg)
- FISH-FLEX FORTE (Cephalexin 500mg)
- FISH-ZOLE (Metronidazole 250mg)
- FISH-PEN (Penicillin 250mg)
- FISH-PEN FORTE (Penicillin 500mg)
- FISH-CYCLINE (Tetracycline 250mg)

- FISH-FLOX (Ciprofloxacin 250mg)
- FISH-CIN (Clindamycin 150mg)
- BIRD BIOTIC (Doxycycline 100mg) - used in birds but the antibiotic is the sole ingredient
- BIRD SULFA (Sulfamethoxazole 400mg/Trimethoprin 80mg), also used in birds

These medications are available without a prescription from veterinary supply stores and online sites everywhere. They come in lots of 30 to100 tablets for less than the same prescription medication at the local pharmacy. If you so desired, you could get as much as you need to stockpile for use in austere settings. These quantities would be close to impossible to obtain even from the most sympathetic physician.

Of course, anyone could be allergic to one or another of these antibiotics, but it would be a very rare individual who would be allergic to all of them. There is a 10% chance for cross-reactivity between Penicillin drugs and cephalexin (Keflex). If you are allergic to penicillin, you could also be allergic to Keflex. For those who can't take penicillin, there are suitable safe alternatives. Any of the antibiotics below should not cause a reaction in a patient allergic to Penicillin-family drugs:

- Doxycycline
- Metronidazole
- Tetracycline
- Ciprofloxacin
- Clindamycin
- Sulfa Drugs

This one additional fact: We have personally used some (not all) of these antibiotics on our own persons without any ill effects. Whenever we have used them, their effects have been undistinguishable from human antibiotics.

Having said this, we do *not* recommend self-treatment in any circumstance that does not involve the complete long-term loss of access to modern medical care. This is a strategy to save lives in a post-calamity scenario only.

Finding Out More

Although you might think that any antibiotic will work to cure any disease, specific antibiotics are used at specific doses for specific illnesses. The exact dosage of each and every medication in existence is well beyond the scope of this handbook. It's important, however, to have as much information as possible on medications that you plan to store.

This information is available in the Physician's Desk Reference. This book comes out yearly and has just about every bit of information that exists on a particular drug, including photos. Online sources such as drugs.com or rxlist.com are also useful, but you are going to want a hard copy for your library, as a disaster might possibly affect the internet.

The Desk Reference has versions that list medications that require prescriptions as well as those that do not. Under each medicine, you will find the "**indications**", which are the medical conditions that the drug is used for. Also listed will be the dosages, risks, side effects, and even how the medicine works in the body. It's okay to get last year's book; the information doesn't change a great deal from one year to the next.

Using Antibiotics Wisely

Antibiotics are essential tools for success in long-term survival. Unfortunately, the government, the livestock industry, and some physicians and patients are fostering widespread resistance to many of the standard drugs. More than 2 million diagnosed cases of antibiotic resistance were reported in the United States in 2013, leading to 23,000 deaths and costing 30 billion dollars.

This doesn't mean that that antibiotics aren't useful, especially in survival scenarios. In situations where modern medical care isn't available, they will prevent many avoidable deaths. You should have a good supply of these drugs in your storage.

If you use antibiotics for every minor ailment that comes along, however, you will run out very quickly and may contribute to an epidemic of antibiotic resistance caused by overuse. In survival, you are the medical quartermaster; you'll want to wisely dispense that limited and, yes, precious supply of life-saving drugs. You must walk a fine line between observant patient management (doing nothing) and aggressive management (doing everything).

Liberal use of antibiotics is a poor strategy for a few reasons:

- Overuse can foster the spread of resistant bacteria. In the 2011 salmonella outbreak, millions of pounds of antibiotic-laden turkey meat were discarded after 100 people were sent to the hospital with severe diarrheal disease. The food industry is responsible for 80% of the antibiotic use in the U.S. This is not used to treat sick livestock, but to make healthy livestock grow faster and get to market sooner.

  Consider supporting farmers who raise antibiotic-free livestock; this will decrease the further development of resistant bacteria, and, thus, the antibiotics you've stockpiled will be more effective.
- Potential allergic reactions may occur that could lead to anaphylactic shock. Frequent exposure to antibiotics increases the likelihood of developing an allergy to one or more of them.
- Many infections, including most respiratory infections, are viral; antibiotics are completely ineffective in treating them.
- Lastly, being trigger-happy with antibiotics may make diagnosing an illness more difficult. If you give antibiotics before you're sure what medical problem you're actually dealing with, you might "mask" the condition. In other words, symptoms could be temporarily improved that would have helped you figure out what disease your patient has. This could cost you valuable time in determining the correct treatment.

You can see that judicious use of antibiotics, under your close supervision, is necessary to fully utilize their benefits. In survival settings, discourage your group members from using these drugs without first consulting you. In normal times, seek a qualified medical professional.

It should be noted that the director of the CDC (Centers for Disease Control) has advocated an increased "stewardship" of veterinary antibiotics due to the epidemic of antibiotic resistance. Aquarium and avian antibiotics may, one day, be removed from availability to the average person. Consider stockpiling these now while you can.

Other Medicines

Many other important medications for those with chronic medical issues, such as heart disease or high blood pressure, will require a prescription. These medications are not available in aquarium supply houses, so how can you work to stockpile them?

Many health insurance plans allow you to come a little early each month to fill your prescriptions. If this is the case, you should always go on the first day possible. Over time, you will accumulate a supply.

A much more controversial strategy is asking your physician to prescribe a higher dose than the amount you usually take. Many drugs come in different dosages. If your medicine is a 20 milligram dosage, for example, you might ask your doctor to prescribe the 40 mg dosage. You would then cut the medication in half; take your normal dosage and store the other half of the pill. It's very important to assure your physician that you will continue to follow their medical advice and not take more medicine than is appropriate for your condition. Most doctors, honestly, will not take kindly to the request.

Those traveling into areas with questionable water or sanitation issues should ask their physician for preventative antibiotics to take with them. Also, every flu season you should consider asking your doctor for antiviral meds like Oseltamivir (Tamiflu). These medicines are only effective if used in the first 48 hours of symptoms.

Consider having a serious and honest discussion with your healthcare provider. Describe your concerns about not having needed medications in a disaster situation. You don't have to describe the disaster as a complete societal collapse; any catastrophe could leave you without access to your doctor for an extended period. A letter at the end of this book may help if given to your local physician. A printer-friendly version can be found on the survival medicine website www.doomandbloom.net.

Alternative therapies such as herbal supplements and essential oils should be stockpiled as well. Honey, onion, silver, and garlic have known antibacterial actions; be sure to integrate all medical options, traditional and alternative, and use every tool at your disposal to keep your community healthy. If you don't, you're fighting with one hand tied behind your back.

Remember that essential oils and other traditional medicines will eventually run out in a long term collapse. Begin your medicinal garden now and get experience with the use of these beneficial plants. There is a learning curve, and you don't want to go through it in tough times. Basic medicinal gardening is discussed earlier in this book.

If we ever find ourselves without modern medical care, we will have to improvise medical strategies that we perhaps might be reluctant to consider today. Without hospitals, it will be up to the medic to nip infections in the bud. That responsibility will be difficult to carry out without the weapons to fight disease. Accumulate equipment and medications and never ignore avenues that may help you gain access to them.

HOW TO USE ANTIBIOTICS

There are many antibiotics, but what antibiotics accessible to the average person would be good additions to your medical storage? When do you use a particular drug? In this section, we'll discuss antibiotics (all available in veterinary form without a prescription) that you will want in your medical arsenal:

• Amoxicillin	250mg/500mg (FISH-MOX, FISH-MOX FORTE)
• Ciprofloxacin	250mg/500mg (FISH-FLOX, FISH-FLOX FORTE)
• Cephalexin	250mg/500mg (FISH-FLEX, FISH-FLEX FORTE)
• Metronidazole	250mg (FISH-ZOLE)
• Doxycycline	100mg (BIRD-BIOTIC)
• Ampicillin	250mg/500mg (FISH-CILLIN, FISH-CILLIN FORTE)
• Sulfamethoxazole	400mg/Trimethoprim 80mg (BIRD-SULFA)
• Clindamycin	150mg (FISH-CIN)
• Azithromycin	250mg (Aquatic Azithromycin)
• Erythromycin	250mg/500mg (FISH-MYCIN)

There are various others that you can choose, but these selections will give you the opportunity to treat many illnesses and have enough variety so that even those with Penicillin allergies will have options.

Other than allergies, there are other times when a particular antibiotic (or other drug) should not be used. Many medications, for example, are not recommended for use during pregnancy. Sometimes, this is because lab studies have shown birth defects in animal fetuses exposed to the drug. Other times, it is because no studies on pregnant women or animals have yet been performed.

There are additional circumstances where a particular medication should not be used. There may be warnings about mixing one drug with another because there may be a dangerous interaction between them. For example, taking the antibiotic Metronidazole (Fish-Zole) and drinking alcohol will make you vomit. Some drug interactions may cause the effect of one of them to become stronger or weaker. A certain medicine, for example, may decrease the effect of another when taken together. Also, some drugs should be avoided due to their side effects.

It should be noted that each physician may use a specific antibiotic for different purposes or to treat different infections. There is always some variance when you receive opinions about treatment from different caregivers. It's certain that some will not agree with everything you see written in this book.

Amoxicillin

Let's discuss how to approach the use of antibiotics by using an example. Amoxicillin (veterinary equivalent: FISH-MOX, FISH-MOX FORTE, AQUA-MOX): comes in 250mg and 500mg doses, usually taken 3 times a day. Amoxicillin is the most popular antibiotic prescribed to children, usually in liquid form. It is more versatile and better absorbed and tolerated than the older Pencillins, and is acceptable for use during pregnancy. Ampicillin (Fish-Cillin) and cephalexin (Fish-Flex) are related drugs.

Amoxicillin may be used for the following diseases:

- Anthrax (Prevention or treatment of the cutaneous variety)
- Chlamydia (sexually transmitted infection)
- Urinary Tract (bladder or kidney infections)
- Helicobacter pylori (causes stomach ulcers)
- Lyme Disease (transmitted by ticks)
- Otitis Media (middle ear infection)
- Pneumonia (lung infection)
- Sinusitis (sinus infection)
- Skin or Soft Tissue Infection (cellulitis, boils)
- Actinomycosis (causes abscesses in humans and livestock)
- Bronchitis (airway infection)
- Tonsillitis/Pharyngitis (Strep throat)

You can see that Amoxicillin is a versatile drug. It is even safe for use during pregnancy, but all of the above is a lot of information. How do you determine what dose and frequency would be appropriate for which individual? Let's take an example: Otitis media is a common ear infection often seen in children. Amoxicillin is one of the "**drugs of choice**" for this condition. That is, it is recommended to be used *first* when you make this particular diagnosis. The drug of choice for a particular ailment can change, over time, based on new scientific evidence.

Before administering this medication, however, you would want to determine that your patient is not allergic to Amoxicillin. The most common form of allergy would appear as a rash, but diarrhea, itchiness, and even respiratory difficulty could also manifest. If you see any of these symptoms, you should discontinue your treatment and look for other options. Antibiotics such as Azithromycin (Aquatic Azithromycin) or Sulfamethoxazole/Trimethoprim (Bird-Sulfa) could be a "**second-line**" solution in this case. Remember that some "allergies" are actually just a side effect that is commonly seen in anyone who takes the medicine, as previously discussed in this book.

Once you have identified Amoxicillin as your treatment of choice to treat your patient's ear infection, you will want to determine the dosage. As Otitis Media often occurs in children, you might have to break a tablet in half or open the capsule to separate out a portion that would be appropriate. For Amoxicillin, you would give 20-50mg per kilogram (2.2 pounds) of body weight (20-30mg/kg for infants less than four months old). This formula would be useful if you have to give the drug to a toddler less than 30 pounds.

A common older child's dosage would be 250mg and a common maximum dosage for adults would be 500 mg three times a day. Luckily (or by design), these dosages are exactly how the commercially-made aquatic medication comes in the bottle. Take this dosage orally 3 times a day for 10 to 14 days (twice a day for infants). .

If your child is too small to swallow a pill whole, you could make a mixture with water (called a "**suspension**"). To make a liquid suspension, crush a tablet or empty a capsule into a small glass of water and drink it; then, fill the glass again and drink that (particles may adhere to the walls of the glass). You can add some flavoring to make it taste better.

Do not chew or make a suspension out of time-released capsules of any medication; you will wind up losing some of the gradual release effect and perhaps get too much into your system at once. These medications should be plainly marked "Time-Released".

You will probably see improvement within 3 days, but don't be tempted to stop the antibiotic therapy until you're done with the entire 10-14 days. Sometimes, you'll kill most of the bacteria but some colonies may persist and multiply if you prematurely end the treatment. This is one way that antibiotic resistance develops. In a long-term survival situation, however, you might be down to your last few pills and have to make some tough decisions.

Ciprofloxacin

A useful option is Ciprofloxacin (veterinary equivalent: FISH-FLOX). Ciprofloxacin is an antibiotic in the fluoroquinolone family. It kills bacteria by inhibiting the reproduction of DNA and bacterial proteins. This drug usually comes in 250mg and 500mg doses.

Ciprofloxacin (brand name Cipro) can be used for the following conditions:

- Urinary tract infections, especially in females
- Prostate infections
- Pneumonia and other lower respiratory infections
- Acute sinusitis
- Skin infections (cellulitis)
- Bone and joint infections
- Infectious diarrhea
- Typhoid fever caused by Salmonella
- Inhalational Anthrax (as opposed to skin Anthrax)

In most cases, you should give 500mg twice a day for 7-14 days, with the exception of bone and joint infections (4-6 weeks) and Anthrax

(60 days). You can get away with 250mg doses for 3 days for most mild urinary infections. Generally, you would want to continue the medication for 2 days after improvement is noted.

Unlike Amoxicillin, many antibiotics may not be safe for use in certain situations. For example, Ciprofoxacin has not been approved for use during pregnancy. It is, however, acceptable for those allergic to Penicillin.

Taking Cipro is not without risks. Among its side effects, Cipro has been reported to occasionally cause weakness in muscles and tendons. It may also cause joint and muscle complications in children, so it is restricted in pediatric use only to the following conditions:

- Urinary tract infections due to E. coli (the most common type)
- Inhalational anthrax

In children, the dosage is measured by multiplying 10mg by the weight in kilograms (1 kg = 2.2 lbs.). The maximum dose should not exceed 400mg total twice a day, even if the child weighs more than 100 pounds. Ciprofloxacin should be taken with 8 ounces of water.

Cephalexin

Cephalexin (veterinary equivalent: Fish-Flex, Fish-Flex Forte) is an antibiotic in the Cephalosporin family. It is different from but cross-reactive with the Penicillin family; 10% or more of Penicillin-allergic patients will also be allergic to Cephalosporins.

Cephalexin works by interfering with the bacteria's cell wall formation. This causes the defective wall to rupture, killing the bacteria. This antibiotic is useful in the treatment of:

- Cystitis (bladder infections)
- Otitis media (ear infections)
- Pharyngitis (sore throats)
- Skin or soft tissue infection (cellulitis))
- Osteomyelitis (infections of bone and marrow)
- Prostatitis (prostate infections)

- Pyelonephritis (kidney infections)
- Upper respiratory tract infections caused by bacteria

Cephalexin is also used as a preventative before surgical procedures in people who are at risk for heart valve infections. It is one of the few antibiotics which is thought to be safe to use during pregnancy.

Cephalexin is marketed in the U.S. under the name Keflex.

To use this medication, you would normally give 250mg (Fish-Flex) or 500mg (Fish-Flex Forte) every 6 hours for 7-14 days. Severe bacterial infections may require an additional week of treatment. Infections of the bone (osteomyelitis) are particularly dangerous and require 4-6 weeks of therapy.

Pediatric dosages are calculated using 12.5 to 25 mg per kilogram of body weight orally every 6-12 hours (never exceed adult dosages).

Doxycycline

Another useful antibiotic in a collapse would be Doxycycline (veterinary equivalent: Bird-Biotic). Doxycycline is a member of the Tetracycline family, and is also acceptable in patients allergic to Penicillin. It prevents reproduction by inhibiting the manufacture of bacterial proteins. Doxycycline is marketed under various names, including Vibramycin and Vibra-Tabs. The veterinary version is found in capsules and powder packets of 100 mg.

Doxycycline is an extraordinarily versatile drug. Indications for its usage include the following:

- E. coli, Shigella and Enterobacter infections as causes of diarrheal disease
- Chlamydia (sexually transmitted disease)
- Lyme disease (tick-borne)
- Rocky Mountain spotted fever (tick-borne)
- Anthrax
- Cholera
- Plague (from fleas on rats)

- Gum disease (gingivitis)
- Folliculitis (boils)
- Acne and other inflammatory skin diseases, such as hidradenitis (seen in armpits and groins)
- Some lower respiratory tract (pneumonia)
- Some urinary tract infections
- Upper respiratory infections caused by Strep
- Methicillin-resistant Staph (MRSA) infections
- Malaria (prevention)
- Some parasitic worm infections (kills bacteria in their gut needed to survive)

In the case of Rocky Mountain spotted fever, doxycycline is indicated even for use in children. Otherwise, doxycycline is not meant for those under the age of eight years. It has not been approved for use during pregnancy.

The recommended Doxycycline dosage for most types of bacterial infections in adults is 100 mg to 200 mg per day for 7-14 days. For chronic (long-term) or more serious infections, treatment can be carried out for a longer time. When appropriate, children will receive 1-2 mg per pound of body weight per day. For Anthrax, the treatment should be prolonged to 60 days. As prevention against malaria, adults should use 100 mg per day.

You may have read that drugs in the tetracycline family have been reported to cause kidney toxicity. Tetracycline incited considerable concern due to this in the 1960s, shortly after its introduction. People, particularly children, developed kidney dysfunction after receiving outdated drugs.

In these cases, the cause was found to be due to a degradation product of the drug called anhydro-4-epitetracycline. This no longer seems to be an issue after a new formulation substituted citric acid for lactose, at least according to a 1991 report from the World Health Organization. Kidney issues are rare in patients who take doxycycline as long as they started out with normal renal function.

Although antibiotics may be helpful in diarrheal disease, always start with hydration and symptomatic relief unless confronted with very high fevers or failure to improve over time. The problem is that one of the most common side effects of antibiotics is...diarrhea!

Azithromycin

Another antibiotic available in an aquatic equivalent is Azithromycin 250mg. Azithromycin is a member of the macrolide (Erythromycin) family and can be found as "Aquatic Azithromycin". It works by stopping the growth and multiplication of bacteria. We prefer it to aquatic Erythromycin powder (Fish-Mycin) as Azithromycin is available in a capsule; thus, it is more easily administered.

Azithromycin can be used to treat various types of:

- Bronchitis
- Pneumonia
- Ear infections
- Skin infections
- Throat infections (some)
- Sinusitis
- Tonsillitis
- Typhoid fever
- Gonorrhea
- Chlamydia
- Whooping cough
- Lyme Disease (early stages)

Azithromycin is taken 250mg or 500mg once daily for a relatively short course of treatment (usually five days). The first dose is often a "double dose," twice the strength of the remaining doses. This method of taking the drug is packaged in the U.S. as "Z-Pak".

For acute bacterial sinusitis, azithromycin may be taken once daily for three days. If you are taking the 500mg dosage and have side effects such as nausea and vomiting, diarrhea, or dizziness, drop down to 250 mg. Azithromycin is not known to cause problems in pregnant patients and can be used by those allergic to Penicillin.

Clindamycin

Clindamycin (Fish-Cin) is part of the family of drugs called Lincomycin antibiotics. It, like Azithromycin, works by slowing or stopping the growth of bacteria. It works best on bacteria that are **anaerobic**, which means that they thrive in the absence of oxygen. It can be used to treat:

- Acne
- Dental infections
- Soft tissue infections (cellulitis)
- Peritonitis (inflammation of the abdominal lining)
- Pneumonia and lung abscesses
- Uterine infections (such as after miscarriage or childbirth)
- Blood infections (septicemia, although IV meds are more effective)
- Pelvic infections
- MRSA (Methicillin-resistant Staph. Aureus infections)
- Parasitic infections (Malaria, Toxoplasmosis)
- Anthrax

Clindamycin is given in 150 mg or 300 mg doses every 6 hours with a glass of water. It should be used with caution in individuals with a history of gastrointestinal disease as it can cause diarrhea during treatment. Sometimes, a very serious "**colitis**" (infection of the intestine) can develop.

This drug is, like Azithromycin, pregnancy category B, which means that no ill effects have been determined in animal studies. With most drugs, testing cannot be done ethically on pregnant humans, so very few drugs are willing to say that they are completely safe during pregnancy.

Clindamycin is acceptable for use in patients with Penicillin allergies. This is not to say that you might not have a different allergy to clindamycin or any other antibiotic.

Metronidazole

Metronidazole (aquatic equivalent: Fish-Zole) 250mg is an antibiotic in the Nitroimidazole family that is used primarily to treat infections caused by anaerobic bacteria and protozoa.

"**Anaerobes**" are bacteria that do not depend on oxygen to live. "**Protozoa**" are single-cell organisms with animal-like behavior. Many can propel themselves from place to place by the means of a tail-like "hair" called a "flagellum" that they whip around to move randomly in water.

Metronidazole works by blocking some of the functions within bacteria and protozoa, resulting in their death. It is better known by the U.S. brand name Flagyl and usually comes in 250mg and 500mg tablets. Metronidazole is used in the treatment of these bacterial diseases:

- Diverticulitis (an intestinal infection seen in older individuals)
- Peritonitis (infection due to ruptured appendix, etc.)
- Some pneumonias
- Diabetic foot ulcer infections
- Meningitis (infection of the spinal cord and brain lining)
- Bone and joint infections
- Colitis due to Clostridia bacteria (sometimes caused by taking Clindamycin!)
- Endocarditis (heart infection)
- Bacterial vaginosis (common vaginal infection)
- Pelvic inflammatory disease (infection in women which can lead to abscesses and infertility) – used in combination with other antibiotics
- Uterine infections (especially after childbirth and miscarriage)
- Dental infections (sometimes in combination with amoxicillin)
- H. pylori infections (causes peptic ulcers)
- Some skin infections

And these protozoal infections:

- Amoebiasis: dysentery caused by Entamoeba species (contaminated water/food)
- Giardiasis: infection of the small intestine caused by Giardia species (contaminated water/food)
- Trichomoniasis: Sexually-transmitted vaginal infection with greenish-gray, frothy, foul discharge.

Amoebiasis and Giardiasis can be caught from drinking what appears to be the purest mountain stream water. Never fail to sterilize all water, regardless of source, before drinking it.

Metronidazole is used in different dosages to treat different illnesses. Here are the dosages and frequency of administration for several:

- Amoebic dysentery: 750 mg orally 3 times daily for 5-10 days. For children, give 35 to 50 mg/kg/day orally in 3 divided doses for 10 days (no more than adult dosage, of course, regardless of weight).
- Anaerobic infections (various): 7.5 mg/kg orally every 6 hours not to exceed 4 grams daily.
- Clostridia infections: 250-500 mg orally 4 times daily or 500-750 orally 3 times daily.
- Giardia: 250 mg orally three times daily for 5 days. For children give 15 mg/kg/day orally in 3 divided doses (no more than adult dosage regardless of weight).
- Helicobacter pylori (ulcer disease): 500-750mg twice daily for several days in combination with antacids like Prilosec (Omeprazole).
- Pelvic inflammatory disease (PID): 500 mg orally twice daily for 14 days in combination with other drugs, perhaps doxycycline or azithromycin.
- Bacterial Vaginosis: 500mg twice daily for 7 days
- Vaginal Trichomoniasis: 2 g single dose (4 500mg tablets at once) or 1 g twice total.

Like all antibiotics, Metronidazole has side effects which you can review by picking up a Physician's Desk Reference or going to drugs.com or rxlist.com. One particular side effect has to do with alcohol: Drinking alcohol while on Metronidazole will very likely make you vomit. Metronidazole should not be used in pregnancy but is acceptable in those allergic to Penicillin.

Sulfa Drugs

Sulfamethoxazole 400mg/Trimethoprim 80mg (avian equivalent: Bird-Sulfa) is a combination of two medications in the Sulfonamide family.

This drug is well-known as its U.S. brand names Bactrim and Septra. Our British friends may recognize it by the name Co-Trimoxazole.

Sulfamethoxazole acts as an inhibitor of an important bacterial enzyme. Trimethoprim interferes with the production of folic acid in bacteria, which is necessary to produce DNA. The two antibiotics together are stronger in their effect than alone (at least in laboratory studies), so are used together.

Sulfamethoxazole 400mg/Trimethoprim 80mg is effective in the treatment of the following:

- Some upper and lower respiratory infections (chronic bronchitis and pneumonia)
- Kidney and bladder infections
- Ear infections
- Intestinal infections caused by E. coli and Shigella bacteria (a cause of dysentery)
- Skin and wound infections
- Traveler's diarrhea
- Acne

The usual dosage is one tablet twice a day for most of the above conditions in adults for 10 days (less in traveler's diarrhea).

The recommended dose for pediatric patients with urinary tract infections or acute otitis media is 8 mg/kg trimethoprim and 40 mg/kg sulfamethoxazole per 24 hours, given in two divided doses every 12 hours for 10 days. 1 kilogram equals 2.2 pounds. This medication should not be used in infants 2 months old or younger.

In rat studies, the use of this drug was seen to cause birth defects; therefore, it is not used during pregnancy. Sulfamethoxazole 400mg/Trimethoprim 80mg is well known to cause allergic reactions in some individuals. These reactions to sulfa drugs are almost as common as Penicillin allergies.

Ampicillin

Ampicillin (veterinary equivalent: Fish-Cillin) is a member of the penicillin family. It interferes with the ability of bacteria to make cell walls. Ampicillin can be used to treat a number of infections:

- Respiratory tract Infections (bacterial bronchitis)
- Throat infections
- Ear infections
- Cellulitis
- Meningitis
- Urinary tract infections
- Typhoid fever (Salmonella)
- Dysentery (Shigella)

Ampicillin is usually given to adults in doses of 500mg 4 times a day for 7-10 days. A common pediatric dosage formula is 6.25 to 12.5 mg/kg every 6 hours (maximum 2 to 3 g/day).

Ampicillin is acceptable for use during pregnancy. Like most antibiotics, it has stronger effect in intravenous form, and can be used IV in some cases of septicemia (blood infection) and endocarditis (heart infection).

Erythromycin

Erythromycin (Fish-Mycin) belongs to the same family of antibiotics as Azithromycin. Macrolide antibiotics retard the growth of bacteria by lowering the production of proteins needed to survive. Erythromycin will work for:

- Intestinal infections like Campylobacter (previously discussed)
- Upper and lower respiratory infections
- Pharyngitis
- Skin Infections (cellulitis)
- Ear Infections
- Sexually Transmitted Diseases, such as: Chlamydia, Syphilis, Gonorrhea, Chancroid, and Lymphogranuloma Venereum.

- Whooping Cough
- Heart infections (endocarditis)

The standard adult dosage is 500 mg every 4 hours for 7-14 days. Pediatric dosages are calculated by weight: 50 mg/kg/day divided into four 6-hour doses for 2 weeks.

Although Erythromycin is acceptable for both pregnant women and those allergic to Penicillin, many drugs will interact with it. These include blood pressure meds, cholesterol-lowering meds, and other antibiotics.

Anti-Fungal Drugs

Not every medication you use to treat infection are meant to kill bacteria. Viruses and fungi can also cause infection, and you will have to stockpile drugs that are effective against these organisms. Common fungal infections like ringworm, athlete's foot, and jock itch will be rampant in wet climates or in situations where you might not be able to change socks or underwear routinely.

Clotrimazole (Lotrimin) is a good choice as an antifungal, as it comes in cream or powder, and doesn't require a prescription. Medications like **Miconazole** (Monistat) would be useful for vaginal yeast infections. Oral antifungals exist as well, such as **Fluconazole** (Diflucan). These drugs may be more convenient than creams or powders, but require a prescription.

Like some antibiotics, some anti-fungal drugs come in veterinary equivalents. **Ketoconazole** is a common anti-fungal that can be obtained in its aquatic version (Fish-Fungus 200mg). It kills certain fungi by interfering with the formation of the fungal cell membrane.

Ketoconazole tablets are indicated for the treatment of **systemic** (throughout the body) fungal infections. It is only used for local infections when severe and other anti-fungal medications fail due to the risk of liver malfunction and other adverse effects. In other words, although you might find Ketoconazole in veterinary form, stick with the other anti-fungals if at all possible. Ketoconazole is used for:

- Systemic candidiasis (same fungus as in vaginal infections)
- Oral thrush (mouth infections, usually in infants)
- Candiduria (fungus in the urine)
- Fungal lung infections (various species)

Anti-Viral Drugs

Finally, antiviral drugs would be useful to have. Many infections, especially respiratory, that we assume to be bacterial in nature are more likely to be viral. Antibiotics have no significant effect on viruses; despite this, many patients will demand an antibiotic prescription from their doctors as soon as they feel the first symptom. The problems that arise from overuse are discussed earlier in this section.

One of the most popular anti-viral influenza drugs is called Tamiflu **(oseltamvir)**. Tamiflu gives effective relief against symptoms of influenza and decreases the amount of time your patient is ill. It can be taken upon exposure to the infection, even before symptoms have begun.

If Tamiflu is taken once exposed and before symptoms occur, it might even prevent the illness altogether. This may be a wise strategy if family members are ill with the flu and you haven't gotten it yet.

Taken in the first 48 hours of a flu-like syndrome, Tamiflu may decrease the severity and duration of symptoms. Unfortunately, if taken after this time, it won't have much effect. You should know that Tamiflu is specifically meant to treat influenza, and won't help in other viral illnesses, such as Herpes or Ebola.

The adult preventative dose of Tamiflu is 75 mg once daily for 10 days. To treat those already ill, take 75mg twice a day for 5 days. For children, follow the above regimen in the following doses:

- 15 kg (33 lbs.) or less: 30 mg dosage
- 16-23 kg (34-51 lbs.): 45 mg dosage
- 24-40 kg (52-88 lbs.): 60 mg dosage
- Above 40 kg (89 lbs. or more): adult dosage

Other anti-viral drugs such as Acyclovir or Famcyclovir are usually used to treat common herpes-virus related conditions, such as:

Shingles (painful skin eruption)
Adults: 800 mg every 4 hours for 5 to 10 days
Children under 40 kg (and older than 2 years):
20 mg/kg 4 times a day for 5 days.

Varicella (chickenpox)
Adults: 800 mg 4 times a day for 5 days
Children under 40 kg (and older than 2 years):
20 mg/kg orally 4 times a day for 5 days

Oral/genital Herpes (painful cold or genital sores)
Adults: 200 mg every 4 hours for 10 days or 400 mg 3 times a day for 7-10 days
Children under 40 kg (and older than 2 years):
40 to 80 mg/kg a day in 3 to 4 divided doses for 5 to 10 days. Max dose: 1 g per day

Don't forget that natural products such as Garlic and Honey may have significant properties against certain infections. Garlic, for example, is thought to have anti-bacterial, anti-fungal, and anti-viral effects. Many people report significant antibacterial/antiviral effects with colloidal silver, as well. Before there were antibiotics, there silver was used to prevent infection; it is still used in some topical creams.

EXPIRATION DATES

The diligent medic will be successful in accumulating various medicines that will help keep his family healthy. What happens, however, when all these stockpiled drugs pass their expiration date"? The short answer is: In most cases, not very much.

Since 1979, pharmaceutical companies have been required to place expiration dates on their medications. But what does that date signify? Officially, the expiration date is the last day that the company will certify that their drug is fully potent. Some believe this means that the medicine in question is useless or in some way dangerous after that date.

This is a false assumption, at least in the vast majority of those medicines that come in pill or capsule form. Expiration dates pertain to the strength of the medication and not whether it causes strange or dangerous effects afterward. You will not grow a third eye in the middle of your forehead or be poisoned simply because a drug has "expired".

An exception to this was thought to be tetracycline. A report of kidney damage after taking expired tetracycline was published in the Journal of the American Medical Association in 1963. Since that time, the formulation for the drug has changed, and we could find no similar recent reports in the medical literature.

We did, however, find a study that used expired Doxycycline, a member of the Tetracycline family, in dialysis patients without ill effects. Doxycycline is preferable over Tetracycline as it is a newer generation drug, and might have less resistance issues. For this reason, stockpile doxycycline instead of tetracycline.

Years ago, the U.S. military commissioned a study regarding expiration dates. Consider their situation: In warehouses all over the country, they had over one billion dollars invested in medications. Every two years or so, they were faced with the challenge of disposing of huge quantities.

The study, which was conducted by the Food and Drug Administration, revealed that 90% of medications tested were acceptable for use 8-15 years after the expiration date. The FDA tested over

100 medications, prescription and non-prescription, and published its findings in 2000. The issues continues to be studied today.

The exceptions were mostly in liquid form (some pediatric antibiotics, insulin, among others). These lose their potency very soon after the date on the package. Possible signs of spoilage of a liquid medicine is a change in the color of the liquid or the appearance of solid material at the bottom.

More recently, a program called the **Shelf Life Extension Plan** evaluated a number of expired medications stockpiled for use in peacetime disasters. They found, as the previous study did, that almost all medications in pill or capsule form were still good 2-10 years after their expiration dates. A short summary of Shelf Life Extension Plan data:

"STUDY ABSTRACT: The American Medical Association has questioned whether expiration dating markedly underestimates the actual shelf life of drug products. Results from the Shelf Life Extension Program (SLEP) have been evaluated to provide extensive data to address this issue. The SLEP has been administered by the Food and Drug Administration for the United States Department of Defense (DOD) for 20 years.

This program probably contains the most extensive source of pharmaceutical stability data extant. This report summarizes extended stability profiles for 122 different drug products (3005 different lots). The drug products were categorized into five groups based on incidence of initial extension failures and termination failures (extended lot eventually failed upon re-testing).

Based on testing and stability assessment, 88% of the lots were extended at least 1 year beyond their original expiration date for an average extension of 66 months, but the additional stability period was highly variable. **The SLEP data supports the assertion that many drug products, if properly stored, can be extended past the expiration date.**"

A PDF file of the entire study, published July 2006 in *The Journal of Pharmaceutical Sciences*, is available online at: http://ofcaems.org/ds-Stability_Profiles.pdf

Even more incredibly, in 2012, researchers at the University of California (San Francisco) School of Pharmacy found cases of 14 different medications in a retail pharmacy in their original, unopened packaging. These cases were labeled with expiration dates 28-40 years old.

When analyzed, 12 of the 14 active ingredients persisted in concentrations that were 90% or greater of the amount indicated on the label. These results were conclusive enough for inclusion in the prestigious journal "Archives of Internal Medicine" (October 2012).

As a result of all these findings, even the government has changed their stance on expiration dates. During a recent flu epidemic, a 5 year extension was issued for the use of expired Tamiflu, a drug used to prevent and treat Swine Flu and other influenzas. The antibiotic Doxycycline and radiation exposure drug Potassium Iodide have also received extensions.

Despite this, you'll see quotes from academic types that say medications are dangerous when expired and should be tossed. These opinions are fine in normal times, but foolhardy if you're preparing for uncertain times. Let's say a loved one is fading from an infection. Something bad has happened; you're off the grid with little or no hope of getting to modern medical care. You have an expired bottle of antibiotics. Are you going to use the expired drug or not? Exactly.

You should make efforts to stockpile medications in pill or capsule form, but not as liquids. The SLEP data found most of the failures among drugs that were in liquid form. Medications in pill or capsule form lasted the longest, although potency may fade over time if stored poorly.

Proper storage of medications involve three factors: heat, humidity, and light. Make certain that your supplies are stored in a cool, dry, dark place. The effective life of a drug usually is in inverse relation to the temperature it is stored at. In other words, a drug stored at 50 degrees Fahrenheit will last longer than one stored at 90 degrees Fahrenheit. Freezing drugs, however, is not necessary and sometimes may decrease the effectiveness.

Sunlight can damage the activity of certain drugs, so using opaque or "smoky" containers is preferable to clear containers. This is why many medications come in amber-colored bottles. Place them in a dark place for long-term storage.

Humidity will also affect medications, and could even cause mold and mildew to form, especially on natural remedies such as dried herbs and powders. Many will vacuum-pack medications to extend shelf life.

Planning ahead, we must consider all alternatives in the effort to stay healthy in hard times. Don't ignore any option that can help you achieve that goal, even expired medicines. We encourage everyone to conduct their own study into the truth about expiration dates; come to your own conclusions after studying the facts.

AN OPEN LETTER TO DOCTORS ABOUT MEDICAL PREPAREDNESS

In this book, we recommended a frank discussion with your physician about the importance of being medically prepared for emergency situations, both short and long term. Many, however, will not know how to broach the subject, in fear of being ridiculed by the medical establishment.

Therefore, we have written a letter specifically meant for healthcare providers to introduce them to the concerns of the preparedness community. This is a letter that any person concerned about disaster situations can present to their physician. It addresses issues associated with situations such as the aftermath of a major storm or other disasters. Feel free to present it to your family physician if you think it would be beneficial to have them better understand preparedness issues.

To my fellow physicians:

I am a Fellow of both the American College of Surgeons and the American College of OB/GYN, recently retired, and I am writing this letter in an effort to inform you about the importance of improving the level of medical preparedness in your patient population.

We live in uncertain times, and more and more people are becoming concerned about what would happen in the event of a major disaster. From tornadoes to wildfires to national emergencies, there are circumstances where medical personnel may be overwhelmed by the number of victims requiring medical aid. In these situations, many of your patients will be unable to reach you. They may find themselves as the sole resource available to care for sick or injured members of their families.

In the aftermath of Hurricane Katrina in 2005, disaster medical assistance teams (DMATs) were formed from many areas in the country and converged upon New Orleans. They were immediately overwhelmed by the number of victims requiring medical help. In such a scenario, it stands to reason that your patients would benefit from a concerted effort on your part to help them become prepared to deal with likely problems they would face.

In an era of high technology, we may have expectations that our resources will always be sufficient to meet our emergency needs. Recent history has proven otherwise, and it may be time for us, as physicians, to increase the amount of education we provide for our patients. In this way, they can function as assets to their family if you or emergency medical personnel are not available.

Few medical offices provide information regarding the types and quantities of medical supplies that are recommended for the average household. Consider your area's likely needs for the disasters that might befall it, and print lists of items that you would advise your patients to have in their homes.

As well, provide resources for classes that your patients can take so that they will have the medical education necessary to deal with possible emergencies during these events. Direct them to sites recommended by the federal government for emergency preparedness, such as www.ready.gov; they will find free informational booklets that will help to increase their chances of surviving natural calamities and other disasters.

For your individual patients, especially those with chronic medical problems, you might consider providing the opportunity for them to keep a supply of needed medications by offering them an extra prescription to fill. In this manner, you can assure that your patients will have enough medicine to get them through situations which prevent them from contacting you in times of trouble.

I'm not asking you to abandon your responsibility by throwing prescriptions at them; I'm simply suggesting that they would benefit from having some extra supplies available to deal with unforeseen circumstances. Also, consider listing recommended over-the-counter medications that would be useful to have on hand.

Our purpose as physicians is to improve the health of our people while doing no harm. Many doctors dedicate their entire lives to this purpose, and we must work to preserve the well-being of our patients in difficult times. The worst nightmare of your patients is the inability to reach you in a major disaster; help them become better prepared to deal with medical emergencies with education, compassion, and understanding.

Thank you for all you do to keep your patients healthy, and for your time and attention in reading this letter.

Joseph Alton, M.D., F.A.C.S., F.A.C.O.G.

This open letter is available to print out at: www.doomandbloom.net.

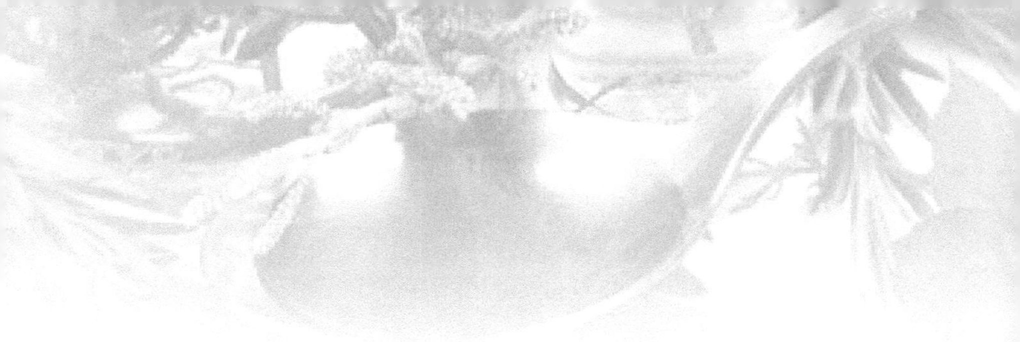

SECTION 10

✚ ✚ ✚

REFERENCES

Certainly, you have accumulated a reasonable amount of medical supplies to prepare you for the role of survival medic. If you have been prudent, you have taken emergency courses offered by your municipality and availed yourself of other hands-on teaching resources. Now, it is time to build your survival print and video libraries.

This book has taken an unusual route in assuming that no modern medical care or facilities will be available to you. Although we have attempted to be comprehensive in our approach, there is still much to learn. In power-down situations, you should have a number of printed medical books that you can refer to in times of trouble. In this section, we have given you a list that will be welcome assistance in your efforts to keep your people healthy. Realize, however, that they are written in the mindset of normal times.

While you have power, you should also avail yourself of the many resources available on the internet. For many procedures, there is no substitute to seeing something done in real time, such as placing a cast. Make every effort to download how-to videos on various medical subjects. No prepared individual should be without a source of power in hard times, so have a solar cell or other rechargeable method that will allow you to review downloaded references.

Arm yourself with an arsenal of medical knowledge. We refer to our library constantly to stay current on the options available to us, and so should you.

PRINT REFERENCES

We mentioned earlier that some reference books will be necessary for any aspiring medic. A printed medical library will still be there in a collapse situation, even if the internet, television, and other media are not. There are many good written resources for handling medical problems; these are but a few:

Stedman's Medical Dictionary
(a must for any medic)

Gray's Anatomy for Students
(yes, the television show's title was taken from this book)

The Physician's Desk Reference
(tells you indications, dosages, and risks of just about every medicine with images; comes our yearly, but any recent edition will serve your needs)

The Merck Manual
(good pocket reference on many common medical problems)

The Mayo Clinic Family Health book
(exhaustive and thorough with lots of photos)

Clinical Physiology Made Ridiculously Simple
by Stephen Goldberg, M.D. (all the basics on how the body works)

American College of Emergency Physicians First Aid Manual
(excellent first aid book)

Where there is No Doctor
by David Werner (third-world medicine)

Where there is no Dentist
by Murray Dickson (third-world dentistry)

A Comprehensive Guide to Wilderness and Travel Medicine
by Eric Weiss, M.D. (helpful pocket version)

Wilderness Medicine
by William W. Forgey, M.D. (outdoor survival)

Encyclopedia of Herbal Medicine
by Andrew Chevallier (talks about how medicinal plants work; information on every herb)

Prescription for Herbal Healing
by Phyllis A. Balch, CNC (extensive herbal remedy book)

Essential Oils Desk Reference
by Essential Science Publishing (exhaustive listings with photos)

National Geographic Guide to Medicinal Herbs
by Andrew Weil, MD (especially good identifying images)

Principles of Surgery
by Schwartz et al (for the very, very ambitious)

Tactical Medicine Essentials
by the American College of Emergency Physicians (for high-risk situations)

Varney's Midwifery or **Varney's Pocket Midwife**
(you never know when you'll need it)

If you have all these books in your medical library, you will have as much information at your fingertips as you'll need to keep your loved ones healthy in times of trouble.

VIDEO RESOURCES

This book has, hopefully, provided a lot of reading material to help you learn. In modern times, however, we learn as much by audiovisual means as we do the written word. One of the best resources available to information seekers is the online video. This phenomenon has placed a veritable library at your fingertips with regards to medical information. Even better than a library, you can actually see important medical procedures being performed. They range from a short blurb of a minute or so to a full one hour medical school lecture. The next few pages are essentially an entire second book filled with medical knowledge.

We have endeavored to find a representative video for just about every subject covered in this book. Different sources are listed, so that you can see the many options available for health information in all fields. The source is listed in parentheses after the title of the video, along with a short comment. Search YouTube.com for the title exactly as listed. If more than one video exists with the same title, look to see the source.

We don't agree with everything said on every video; do your own research and make you own decisions. Remember that these videos are written with modern medicine in mind. Many of them end with "and head for the hospital" or "see your doctor as soon as possible". Few if any are considering a societal collapse in their presentations, but they will provide you with an excellent base of knowledge from which to move forward:

7.Medical Interview -Review of Systems (by tvmariel)
(One of various videos, it shows a doctor conducting a leisurely interview with a patient before an exam. Watch as many as you can.)

01. Physical Exam-Introduction & Vital Signs (by tvmariel)
(Just one of many videos, it shows a doctor performing portions of the physical exam. Watch them all.)

1. Introduction - Lung Sounds Collection (by Dr. Prodigious)
(The first of a series of over 20 different short recordings of normal and abnormal lung sounds explained by a doctor)

Survival Medicine Gauze by Nurse Amy

(by DrBones NurseAmy)
(Review of all the different dressing materials)

An essential oil video (I can't verify all the claims made here; do you own research and decide for yourself.)

Using Colloidal Silver (by Chris Hyslop)
(All about how to use this alternative)

The Dangers of Colloidal Silver (by pogue972)
(Taking too much colloidal silver did this to a man, who later passed away from a heart attack at 62 years old)

Jacket Stretcher Wilderness First Aid Paul Tarsitano 1 of 3
Rope and Stick Stretcher Paul Tarsitano 2 of 3
Tarp Stretcher Wilderness First Aid Paul Tarsitano 3 of 3
(all by pault1960)
(3 videos by an expert in improvised patient transport)

Carrying the Injured (1933) (by wellcomefilm)
(Amazing old video with various patient carry techniques)

Extremities Lift and Carry (Pocket Tools Training - NCOSFM) (by ncosfm)

Blanket Drag (Pocket Tools Training – NCOSFM (by ncosfm)
(Just two of a series on patient transport by same author)

Life Saving Technique | The Fireman's Carry. (by Daniel Shaw)
(How to perform a one-man carry)

Sterility in Survival (by DrBones NurseAmy)
(The authors explain how to clean and sterilize instruments in austere settings)

Survival Sanitation with Dr. Bones (by DrBones NurseAmy)
(The authors discuss safe waste disposal in austere settings)

School Nurses Talk Head Lice (by NPSschoolnurses)
(Lice advice from those who should know)

Bed Bugs Part 1: What are they? (by UMDHGIC)

(First of a 3-part series all about bedbugs)

How to properly remove a tick (by University of Manitoba)
(simple removal procedure with fine tweezers)

Symptoms, Prevention and Treatment of Lyme Disease (by Columbia Association)
(All about Lyme disease)

Mt. Everest Dental Extraction at Base Camp (by cristenhfdg)
(Tooth extraction in an austere environment)

How to INSTANTLY CURE A TOOTHACHE at home remedy (by askmydentisttv)
(Dentist teaches you how to make temporary filling cement)

Respiratory Infection Health Byte (by livestrong)
(Basics of upper and lower respiratory infections)

How pneumonia affects the lungs (by Bupalhealth)
(Visuals of lung anatomy and pneumonia)

The Top 8 Signs of Dehydration (by ActiveBeat)
(Identifying water loss)

How To Treat Diarrhea (by howcast)
(General information)

How to Treat Someone for Food Poisoning | First Aid Training (by Howcast)
(simple treatment information)

Appendicitis: How To Recognize the Symptoms (by The Dr. Bob Show)
(How to identify early to late stage appendicitis)

Appendectomy (Stab Appendectomy) by Dr. Irfan Ahmad Nadeem
(by ianadeem)
(An appendectomy performed under local anesthesia; it *can* be done)

urinary tract infection (by Neil Baum, M.D., urology)
(Plain English basic of urinary tract infections)

How to Treat Heatstroke (by howcast)
(Just what the title says)

Hypothermia Treatment Scenario (by remote medical international)
(Treating exposure in the wilderness)

Hypothermia with Dr. Bones (by DrBones NurseAmy)
(Dr. Alton's alter ego discusses strategies for hypothermia)

Altitude Sickness with Dr. Bones (by DrBones NurseAmy)
(Dr. Alton's alter ego discusses acute mountain sickness)

First Aid - injury management1 (by businessrecovery)
(Basics about wounds and wound infections)

Blister Treatment/ Survival Medicine By Nurse Amy (by DrBones NurseAmy)
(Simple ways to treat a blister.)

First Aid - Severe bleeding (by businessrecovery)
(Step by step)

How to Treat Gunshot & Knife Wounds (by sootch00)
(Just in case)

The Emergency Bandage (aka The Israeli Bandage) (by PerSysMedical)
(Best trauma bandage)

Combat Gauze LE - Wound Packing and Soak Through procedures (by FDL Group)
(Hemostatic agents in action on mannikin)

Celox Haemostatic Agent (by Medtree)
(Hemostatic agent in action on live pig; not for the squeamish)

Ballistic Trauma Basics in Survival (by DrBones NurseAmy)
(The authors explain how bullets cause tissue damage)

Sucking Chest Wound: How to Treat an Open Pneumothorax Part 3 (by medicaltactics)
(An improvised chest seal is applied to a gunshot wound)

How to Suture With Dr. Bones (by DrBones NurseAmy)
(Learn how to put stitches into a pig's foot.)

How to Staple Skin with Dr. Bones (by DrBones NurseAmy)
(Learn how to put staples into a pig's foot.)

Surgical Debridement (by nucleus medical media)
(Removing dead tissue from a wound)

How to Prevent & Treat Foot Blisters | Foot Care (by Howcast)
(Strategies to deal with blisters)

First Aid Tips: How to Treat a Burn in the Wilderness (by ehow)
(Fire captain discussing burn injuries in the wild)

Burns - First Aid (by ProCPR)
(Basic treatment explained)

Snakebite: Survival Medicine with Dr. Bones (by DrBones NurseAmy)
(All you need to know)

Black Widow spider bite - Day 3 (by varvelle)
(Classic appearance on an actual victim)

First aid – Anaphylaxis (by Premium Health)
(Quick video on anaphylactic shock)

Dermatology Treatments : How to Diagnose Skin Rashes (by ehowhealth)
(Some common skin rashes explained)

Abdominal wall cellulitis (by theedexitvideo)
(Example of cellulitis and abscess drainage procedure)

Symptoms of Tension vs. Migraine Headache (by FYInowhealth)
(List of symptoms of each)

Practical First Aid #18 - Sprains and Strains (by FlemingMedical)
(Quick overview and wrapping technique)

Sprains Fractures and Dislocations (by uctelevision)

(Full 1 hour medical school lecture with lots of great info- early portion includes an easy quiz)

Symptoms and Treatments of Hypothyroidism (by mercola)
(Discussion of this common thyroid condition)

Diabetes Overview (by answerstv)
(Comprehensive discussion)

Understanding High Blood Pressure (HBP #1) (by healthguru)
(All the facts in plain English)

Chest pain vs. heart attack - ask the doctor (by wptvnews)
(Different causes of chest pain)

Heartburn, Acid Reflux, GERD-Mayo Clinic (by Mayo Clinic)
(Description with images)

Understanding Epilepsy (Epilepsy #1) (by healthguru)
(Why seizures happen, go on to Epilepsy #2 to see each one live)

Understanding Arthritis (Arthritis #1) (by healthguru)
(Osteoarthritis and rheumatoid arthritis overview)

Healthbeat - Kidney Stones (by koattv)
(Advice to avoid recurrences)

Gallstones Health Byte (by livestrong)
(Causes, types, symptoms)

How to Give the Heimlich Maneuver | First Aid Training (by Howcast)
(Excellent demonstration)

CPR Training Video New 2010 / 2011 Guidelines - Preview Safetycare Cardiopulmonary Resuscitation
(by safetycare)
(Excellent preview but not a substitute for a full course)

Eye Care & Vision Problems : How to Get Rid of Bloodshot Eyes (by ehowhealth)
(Discussion of eye allergies)

Pink Eye - 10 Tips To Identify, Prevent, and Treat Conjunctivitis (by myfamilydoc) (an eye doctor talks about eye infections and more)

How to Treat a Nosebleed | First Aid Training (by Howcast)
(Title says it all)

Ears 101 : How to Relieve an Ear Ache (by ehowhealth)
(Common infections and treatment; part of a series)

Prenatal Care: Early Pregnancy Visits (by march of dimes)
(Explains prenatal care and shows an actual visit)

Baby delivery (by saalie100)
(Typical hospital delivery – note that an episiotomy is performed, which we don't recommend unless absolutely necessary. Also, cord does not have to be cut immediately and the baby should be placed on mother's stomach almost immediately for bonding purposes)

Anxiety Overview (by answertv)
(All the basics)

Signs, Symptoms, and Treatment of Depression (by nimhgov)
(Again, all the basics)

Mass Casualty Incident- S.T.A.R.T. Triage Part 1 (by DrBones NurseAmy)
(Dr. Alton discusses your plan of action in mass casualty events)

Trephining a nail to drain subungual haematoma (by John Yannopapas)
(Treating a nailbed injury)

The Effects of Sleep Deprivation (by roperstfrancis)
(Personal story of a sleep deprivation patient)

Fish Antibiotics in a Collapse by Dr. Bones (by drbones nurse amy)
(Alternative options for stockpiling antibiotics)

Do Expiration Dates Matter in Survival? (by drbones nurseamy)
(What expiration dates really mean)

GLOSSARY OF MEDICAL TERMINOLOGY

ABRASION:	area of skin scraped off down to the dermis
ABSCESS:	collection of pus and inflamed tissue
ACID REFLUX:	Pain and burning caused by stomach acid traveling up the esophagus
ADRENALINE:	name for epinephrine outside the U.S.
AIRWAY:	breathing passage
ALLERGEN:	a substance that triggers hypersensitivity
ALLERGY:	exaggerated physical reaction to a substance
ALVEOLI:	air sacs in the lung that absorb oxygen
AMNIOTIC FLUID:	liquid inside the pregnant uterus
AMBU-BAG:	CPR breathing unit (brand name)
ANAEROBE:	organism that doesn't require oxygen to survive
ANALGESIA:	pain relief
ANAPHYLAXIS::	hypersensitivity to a substance due to antibodies after an initial exposure
ANAPHYLACTIC SHOCK:	life-threatening organ failure as a result of hypersensitivity to a substance
ANGINA:	heart pain caused by lack of oxygen
ANTIBIOTIC:	substances that kill bacteria in living tissue

ANTIBODY:	substances produced by the body that respond to toxins
ANTICOAGULANT:	substances that stop clotting
ANTIEMETIC:	substances that stop vomiting
ANTIHISTAMINE:	drugs that relieve minor allergies
ANTIINFLAMMATORY:	substances that limit inflammation
ANTISEPTIC:	anything that limits the spread of germs on living surfaces
ANTISPASMODIC:	decreases blood vessel constriction
ANTIVENIN:	substance that inactivates snake or insect venom
ANTIVIRAL:	substances that kill viruses
APPENDICITIS:	inflammation of the appendix
ARTERY:	blood vessel that carries oxygen to the tissues
ARTHRITIS:	inflammation of the joints
ASCITES:	fluid accumulation in the abdomen
ASPHYXIANT:	substance that deprives the body of oxygen
ASPIRATION:	inhalation of fluids into the airways
ASTHMA:	shortness of breath caused by a narrowing of airways, often due to an allergic reaction
ASYMPTOMATIC:	without signs or symptoms
ATHEROSCLEROSIS:	blockage of the coronary arteries
AUSTERE:	plain, remote, off-grid
AUTOIMMUNE:	a response of the body against its own tissues

AVULSION:	tissue torn off by trauma
BAG VALVE MASK:	CPR breathing apparatus
BANDAGE:	wound covering
BETADINE:	iodine antiseptic solution
BILE:	fluid found in the gall bladder
B.R.A.T. DIET:	diet used to treat dehydration consisting of bananas, rice, applesauce and dry toast
BRAXTON-HICKS:	contractions that do not result in active labor
BRONCHITIS:	inflammation of the airways
BRONCHUS:	main respiratory airway
BRUISE:	injury that does not break the skin but causes bleeding due to damaged blood vessels
CALDERA:	a basin formed by the explosion of a volcano
CAPILLARY:	tiny blood vessel that connects arteries to veins throughout the body
CARDIAC:	relating to the heart
CARTILAGE:	fibrous connective tissue found in various parts of the body, such as the joints, outer ear, and larynx.
CATARACT:	a clouding of the lens of the eye
CELLULITIS:	inflammation of soft tissues
CHIN-LIFT:	CPR technique that improves airflow
CHOLECYSTITIS:	inflammation of the gall bladder
CHOLELITHIASIS:	gall stones

CIRRHOSIS:	chronic liver damage
CLOSED FRACTURE:	broken bone that does not break the skin
COLLAPSE SITUATION:	circumstance where modern medical care no longer exists for the long term
COLOSTRUM:	early breast milk rich in antibodies
CONCUSSION:	loss of consciousness caused by trauma to the cranium
CONJUNCTIVITIS:	inflammation of the eye membrane
CONTRECOUP:	injury to the brain opposite to the site of impact
CORNEA:	clear covering over the iris
COSTOCHONDRITIS:	chest pain caused by inflammation of the rib joints
COTYLEDONS:	segments of the placenta
COUP:	injury to the brain at the site of impact
CPR:	cardio-pulmonary resuscitation
CROWNING:	late stage of labor when the baby's head start to emerge from the vagina
CURETTAGE:	scraping dead pregnancy tissue from the uterus after a miscarriage
CYANOSIS:	blue color caused by lack of oxygen
DEBRIDEMENT:	removal of dead tissue from a wound
DEHYDRATION:	loss of body water content
DERMATITIS:	inflammation of the skin
DERMIS:	deep layer of the skin
DIABETES:	disease in which the body fails to produce enough Insulin to control

	blood sugar levels (type 1) or is resistant to the Insulin it produces (Type 2)
DIAGNOSIS:	Identification of a medical condition
DILATION:	the act of making more open
DISCHARGE:	drainage from a surface or wound
DISINFECTANT:	substance that kills germs on non-living surfaces
DISLOCATION:	traumatic movement of a bone out of its joint
DISTAL:	away from the torso
DIURETIC:	substance that increases urine flow
DRESSING:	wound covering
DRUG OF CHOICE:	best drug for a particular illness
DUODENUM:	part of the bowel after the stomach
DYSENTERY:	dangerous diarrheal disease
ECLAMPSIA:	seizures caused by elevated blood pressures during a pregnancy
ECTOPIC PREGNANCY:	pregnancy that implants outside of the womb
EDEMA:	fluid accumulation
ELAPID:	family of venomous "coral" snakes
ELECTROLYTES:	elements found in body fluids
ENDEMIC:	disease native to an area or species
EPIDEMIC:	disease that spreads community-wide
EPIDERMIS:	superficial layer of the skin
EPILEPSY:	convulsive disorder

EPINEPHRINE:	hormone used to treat severe allergic reactions (known as adrenaline outside the US)
EPISTAXIS:	bleeding from the nose
ERYTHEMA:	redness due to inflammation
ESOPHAGUS:	tube that runs from the back of the mouth to the stomach
ESSENTIAL OILS:	highly concentrated liquids of various mixtures of natural compounds obtained from plants.
EXPECTORANT:	substance that loosens congestion
FALLOUT:	particulate radioactive matter in the air
FAULT:	a fracture in base rock
FRACTURE:	a broken bone
FROSTBITE:	frozen tissue, usually in extremities
GALL BLADDER:	organ near the liver that stores bile
GANGRENE:	death of tissue due to lack of circulation
GASTROENTERITIS:	inflammation of the stomach/intestine
GINGIVITIS:	inflammation of the gums
GLAND:	organ that produces hormones
GLUCOSE:	blood sugar
GRAND MAL SEIZURE:	generalized convulsion in epileptics
GRANULOMA:	nodule formed by immune system's attempt to wall off an infection or a foreign object
HEARTBURN:	chest pain caused by stomach acid
HEAT STROKE:	symptoms caused by overheating

HEIMLICH MANEUVER:	action taken to remove foreign object from the airways
HEMOGLOBIN:	red blood cell component that carries oxygen to the tissues
HEMORRHAGE:	blood loss
HEMORRHOID:	varicose vein near the anus
HEMOPTYSIS:	coughing up blood
HEMOSTATIC AGENT:	substance that stops bleeding
HEPATITIS:	inflammation of the liver
HERNIA:	weakness in the body wall
HESITANCY:	difficulty starting a urine stream
HISTAMINES:	substances formed in allergies that cause physical symptoms
HIVES:	bumpy red rash caused by allergies
HORMONE:	substance produced by a gland that affects body functions
HYDRATION:	addition of water to the system
HYGIENE:	cleanliness as health strategy
HYPEROPIA:	farsightedness
HYPERTENSION:	high blood pressure
HYPERTHERMIA:	heat stroke or heat exhaustion
HYPERTHYROIDISM:	condition caused by high thyroid levels
HYPHEMA:	bleeding into the white of the eye
HYPOGLYCEMIA:	low blood glucose levels
HYPOTHERMIA:	syndrome caused by heat loss

HYPOTHYROIDISM:	condition caused by low thyroid levels
IATROGENIC:	caused by the healthcare provider
IDIOPATHIC:	of unknown cause
IMMOBILIZATION:	prevention of movement
IMMUNITY:	protection against a disease
IMPETIGO:	skin infection with weeping sores
INFARCTION:	death of heart tissue due to lack of oxygen
INFLAMMATION:	reaction to injury characterized by redness, swelling, discharge, pain and heat
INFLUENZA:	viral respiratory illness
INTEGRATED CARE:	treatment using different medical methods
INTOXICATION:	state of being poisoned
INTRAVENOUS:	inside the vein
IRIS:	colored portion of the eye
IRRIGATION:	forceful application of fluid to a wound to clean out debris, blood clots, and dead tissue
IRRITANT:	substance that causes inflammation of tissue
ISCHEMIC:	lacking oxygen due to circulatory failure
JAUNDICE:	yellowing of the skin and eyes due to liver malfunction
KETOACIDOSIS:	life-threatening condition related to failure of blood glucose control
KILOGRAM:	2.2 pounds
LACERATION:	penetration of both skin layers by injury

LARYNX:	the voice box
LASIK:	laser surgery to correct vision
LETHARGY:	extreme fatigue or drowsiness
LIGAMENT:	supportive tissue that connects bones
LITER:	0.264 gallons
LOCALIZED:	isolated to an area
LYMPHATICS:	drainage system for body fluids
MASS CASUALTY INCIDENT:	more victims than available help
MCBURNEY'S POINT	area in right lower abdomen corresponding to the pain in appendicitis
MENINGITIS:	inflammation of the brain/spinal cord
MENSTRUATION:	periodic blood flow from the uterus
MIGRAINE:	headaches caused by vascular Spasms
MISCARRIAGE:	early pregnancy loss
MOLESKIN:	protective material for blisters
MURPHY'S SIGN	pain below the lowest rib on the right, usually caused by gallbladder disease
MYOPIA:	nearsightedness
NEUROLOGIC:	pertaining to the nervous system
OPEN FRACTURE:	broken bone that pierces the skin
OPTHALMOSCOPE:	instrument used to look into the eyes
OTITIS:	inflammation of the ear

OTOSCOPE:	instrument used to look into ear canal
OVARY:	female organ that produces eggs
PALPATION:	to feel with the hands
PALPITATIONS:	sensation of dread caused by a rapid heart rate
PANDEMIC:	epidemic that spans across different regions
PATHOGEN:	something that causes disease
PEDIATRIC:	pertaining to children
PELVIC:	pertaining to the bones that provide support for legs and spine
PEPTIC:	relating to stomach acid
PERCUSSION:	to tap on the body to identify hollow and solid areas; for example, when searching for a tumor.
PERINEUM:	area between the vagina and anus
PERIOSTEUM:	outside lining of the bone
PETIT MAL SEIZURE:	epilepsy characterized by loss of awareness without generalized convulsive behavior
PHARYNX:	the throat
PHLEBITIS:	inflammation seen in varicose veins
PHLEGM:	mucus discharge from the respiratory tract
PIT VIPER:	snake in the rattlesnake family
PNEUMONIA:	an infection of the lungs
PNEUMOTHORAX:	free air in the lung cavity affecting breathing

POST-ICTAL STATE:	semi-conscious state after experiencing a grand mal seizure
POTABLE:	safe to drink
PRE-ECLAMPSIA:	pregnancy-induced hypertension
PROGNOSIS:	likely outcome of a medical condition
PRONE:	lying face down
PROPHYLAXIS:	preventative measures
PROXIMAL:	closer to the torso
PROTOZOA:	microscopic organisms that sometimes act as parasites
PULMONARY:	relating to the lungs
PRESSURE POINTS:	areas where pressure on blood vessels stops bleeding to distal areas
PRURITIS:	itchiness
PULMONARY:	relating to the lungs
PUS:	inflammatory discharge caused by the body's response to infection
PYELONEPHRITIS:	inflammation of the kidney
QUADRANT:	body area divided into quarters
REBOUND:	pain elicited by pressing, then made worse by releasing the pressure on a part of the body
REFLUX:	acid traveling up the esophagus
RELAPSE:	recurrence of a disease's symptoms
RENAL:	relating to the kidneys
RESPIRATORY:	relating to breathing

RHYTHM METHOD:	method of determining fertile periods by tracking menstrual cycles
SALINE:	salt water solution used for IV fluids and irrigating wounds
SEBORRHEA:	oily, itchy rash on scalp and face
SEDATION:	to relax or put to sleep
SEIZURE:	convulsion
SHOCK:	life-threatening syndrome caused by multiple organ failure or malfunction
SOFT TISSUE:	muscle, tendons, ligaments, skin, fat
SPRAIN:	damage to a ligament caused by hyperextension
SPHYGNOMANOMETER:	instrument used to measure pressure
STERILE:	free of germs
STERNUM:	breastbone
STETHOSCOPE:	instrument used for listening to heart, lungs, and for evaluating blood pressure
STRAIN:	damage to a muscle or tendon
STROKE:	brain hemorrhage with paralysis
STYE:	infection on the edge of the eyelid
SUBCUTANEOUS:	under the skin
SUPERCELL:	a thunderstorm that spawns tornadoes
SUPINE:	lying face up
SUSPENSION:	a drug mixed in a liquid
SUTURE:	wound closure with needle and thread
SYNDROME:	collection of symptoms

SYSTEMIC:	condition affecting the entire body
TACHYCARDIA:	elevated heart rate
TENDON:	connection of a muscle to a bone
THERMOREGULATORY:	related to body temperature
THROMBOSIS:	a blood clot in the circulatory system
TINCTURE:	plant extract made by soaking herbs in a liquid (such as water, alcohol, or vinegar) for a specified length of time, then straining and discarding the plant material.
TINNITUS:	ringing in the ears
TOURNIQUET:	item that uses pressure to stop bleeding from a wound
TRACHEOTOMY:	procedure meant to open an airway when no other method is possible
TRAUMA:	injury caused by impact
TREPHINATION:	drilling a hole into a nail to expel blood
TRIAGE:	to sort by priority
TUMOR:	a growth in or on the body
TYMPANIC MEMBRANE:	eardrum
ULCER:	damage to the wall of the skin, stomach or intestine due to pressure, acid or disease
ULTRAVIOLET:	invisible light waves that damage skin or eyes
UMBILICAL:	relating to the "belly button"
URGENCY:	sudden desire to urinate
URTICARIA:	allergic rash

UTERUS: womb

VARICES: enlarged and dilated veins

VASCULAR: relating to blood vessels

VEIN: blood vessel that carries de-oxygenated blood back to the lungs

VERTIGO: dizziness

WHEEZING: high pitched noises heard while breathing during an asthma attack

INDEX

B

CONTACTS

DOCTOR: ______________________________

DENTIST: ______________________________

FIRE DEPT: ______________________________

POLICE: ______________________________

GROUP MEDIC: ______________________________

GROUP MEMBERS: ______________________________

NOTES

NOTES

NOTES

NOTES

NOTES

Made in United States
Cleveland, OH
18 October 2026

46341968R10378